Tumors of the Liver and Intrahepatic Bile Ducts

Atlas
of
Tumor Pathology

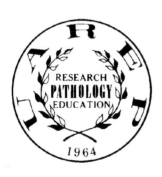

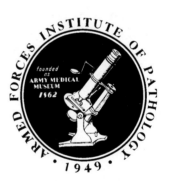

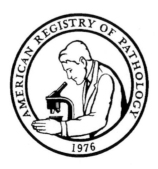

ATLAS OF TUMOR PATHOLOGY

Third Series
Fascicle 31

TUMORS
OF THE LIVER
AND INTRAHEPATIC BILE DUCTS

by

KAMAL G. ISHAK, M.D., Ph.D.
Chairman, Department of Hepatic and
Gastrointestinal Pathology
Armed Forces Institute of Pathology
Washington, D.C.

ZACHARY D. GOODMAN, M.D., Ph.D
Chief, Division of Hepatic Pathology,
Department of Hepatic and Gastrointestinal Pathology
Armed Forces Institute of Pathology
Washington, D.C.

J. THOMAS STOCKER, M.D.
Colonel, Medical Corps, United States Army
Professor of Pathology
Uniformed Services University of Health Sciences
Bethesda, Maryland

Published by the
ARMED FORCES INSTITUTE OF PATHOLOGY
Washington, D.C.

Under the Auspices of
UNIVERSITIES ASSOCIATED FOR RESEARCH AND EDUCATION IN PATHOLOGY, INC.
Bethesda, Maryland
2001

Accepted for Publication
1999

Available from the American Registry of Pathology
Armed Forces Institute of Pathology
Washington, D.C. 20306-6000
www.afip.org
ISSN 0160-6344
ISBN 1-881041-69-7

ATLAS OF TUMOR PATHOLOGY

EDITOR
JUAN ROSAI, M.D.
Dipartimento di Patologia
Istituto Nazionale Tumori
20133 Milano, Italy

ASSOCIATE EDITOR
LESLIE H. SOBIN, M.D.
Armed Forces Institute of Pathology
Washington, D.C. 20306-6000

EDITORS' NOTE

The Atlas of Tumor Pathology has a long and distinguished history. It was first conceived at a Cancer Research Meeting held in St. Louis in September 1947 as an attempt to standardize the nomenclature of neoplastic diseases. The first series was sponsored by the National Academy of Sciences-National Research Council. The organization of this Sisyphean effort was entrusted to the Subcommittee on Oncology of the Committee on Pathology, and Dr. Arthur Purdy Stout was the first editor-in-chief. Many of the illustrations were provided by the Medical Illustration Service of the Armed Forces Institute of Pathology, the type was set by the Government Printing Office, and the final printing was done at the Armed Forces Institute of Pathology (hence the colloquial appellation "AFIP Fascicles"). The American Registry of Pathology purchased the Fascicles from the Government Printing Office and sold them virtually at cost. Over a period of 20 years, approximately 15,000 copies each of nearly 40 Fascicles were produced. The worldwide impact that these publications have had over the years has largely surpassed the original goal. They quickly became among the most influential publications on tumor pathology ever written, primarily because of their overall high quality but also because their low cost made them easily accessible to pathologists and other students of oncology the world over.

Upon completion of the first series, the National Academy of Sciences-National Research Council handed further pursuit of the project over to the newly created Universities Associated for Research and Education in Pathology (UAREP). A second series was started, generously supported by grants from the AFIP, the National Cancer Institute, and the American Cancer Society. Dr. Harlan I. Firminger became the editor-in-chief and was succeeded by Dr. William H. Hartmann. The second series Fascicles were produced as bound volumes instead of loose leaflets. They featured a more comprehensive coverage of the subjects, to the extent that the Fascicles could no longer be regarded as "atlases" but rather as monographs describing and illustrating in detail the tumors and tumor-like conditions of the various organs and systems.

Once the second series was completed, with a success that matched that of the first, UAREP and AFIP decided to embark on a third series. A new editor-in-chief and an associate editor were selected, and a distinguished editorial board was appointed. The mandate for the third series remains the same as for the previous ones, i.e., to oversee the production of an eminently practical publication with surgical pathologists as its primary audience, but also aimed at other workers in oncology. The main purposes of this series are to promote a consistent, unified, and biologically sound nomenclature; to guide the surgical pathologist in the diagnosis of the various tumors and tumor-like lesions; and to provide relevant histogenetic, pathogenetic, and clinicopathologic information on these entities. Just as the second series included data obtained from ultrastructural (and, in the more recent Fascicles, immunohistochemical) examination, the third series will, in addition, incorporate pertinent information obtained with the newer molecular biology techniques. As in the past, a continuous attempt will be made to correlate, whenever possible, the nomenclature used in the Fascicles with that proposed by the World Health Organization's International Histological Classification of Tumors. The format of the third series has been changed in order to incorporate additional items and to ensure a consistency of style throughout. Close cooperation between the various authors and their respective liaisons from the editorial board will be emphasized to minimize unnecessary repetition and discrepancies in the text and illustrations.

To its everlasting credit, the participation and commitment of the AFIP to this venture is even more substantial and encompassing than in previous series. It now extends to virtually all scientific, technical, and financial aspects of the production.

The task confronting the organizations and individuals involved in the third series is even more daunting than in the preceding efforts because of the ever-increasing complexity of the matter at hand. It is hoped that this combined effort—of which, needless to say, that represented by the authors is first and foremost—will result in a series worthy of its two illustrious predecessors and will be a suitable introduction to the tumor pathology of the twenty-first century.

Juan Rosai, M.D.
Leslie H. Sobin, M.D.

ACKNOWLEDGEMENTS

We would like to thank the two anonymous referees who reviewed the chapters of this Fascicle and made many helpful and constructive criticisms. The cooperation and guidance of Drs. Juan Rosai and Leslie Sobin are also much appreciated.

The senior author is most grateful to Ms. Fanny Revelo, for her outstanding secretarial support. He also deeply appreciates the superb photomicrographic support of Ms. Veronica Ferris, M.F.S., Chief, Photography Section, Armed Forces Institute of Pathology, Washington, D.C.

Kamal G. Ishak, M.D., Ph.D.
Zachary D. Goodman, M.D., Ph.D.
J. Thomas Stocker, M.D. COL, MC, USA

DEDICATION

To our families

Contents

TUMORS OF THE LIVER
AND INTRAHEPATIC BILE DUCTS

1
EMBRYOLOGY, HISTOLOGY, AND ANATOMY

EMBRYOLOGY

The development of the liver (3–7,9) begins with the appearance of the hepatic diverticulum, which buds from the ventral foregut at the end of the third week of gestation. The diverticulum grows into the primitive septum transversum; the liver forms from the endodermal cells of the diverticulum and the mesenchyme that is already present.

The embryonic and fetal liver is a vascular and hematopoietic organ composed of a complex venous-sinusoidal plexus, cords of hepatocytes, abundant hematopoietic precursors (fig. 1-1), and macrophages (Kupffer cells), which are also of hematopoietic origin. Most of its blood supply is from the umbilical vein, which is well developed by the seventh week of gestation, with a much smaller amount of blood delivered by the portal vein and hepatic artery. Many of the func-

tions of the adult liver are performed by the placenta, particularly the clearance of wastes that are excreted in the bile and the absorption and regulation of nutrients. Consequently, a large part of the blood delivered by the umbilical vein bypasses the fetal liver and enters the systemic circulation through the ductus venosus. The fetal liver, however, produces plasma proteins, including alphafetoprotein; stores glycogen, fat, iron, and copper; and synthesizes bile acids. Bile secretion, however, remains minimal until birth.

The definitive intrahepatic bile ducts develop relatively late in fetal life, and the ductal system is not complete until after birth. The lining of the large extrahepatic and major intrahepatic bile ducts is derived from the endoderm of the original hepatic diverticulum. The small ducts that drain the hepatic acini, however, are derived from the embryonic ductal plate. This structure forms from the layer of cells that abuts the

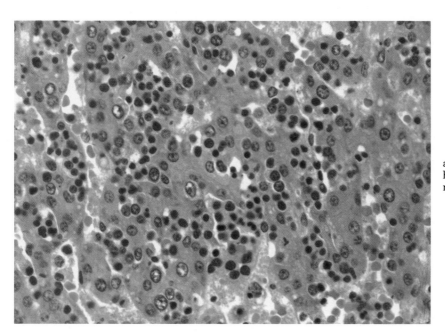

Figure 1-1
FETAL LIVER
There are cords of hepatocytes and sinusoids that contain many hematopoietic precursors and macrophages.

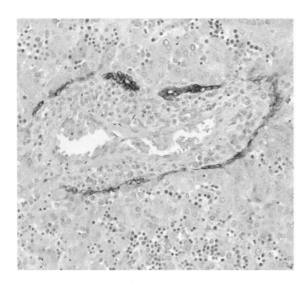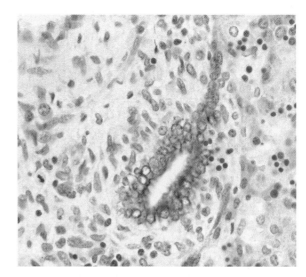

Figure 1-2
FETAL LIVER

Left: The embryonic ductal plate, composed of cytokeratin-rich cells, forms a layer that surrounds the portal area. This immunostain for cytokeratin 18 shows that the ductal plate is discontinuous and in a few places forms a double layer of cells with a small lumen.

Right: Higher magnification of another portal area shows the acinar bile duct forming from the ductal plate, which will eventually disappear as the liver grows.

connective tissue of the small portal tracts. It becomes a cylindrical double layer of biliary-like cells containing abundant cytokeratin 18, which is not present in the hepatocytes at this stage (fig. 1-2, left). A lumen appears in some places, but much of the ductal plate remains an inconspicuous double layer of small cells. Most of the ductal plate is resorbed as the fetal liver develops, but parts develop into bile duct epithelium (fig. 1-2, right), which becomes surrounded by connective tissue as the portal tracts enlarge, allowing the duct to assume its typical position in those tracts. Acinar ducts begin to appear at approximately 20 weeks of gestation and increase in number until, by the 38th week, nearly all portal areas have at least one bile duct. Conversely, hematopoietic cells gradually decrease and are absent in the normal term infant liver.

CELLS OF THE LIVER

Since tumors tend to resemble the normal structures of the tissue in which they arise, a discussion of the types of cells that occur in the normal liver is in order (1,3–7,9).

Hepatocytes. These polyhedral, eosinophilic cells (fig. 1-3) form the bulk of the liver and perform many metabolic functions that are essential for the maintenance of the internal homeostasis of the organism. A unique function of the hepatocyte is bile production and secretion into the bile canaliculi that lie between the hepatocytes in the liver cell plates. Canaliculi are normally inconspicuous, but they can be visualized by electron microscopy or by immunostaining with polyclonal antibodies to carcinoembryonic antigen, due to the presence of a cross-reacting substance, biliary glycoprotein I, which is located in the canalicular membrane (fig. 1-4). Hepatocytes normally contain cytokeratin types 8 and 18, and they are decorated by monoclonal antibody CAM 5.2 as well as antibody Hep Par 1 (antihepatocyte, Dako®), which is directed against an unidentified hepatocyte antigen (10). Other cytokeratins may appear in various pathologic conditions. Hepatocytes may contain glycogen, hemosiderin, or lipofuscin granules, and a variety of plasma proteins, which can be demonstrated by appropriate immunostains, but none of these is always present or absolutely specific when identifying cells with hepatocellular differentiation.

Endothelial Cells. The cells that line the veins and arteries of the portal triads and terminal hepatic venules (central veins) are identical to

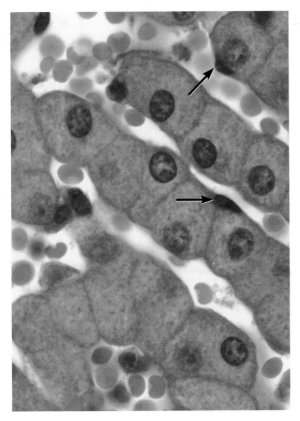

Figure 1-3
HEPATOCYTES AND ENDOTHELIAL CELLS

Normal hepatocytes are polyhedral cells arranged in plates that are one cell thick. They have granular, eosinophilic cytoplasm and usually one nucleus. The sinusoids between the hepatocytes are lined by inconspicuous endothelial cells (arrows).

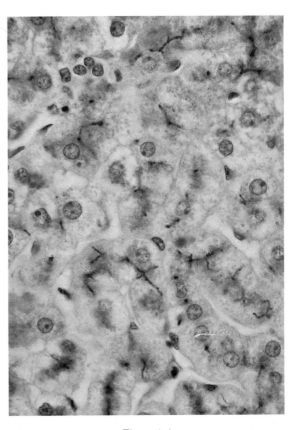

Figure 1-4
HEPATOCYTES

Bile canaliculi between the hepatocytes are demonstrated with immunostains using polyclonal antibodies to carcinoembryonic antigen, due to cross-reacting biliary glycoprotein I.

those of the endothelium of capillaries and larger vessels of the rest of the body. They are attached to a basement membrane, form a single flattened layer lining the lumen, and stain with antibodies to factor VIII–related antigen (von Willebrand factor), CD34, and CD31. Sinusoidal endothelial cells (fig. 1-3) differ from other endothelial cells. They lack a basement membrane and the endothelial markers of the larger vessels. Sinusoidal endothelial cells are fenestrated, having pores (visible by electron microscopy) that allow plasma to circulate freely between the sinusoidal lumen and the surface of the hepatocytes. The inconspicuous area between the endothelial cells and hepatocytes is called the space of Disse.

Kupffer Cells. In addition to endothelial cells, the hepatic sinusoids are partially lined by macrophages that are a large part of the body's reticuloendothelial system. They are normally inconspicuous, but when stimulated to perform their phagocytic function, they become enlarged and often contain lipofuscin or hemosiderin pigment, the residue of the phagocytosed material. They can also be identified with immunostains for macrophage markers, such as lysozyme (fig. 1-5) or CD68.

Stellate Cells. These specialized mesenchymal cells are located in the perisinusoidal space of Disse, between the sinusoidal endothelial cells and the hepatocytes. At various times they have been called *perisinusoidal lipocytes, fat-storing cells,* or *Ito cells,* but the preferred name, by consensus of those involved in their study, is stellate cells. They store vitamin A in lipid vacuoles, and the presence of lipid droplets allows their identification by electron microscopy. They also are the major source of collagen production,

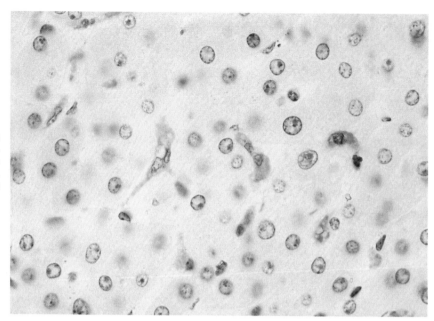

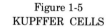

Figure 1-5
KUPFFER CELLS
The sinusoidal macrophages can be distinguished from endothelial cells by the presence of histiocyte markers. This immunostain for lysozyme shows the positive Kupffer cells.

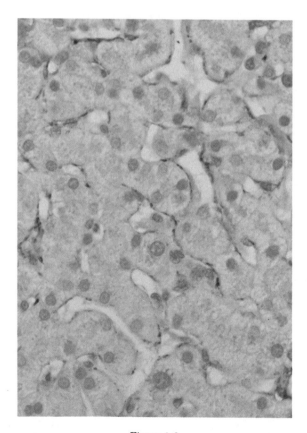

Figure 1-6
STELLATE CELLS
The stellate cells of the perisinusoidal space can be identified with an immunostain for smooth muscle actin.

and in various pathologic conditions transform from fat-storing cells into myofibroblasts and fibroblasts. In humans they are normally inconspicuous by light microscopy, but individuals who consume excess vitamin A have large stellate cells that can be identified by their large fat vacuoles and eccentric nuclei. They can also be identified with immunostains for smooth muscle actin (fig. 1-6) and desmin.

Pit Cells. Large granular lymphocytes, thought to be natural killer cells, can be identified by electron microscopy in the space of Disse. They are inconspicuous by light microscopy.

Biliary Epithelial Cells. The cells that line the acinar (interlobular) and larger ducts are cuboidal and typically have a single nucleus and slightly basophilic cytoplasm (fig. 1-7). They sit on a periodic acid–Schiff (PAS)-positive basement membrane and are surrounded by connective tissue that varies in quantity proportionately with the size of the duct. Bile ducts run parallel to hepatic artery branches, which allows them to be distinguished from ductules. Biliary epithelial cells contain cytokeratin types 7 and 19 as well as types 8 and 18 that are normally found in hepatocytes.

Ductular Cells. Ductules, also called *cholangioles* or *canals of Hering,* are seldom noted in the normal liver, but they can often be found by

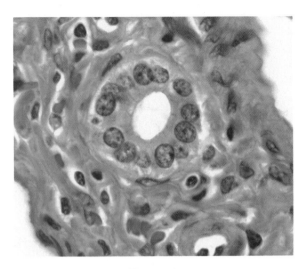

Figure 1-7
BILIARY EPITHELIAL CELLS
This small acinar bile duct is lined by cuboidal cells that are smaller than hepatocytes and have a more basophilic cytoplasm. The nuclei are basally oriented.

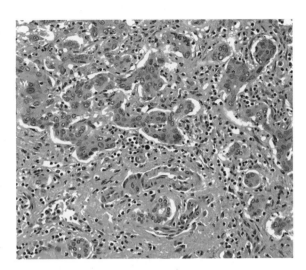

Figure 1-8
DUCTULES
The ductules or cholangioles are normally inconspicuous, but they proliferate in various pathologic conditions and resemble bile ducts. In this case of submassive hepatocellular necrosis, the proliferating ductules will differentiate into hepatocytes in an attempt to repopulate the liver.

careful light microscopic examination. They are very small structures composed of biliary-like cells at the periphery of the portal tracts. A basement membrane may be present, but the structure is not accompanied by an artery, in contrast to the bile duct. Ductules proliferate in many pathologic conditions. Submassive hepatocellular necrosis is typically followed by extensive ductular proliferation (fig. 1-8), as the ductules can differentiate into hepatocytes to repopulate destroyed liver. Hepatocytes can undergo metaplasia into ductules when there is mechanical biliary obstruction or other disorders causing disruption of bile flow, and while this is not strictly "proliferation," the same term is used. Ductules, whether derived from stem cells or from metaplasia of hepatocytes, contain a biliary pattern of cytokeratin including types 7, 8, 18, and 19. When there is ductular proliferation, it may be difficult or impossible to identify the acinar duct among the proliferating ductules, but the ductules tend to be at the edges of the portal areas and lack an accompanying artery. Rodents treated with chemical carcinogens sometimes develop a primary proliferation of small ductular-type cells called "oval cells," which are regarded as hepatic stem cells and which may give rise to carcinomas in these animals. Some investigators have suggested that ductular cells are the human analog of oval cells, but this is not universally accepted.

Peribiliary Gland Cells. The major ducts of the liver have small accessory glands, called peribiliary glands, that are identical to those of the extrahepatic ducts and pancreatic ducts. The cells that compose these structures (fig. 1-9) are unlike those of biliary epithelium, but phenotypically identical to the cells of the Brunner glands of the duodenum and the pyloric and cardiac glands of the stomach (1).

Other Mesenchymal Cells. These are minor constituents of the liver. Smooth muscle cells are found in portal vessels, ligaments of the liver, and supporting tissue in the walls of bile ducts. Fibroblasts and sometimes myofibroblasts are present in the fibrous supporting tissue of portal tracts and in the capsule. Nerves are readily seen in large septa, and nerve fibers, while inconspicuous, reach the smallest portal areas.

Inflammatory Cells. A truly normal liver has few, if any, inflammatory cells, other than the sinusoidal Kupffer cells and pit cells noted above. As the individual progresses through life, however, inflammatory cells tend to increase as the residual of minor injuries that have occurred. The portal areas contain macrophages and a few lymphocytes, and virtually any other inflammatory cell type may be present in response to a disease process.

HISTOLOGIC ORGANIZATION

The microscopic organization of the liver is described in relation to its blood supply and biliary drainage (3–7,9). In traditional histologic terminology, the liver is composed of a honeycomb-like array of hexagonal lobules, each with a central vein and portal triads at alternating corners (fig. 1-10). Blood enters the tissue through small branches of the portal vein and hepatic artery.

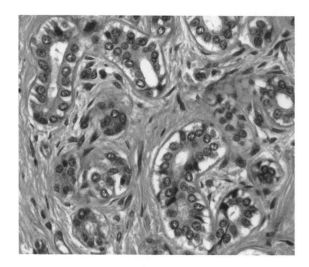

Figure 1-9
PERIBILIARY GLANDS
Small glands in the walls of large bile ducts are composed of small acini of cuboidal cells that resemble bile ducts.

These empty into the sinusoids nearest to the portal areas, and so the periportal (peripheral) part of the lobule has the richest supply of nutrients and oxygen. The part closest to the central vein (centrilobular) receives oxygen-depleted blood and is consequently most susceptible to anoxia and many other types of injury.

An alternative and more physiologic way to view hepatic histology is in terms of the acinus (fig. 1-10). The acini are three-dimensional spherical structures arranged like clusters of grapes around the major branches of the portal tracts. Each acinus has a terminal portal triad at its center. The spherical portion of parenchyma surrounding this is referred to as acinar zone 1; outside of this is zone 2; and at the circulatory periphery, receiving the blood poorest in oxygen and nutrients, is zone 3.

The lobule is a two-dimensional theoretical concept, and since microscopic sections are two-dimensional also, it is easy to think in terms of lobules and lobular landmarks. For most purposes this is adequate, but since the liver exists in three dimensions and, since the three-dimensional acinus more closely approximates the true physiologic functional unit, this is a more accurate way to describe hepatic histology and pathology. Pathologic processes generally follow acinar zones and necessarily lobular zones, but unfortunately, it is difficult to think in three dimensions when looking at a two-dimensional

Figure 1-10
HEPATIC ARCHITECTURE
Two views of the architecture of the liver as seen in microscopic sections. Lobules have a central vein at the center and portal spaces at the corners. A cross section of an acinus superimposed on two lobules shows that zone III tends to be centrilobular, zone II midzonal, and zone I periportal, but all three are crescent shaped and may extend into other parts of the classic lobule.

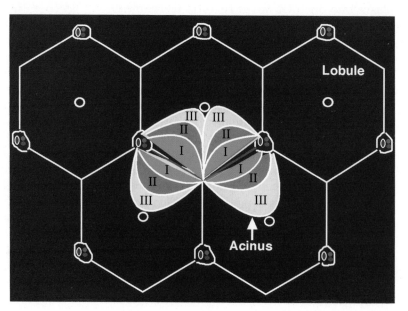

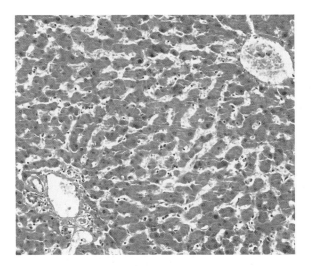

Figure 1-11
HEPATIC ARCHITECTURE
Plates of hepatocytes extend from the portal area (lower left) to the terminal hepatic venule or central vein (upper right). Blood that enters the liver through branches of the portal vein and hepatic artery perfuses the sinusoids and exits through tributaries of the hepatic vein.

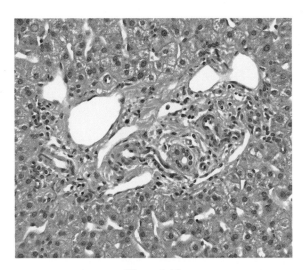

Figure 1-12
PORTAL AREA
A normal small portal area has at least one portal vein branch, one hepatic arteriole, and one bile duct.

section. For most purposes, either lobular or acinar terminology is acceptable.

Cords or, more properly, plates of hepatocytes run in a radial array between the portal areas and central veins (fig. 1-11). The hepatocyte plates are separated by sinusoids lined by endothelial cells and macrophages (Kupffer cells). The sinusoids differ from capillaries in other tissues. Sinusoidal endothelial cells are fenestrated and lack a basement membrane, so that the plasma is in direct contact with the liver cells in the subendothelial space of Disse, where the stellate cells, which store vitamin A and produce collagen, are located. The hepatocytes secrete bile into a network of canaliculi that run within the liver cell plates. These drain toward the portal areas and empty through small ductules into the interlobular bile ducts of the portal triads.

The portal areas (fig. 1-12) have a collagenous supporting stroma within which is at least one interlobular bile duct, one portal vein branch, and one hepatic artery branch. Ductules or canals of Hering can sometimes be found at the edges of portal areas, but are usually inconspicuous in normal liver. The layer of hepatocytes closest to the portal area is called the "limiting plate," a useful landmark in chronic hepatitis.

GROSS ANATOMY

Gross anatomy (2,8,9) plays little role in tumor classification, but it is important in the planning and execution of therapy, especially surgical resection. Traditionally, the liver is considered to have four lobes, based on surface anatomy. The right and left lobes are visible anteriorly, divided by the falciform ligament, while the quadrate lobe, adjacent to the gallbladder fossa, and caudate lobe, partially surrounding the inferior vena cava, are visible on the under surface. The true functional anatomic segments do not correspond very well to these lobes, but rather to eight divisions based on the internal blood supply (fig. 1-13) and designated by Roman numerals. Each segment is supplied by separate major branches of the hepatic artery and portal vein. Venous drainage from the caudate lobe (segment I) is directly into the inferior vena cava, while the other seven segments drain into branches of the hepatic veins and thence into the vena cava. Segments I to IV, which are left of the line from the gallbladder fossa to the vena cava, are considered the functional left lobe, while segments V to VIII are the functional right lobe.

Small lesions can be removed by subsegmental or "wedge" resections, but surgical procedures to remove large tumors are often based on the segmental anatomy, as one or more of the segments can be removed en bloc. Removal of the traditional

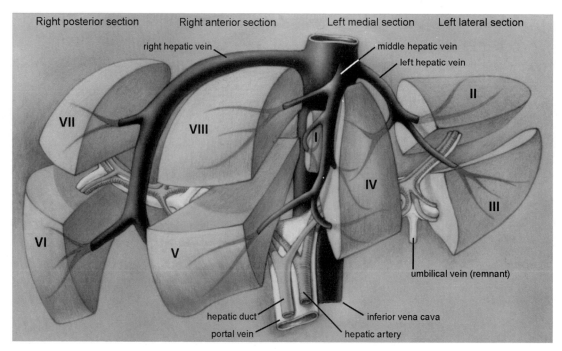

Figure 1-13
SEGMENTAL ANATOMY OF THE LIVER
The segments, designated by Roman numerals, can be resected surgically because each is supplied by a major branch of the hepatic artery and portal vein and drained by a major tributary of the hepatic vein. (Fig. 1-4 from Wanless IR. Physioanatomic considerations. In: Schiff ER, Sorrell MF, Maddrey WC, eds. Diseases of the liver, 8th ed. Philadelphia, JB Lippincott Co, 1999:3-37.)

left lobe (segments II and III) to the left of the falciform ligament is called a left lateral segmentectomy, while removal of the functional left lobe (segments I to IV) is a left lobectomy. A right lobectomy removes the functional right lobe (segments V to VIII) and an extended right lobectomy, or trisegmentectomy, removes the traditional right lobe (segments IV to VIII).

REFERENCES

1. Bhathal PS, Hughes NR, Goodman ZD. The so-called bile duct adenoma is a peribiliary gland hamartoma. Am J Surg Pathol 1996;20:858–64.
2. Bismuth H. Surgical anatomy and anatomical surgery of the liver. World J Surg 1982;6:3–9.
3. Desmet VJ. Intrahepatic bile ducts under the lens. J Hepatol 1985;1:545–59.
4. Jones AL, Aggeler J. Structure of the liver. In: Haubrich WS, Schaffner F, Berk JE, eds. Bockus gastroenterology, 5th ed. Philadelphia: WB Saunders Co, 1995:1813–31.
5. Kahn E, Markowitz J, Aiges H, Daum F. Human ontogeny of the bile duct to portal space ratio. Hepatology 1989;10:21–3.
6. MacSween RN, Scothorne RJ. Developmental anatomy and normal structure. In: MacSween RN, Anthony PP, Scheuer PJ, Burt AD, Portmann BC, eds. Pathology of the liver, 3rd ed. Edinburgh: Churchill Livingstone, 1994:1–50.
7. Ruebner BH, Blankenberg TA, Burrows DA, SooHoo W, Lund JK. Development and transformation of the ductal plate in the developing human liver. Pediatr Pathol 1990;10:55–68.
8. Schwartz SI. Liver. In: Schwartz SI, Shires GT, Spencer FC, Husser WC, eds. Principles of surgery, 6th ed. New York: McGraw-Hill, 1994:1319–66.
9. Wanless IR. Physioanatomic considerations. In: Schiff ER, Sorrell MF, Maddrey WC, eds. Diseases of the liver, 8th ed. Philadelphia: JB Lippincott, 1999:3–37.
10. Wennerberg AE, Nalesnik MA, Coleman WB. Hepatocyte paraffin 1: a monoclonal antibody that reacts with hepatocytes and can be used for differential diagnosis of hepatic tumors. Am J Pathol 1993;143:1050–4.

2
BENIGN HEPATOCELLULAR TUMORS

This chapter deals with the major forms of benign hepatocellular proliferations (Table 2-1), including the three important benign hepatocellular lesions: hepatocellular adenoma (HCA), nodular regenerative hyperplasia (NRH), and focal nodular hyperplasia (FNH). All three lesions arise in a noncirrhotic liver. Benign proliferative lesions occurring in the cirrhotic liver, such as dysplastic nodules, are discussed in the chapter on putative precancerous lesions (chapter 7). Regenerative nodules occurring in livers with submassive necrosis and compensatory hypertrophy of a liver lobe, following atrophy of another lobe, are mentioned briefly.

HCA, NRH, and FNH may occur in both sexes (although HCA is much more frequent in females), and in all age groups (although all three lesions are less common in the pediatric age group). The lesions of NRH are multiple, whereas HCA and FNH are more frequently single. Both NRH and

Table 2-1

TERMINOLOGY OF BENIGN HEPATOCELLULAR PROLIFERATIONS

Entity	Definition
Hepatocellular adenoma	Proliferation of benign hepatocytes without acinar architecture No more than three nodules per liver Normal acinar architecture without parenchymal nodularity in remainder of liver
Hepatocellular adenomatosis	Multiple nodular proliferations of benign hepatocytes without acinar architecture Four or more nodules per liver Normal acinar architecture without parenchymal nodularity in remainder of liver
Nodular regenerative hyperplasia	Diffuse parenchymal nodularity without fibrosis, with preservation of acinar architecture Nodules relatively uniform and small
Nodular regenerative hyperplasia with adenoma-like nodules	One or more nodular proliferations of benign hepatocytes without acinar architecture Diffuse parenchymal nodularity with preservation of acinar architecture and without fibrosis in remainder of liver
Partial nodular transformation	Nodular regenerative hyperplasia-like condition, usually limited to hilar region of liver
Focal nodular hyperplasia	Solitary lesion (may be multiple) with a central or eccentric scar containing an aberrant large artery surrounded by hyperplastic hepatocellular nodules, arising in a normal liver
Compensatory hypertrophy	Enlargement of one lobe of the liver following atrophy of the other lobe secondary to ischemia or biliary obstruction
Postnecrotic regenerative nodule	A large nodule of regenerating hepatocytes that grows following submassive hepatic necrosis of any cause
Multiacinar regenerative nodule (Macroregenerative nodule)	A cirrhotic nodule 5–15 mm in diameter, composed of two cell–thick plates Hepatocytes resemble those in the rest of the liver, but occasionally, low-grade dysplastic areas may be seen
Dysplastic nodule	A nodule of hepatocytes, at least 1 mm in diameter, with dysplasia, low or high grade, usually found in a cirrhotic liver (see chapter 7)

FNH have a vascular basis, while HCA appears to be a true neoplasm induced by contraceptive, and less often, anabolic steroids, or by the glycogenoses or other rare conditions. Rupture is a very serious complication of HCA, regardless of etiology, and may be the initial mode of presentation. More often, patients with HCA come to medical attention because of a mass in the upper abdomen or hepatomegaly. FNH may be symptomatic but is more often diagnosed incidentally at laparotomy or autopsy, or by radiographic imaging. NRH may be manifested by portal hypertension or by symptoms and signs of the underlying disease. Malignant transformation, albeit rare, is a documented complication of HCA.

HEPATOCELLULAR ADENOMA

Definition. HCA is a benign neoplasm composed of cells that closely resemble normal hepatocytes. The lesion arises in a normal liver with the exception of those occurring in patients with the glycogenoses.

Etiology and Epidemiology. Hepatocellular adenomas (frequently called *liver cell adenomas*) typically develop in the setting of a hormonal or metabolic abnormality with the capacity to stimulate hepatocyte proliferation (Table 2-2) (3,4,7,9, 11,20–22,30,33,42,44,47,64,69). In the absence of one of these predisposing conditions, the diagnosis is highly suspect. Exogenous steroid hormone ingestion is undoubtedly the most common such abnormality, and oral contraceptive steroids are the cause of most of these tumors, as demonstrated by epidemiologic case-control studies conducted in the 1970s (20,66). Thus, the tumor nearly always is found in women in the reproductive years, ages 15 to 45, with an incidence estimated to be 3 to 4 per 100,000 long-term contraceptive steroid users per year; an incidence of only 1 per million occurs in nonusers or women with less than 2 years' exposure to contraceptive steroids. The risk increases with duration of contraceptive steroid use and with the potency of the preparation. There is currently a general impression that the incidence of HCA has declined with the use of second and third generation oral contraceptives. In one epidemiologic study from Germany no liver tumors were reported in women who had used third generation oral contraceptives for a 15-year period (61).

Table 2-2

ETIOLOGIC FACTORS AND DISEASES ASSOCIATED WITH HEPATOCELLULAR ADENOMA

Oral contraceptive steroids

Noncontraceptive estrogens, e.g., danazol

Virilizing and feminizing ovarian tumors

Endogenous sex steroids

Klinefelter's syndrome

Antiestrogens, e.g., clomiphene citrate

Anabolic/androgenic steroids

Carbamazepine therapy

Severe combined immunodeficiency

Type Ia glycogenosis

Type III glycogenosis

Hurler's disease

Familial diabetes mellitus

Beta-thalassemia with secondary iron overload

The exact mechanism by which adenomas are produced is not known, but experimental evidence suggests that sex hormones are promotors rather than initiators of hepatocellular neoplasms (59,77). Estrogen, progesterone, and androgen receptors have been found in the tumors by some investigators but not by others (8,13,46). In several cases unresectable masses have been observed to regress after contraceptive steroid use was stopped (6,21). Alternative pathogenetic mechanisms are suggested by the other conditions associated with HCA (Table 2-3). Experimentally, methyl testosterone acts as a weak total hepatocarcinogen when administered long-term to BALB/c mice (72).

Since HCAs nearly always occur in long-term users of oral contraceptives, any cases outside this setting are highly suspect, and may actually be a different benign lesion such as FNH or a well-differentiated hepatocellular carcinoma. Cases of HCA have been reported in men, children, and women not taking oral contraceptives, but these are rare (32,38,64,79), with the exception of cases related to the glycogenoses and to anabolic steroid use. It is important to point out that we consider so-called HCA in cirrhotic livers of patients with

Table 2-3

COMPARISON OF HEPATOCELLULAR ADENOMA (HCA), NODULAR REGENERATIVE HYPERPLASIA (NRH), AND FOCAL NODULAR HYPERPLASIA (FNH)

Lesion	Associated Conditions	Portal Hyper-tension	Liver Weight	Acinar Atrophy	Fibrous Scars/ Septa/ Ductules	Chronic Chole-stasis	Vascular Changes
HCA (S,M)*	Peliosis hepatis, intrahepatic cholestasis, hemosiderosis (AS-related tumors)	–	Increased	–	–	–	–
NRH (M)	Myeloproliferative disorders, connective tissue diseases, drugs, thrombosis of portal vein	+/–	Decreased or normal	+	–	–	Portal venopathy
FNH (S,M)	Cavernous hemangioma, extra-hepatic vascular lesions, brain tumors	–	Normal or increased	–	+	+	Thick arteries in septa

*S = single; M = multiple; AS = anabolic steroid; + = present; +/– = present or absent; – = absent.

some of the inherited metabolic diseases as examples of macroregenerative nodules (1,19).

Clinical Features. In two large series of HCA associated with oral contraceptives the average age was 30 years, and most patients were between 20 and 39 years (12,66). Patients usually come to medical attention when symptoms develop, and only 5 to 10 percent of lesions are found incidentally. Symptoms include abdominal mass (25 to 35 percent of patients); chronic or mild episodic abdominal pain (20 to 25 percent); and acute abdominal pain (30 to 40 percent), due to hemorrhage into the tumor (30 percent) or into the peritoneal cavity (70 percent). Intraperitoneal hemorrhage, the most serious complication of HCA, regardless of etiology, often requires emergency surgery and causes circulatory collapse and death in 20 percent of patients. Pregnancy is a recognized risk factor for rupture of HCA (37,75). Rare manifestations of HCA include systemic AA amyloidosis (15,74), and production of cortisol and adrenocorticotrophic hormone (ACTH) or ACTH-like peptides (39). Levels of serum alpha-fetoprotein are in the normal range. Radiographic imaging studies typically demonstrate a mass with little to distinguish it from other benign and malignant lesions. Radionuclide colloid scans usually show a photopenic area, indicating a lack of functioning Kupffer cells (43).

The majority of adenomas in patients on anabolic steroids have occurred in those with Fanconi's anemia, but "non-Fanconi" cases have been reported, e.g., in patients with other anemias, hypopituitarism, hypogonadism, transsexualism and impotence, and in those on body building regimens (10,16,30,33,69,78). The majority of the patients, with one exception (10), had received 17-alpha alkylated compounds. Patients have ranged from 5 to 68 years of age, with a mean age of 31.2 years (10). Most of the patients had received the anabolic steroids for more than 2 years.

Many cases of HCA have occurred in patients with glycogenosis Ia; a lesser number have been diagnosed in patients with glycogenosis III (4,14, 42,67): in one large series, adenomas were reported in 28 percent and 10 percent of patients with glycogenosis Ia and III, respectively (70). These patients are from 3 to 40 years of age; twice as many cases have been reported in males than in females (14).

Gross Findings. HCA is a solitary nodule, although occasional patients may have more than one (figs. 2-1–2-3). Adenomas related to anabolic androgen therapy and the glycogenoses are usually multiple (fig. 2-4). The liver surrounding the HCA reveals no fibrosis or cirrhosis. Some of the anabolic steroid–related adenomas may be associated with peliosis hepatis, another complication of that therapy. The tumors are globular,

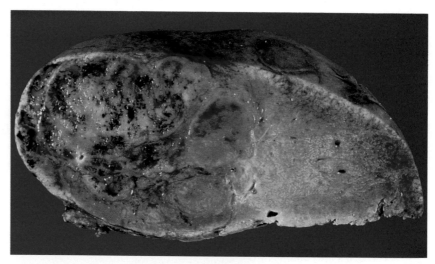

Figure 2-1
HEPATOCELLULAR
ADENOMA
A section of an oral contracep-tive-related tumor that is nonen-capsulated, and demonstrates ill-defined nodularity and multiple hemorrhages.

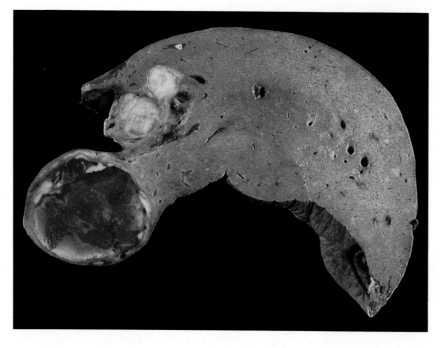

Figure 2-2
HEPATOCELLULAR
ADENOMAS
One of the three oral contracep-tive-related adenomas is totally infarcted.

spherical or ovoid, and may measure up to 30 cm in diameter, although the majority are 5 to 15 cm. They are rarely multilobulated (20). Many adenomas bulge from the surface of the liver and often have large blood vessels running across the surface. A few are pedunculated.

On sectioning, the tumors are firm to soft and well demarcated from the surrounding liver, but are usually unencapsulated (figs. 2-1, 2-2). The color varies from yellow or tan to brown, and there may be green areas indicating bile produc-tion or rarely, a slate gray to black color due to

an excessive amount of lipofuscin. There is often a variegated appearance, with solid areas of light brown to tan tumor tissue alternating with yel-low areas of necrosis; white infarcts surrounded by zones of hyperemia; and cystic, reddish brown hemorrhagic foci (fig. 2-1). Sometimes, irregular scars mark areas of previous necrosis.

Microscopic Findings. HCAs are composed of benign hepatocytes arranged in sheets and cords without an acinar architecture (figs. 2-5, 2-6). A striking feature of some, but not all the tumors associated with anabolic steroid use, is

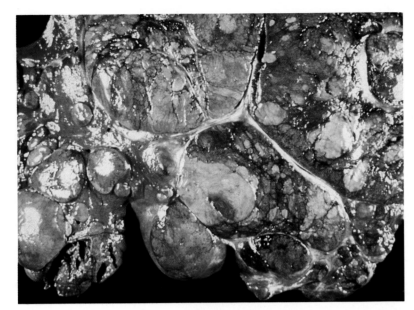

Figure 2-3
HEPATOCELLULAR
ADENOMATOSIS
Multiple adenomas of varied size have a yellowish color due to an increased content of fat. The tumors were of unknown etiology.

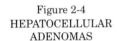

Figure 2-4
HEPATOCELLULAR
ADENOMAS
Two adenomas with extensive hemorrhage in a patient with glycogenosis type I.

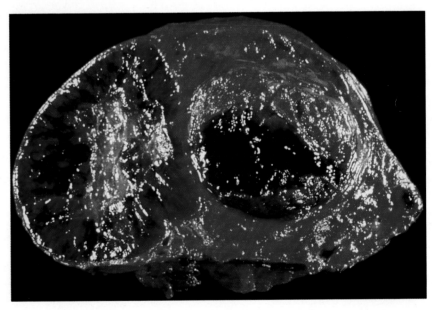

pseudogland formation, with bile-plugging of centrally located canaliculi (fig. 2-7). The tumor cells may be the same size but are usually larger and paler than nontumor hepatocytes in the surrounding tissue, due to increased cytoplasmic glycogen and/or fat (fig. 2-8). However, the cells of tumors occurring in patients with glycogenoses Ia and III typically contain much less glycogen than the non-neoplastic cells (figs. 2-9–2-11). In some cases fat accumulation is quite abundant, and if the lack of an acinar architecture is not noted,

the lesion may be mistaken for non-neoplastic fatty liver. The tumor cell cytoplasm may rarely contain an abundant Dubin-Johnson–like pigment; these "pigmented liver cell adenomas" (28a) were at one time considered to be hepatocellular carcinomas. Mallory bodies may be seen in rare adenomas induced by oral contraceptives (29) or in patients with glycogenosis type Ia (58). Bile is sometimes present in the cytoplasm, intercellular canaliculi, or dilated pseudoglands, particularly at the periphery. The presence of

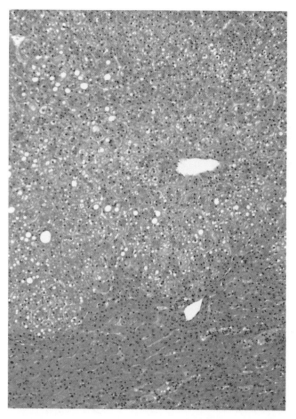

Figure 2-5
HEPATOCELLULAR ADENOMA
Cells of this oral contraceptive-related tumor (top) are larger and paler than the normal hepatocytes (bottom).

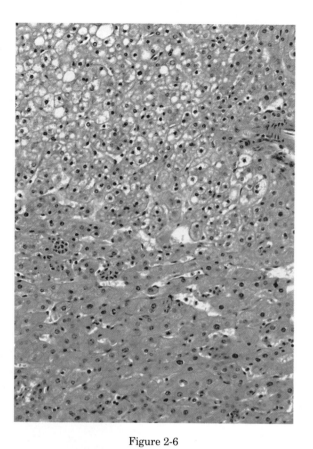

Figure 2-6
HEPATOCELLULAR ADENOMA
Higher magnification of the tumor shown in figure 2-5 shows large cells with a low nuclear/cytoplasmic ratio and a pale or vacuolated cytoplasm.

Figure 2-7
HEPATOCELLULAR
ADENOMA
This anabolic steroid-related tumor reveals pseudogland formation, with bile casts in the lumen of the pseudoglands.

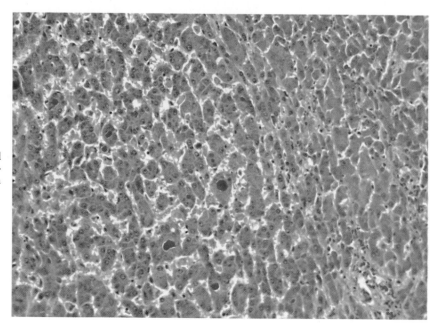

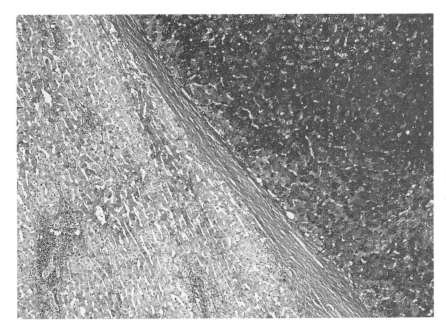

Figure 2-8
HEPATOCELLULAR
ADENOMA
Cells of this oral contraceptive-related tumor (right) contain much more glycogen than those of the adjacent liver (left) (PAS stain).

Table 2-4

**HISTOLOGIC DIFFERENTIAL DIAGNOSIS OF HEPATOCELLULAR
ADENOMA AND HEPATOCELLULAR CARCINOMA**

Feature	Hepatocellular Adenoma	Hepatocellular Carcinoma
Nuclei	Regular	Pleomorphic
Nucleoli	Variable	Often prominent
Mitoses	Absent	Often present
N/C* ratio	Low	High
Cytoplasm	Abundant, with fat and glycogen	Less abundant, variable fat and glycogen
Architecture	Sheets and two cell-thick plates	Trabeculae, pseudoglands, and others
Invasion (vessels, bile ducts)	Absent	Present

*N/C = nuclear/cytoplasmic.

canaliculi can be confirmed by use of a polyclonal carcinoembryonic antigen immunostain. The tumor cells do not express alpha-fetoprotein.

The nuclei of HCAs are typically uniform and regular, the nuclear/cytoplasmic ratio is normal, and mitoses are almost never seen. In most tumors they are normochromatic and contain small amphophilic nucleoli, but moderately pleomorphic cells with multiple or dysplastic nuclei (large cell change) can be seen, especially in patients who have taken contraceptive steroids for more than a decade (figs. 2-12, 2-13) (57). This dysplasia probably merely indicates a tumor that has been

present for some time, but any nuclear pleomorphism should raise the possibility that the lesion is a carcinoma rather than an adenoma (Table 2-4). Many of the tumors complicating anabolic steroid therapy have been misdiagnosed as hepatocellular carcinoma on the basis of prominent dysplasia. The dysplastic cells resemble those of "large cell" dysplasia (or large cell change) occurring in a cirrhotic milieu (see chapter 7), but can be distinguished from malignant cells by their normal nuclear/cytoplasmic ratio.

The typical HCA has no collagenous stroma, and reticulin fibers are usually present. Bile ducts are

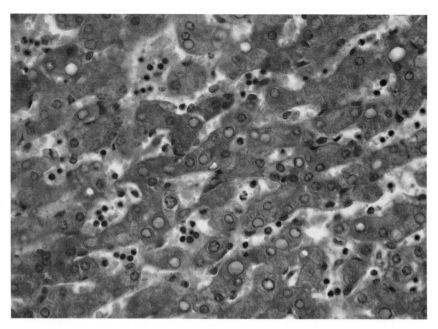

Figure 2-9
HEPATOCELLULAR
ADENOMA

This tumor in a patient with glycogenosis type I shows two cell-thick
plates, and minimal variation in size
and shape of cells and nuclei. Note
the multiple glycogenated nuclei of
the tumor cells and the hematopoietic cells in the sinusoids of the
tumor. (Figures 2-9 through 2-11
are from the same case.)

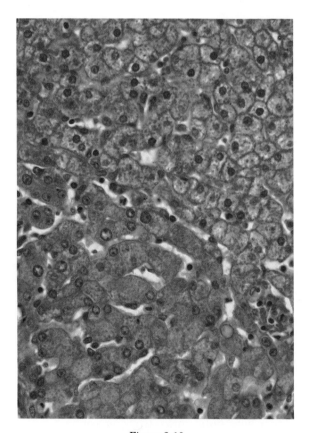

Figure 2-10
HEPATOCELLULAR ADENOMA

The tumor cells (bottom) are arranged in two cell-thick
plates. Note the lighter cytoplasm of the glycogen-laden,
non-neoplastic cells (top).

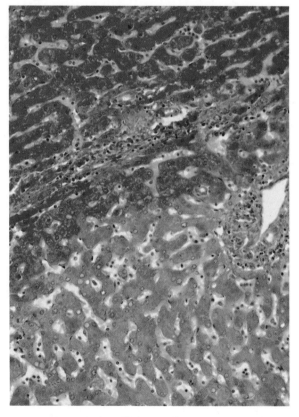

Figure 2-11
HEPATOCELLULAR ADENOMA

The non-neoplastic cells (top) are full of glycogen whereas
the adenoma cells (bottom) contain none (PAS stain).

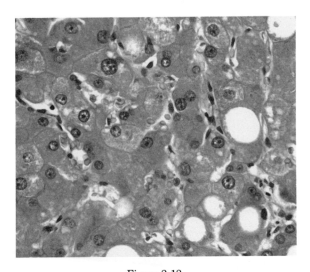

Figure 2-12
HEPATOCELLULAR ADENOMA
Marked variation in the size of the nuclei of an oral contraceptive-related tumor. Some cells contain fat vacuoles and/or bile.

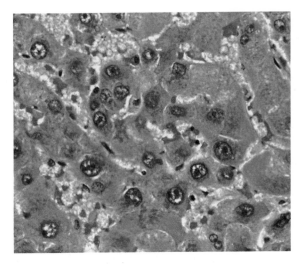

Figure 2-13
HEPATOCELLULAR ADENOMA
Large cell dysplasia of tumor cells.

typically absent. Thin-walled vascular channels are scattered throughout the tumor but large arteries are only seen around the periphery. The sinusoids, with flattened endothelial-lining cells, are usually compressed, thus contributing to the sheet-like appearance. Sometimes the sinusoids are dilated, a finding that can be mistaken for peliosis hepatis. Kupffer cells are present although usually inconspicuous (fig. 2-14), and perisinusoidal lipocytes are rarely seen. Hematopoietic elements are noted in the sinusoidal lumina of some tumors (figs. 2-9, 2-15), and a few tumors have noncaseating granulomas (fig. 2-16) (31,40). Degenerative changes include apoptotic bodies, focal necrosis, a myxoid stroma (27), recent small or large hemorrhages (sometimes erroneously referred to as peliosis hepatis), recent or old infarcts, and areas of scarring containing hemosiderin-laden macrophages from old hemorrhages (figs. 2-17, 2-18). HCAs in patients with type I glycogenosis may have fibrous septa, presumably reflecting long duration, and can be confused with focal nodular hyperplasia (4).

The large vessels, especially arteries, located at the periphery of HCA display characteristic changes which include intimal thickening, accumulation of acid mucopolysaccharide, and thickening and reduplication of the internal elastic

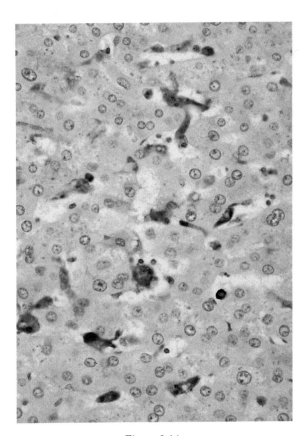

Figure 2-14
HEPATOCELLULAR ADENOMA
Numerous Kupffer cells in an oral contraceptive-related tumor (lysozyme immunostain).

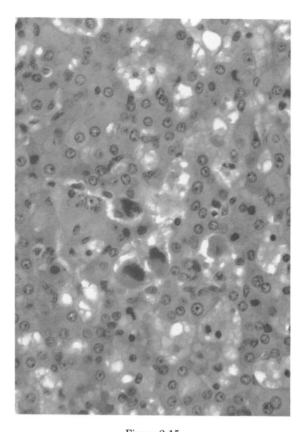

Figure 2-15
HEPATOCELLULAR ADENOMA
Three megakaryocytes in sinusoids of an oral contraceptive-related tumor.

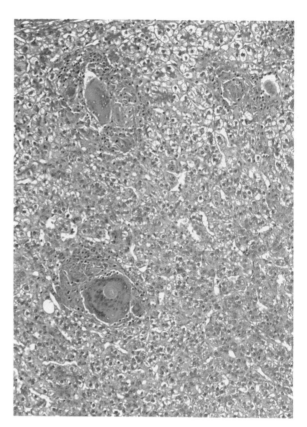

Figure 2-16
HEPATOCELLULAR ADENOMA
Three epithelioid granulomas within an oral contraceptive-related tumor. No granulomas were present in the non-neoplastic parenchyma (not shown).

lamina (fig. 2-19, left). Veins may exhibit marked proliferation of smooth muscle fibers with narrowing or obliteration of the lumen (fig. 2-19, right). In the past we suspected that these changes might represent a contraceptive steroid–related vasculopathy. However, we have found similar vascular lesions around other liver tumors unrelated to contraceptive steroids (although less often), and we now believe this most likely is a nonspecific vascular response rather than a drug-induced lesion. Deep in HCAs, the vessels (usually small paired arteries and veins) are normal in appearance and are not found in collagenized septa.

As already mentioned, the non-neoplastic parenchyma in adenomas related to the use of anabolic steroids may show peliosis hepatis (fig. 2-20). Additionally, there may be intrahepatic cholestasis, another complication of anabolic steroid therapy, as well as hemosiderosis related to the underlying anemia or to multiple blood transfusions.

Ultrastructural Findings. These are not helpful in diagnosis. They include the presence of bile canaliculi with tight junctions and desmosomes, pleomorphism of mitochondria that often contain paracrystalline inclusions, an increased content of glycogen, paucity of Kupffer cells, absence of perisinusoidal lipocytes (which are replaced by myofibroblasts), and capillarization of sinusoids (2,5,36).

Differential Diagnosis. Benign lesions that must be distinguished from HCA are discussed later in this chapter. Distinction from well-differentiated hepatocellular carcinoma can be difficult and sometimes impossible, but can usually be made morphologically (Table 2-4). Recognition of a trabecular growth pattern and cytologic features of malignancy, including high nuclear/cytoplasmic ratios and nuclear irregularities, are most helpful. When a lesion with all the features of HCA has a moderate degree of nuclear irregularity and

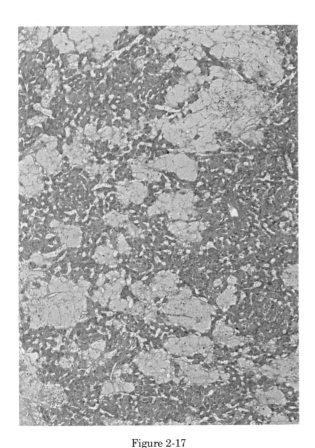

Figure 2-17
HEPATOCELLULAR ADENOMA
Multiple (peliosis-like) foci of hemorrhage in an oral contraceptive-related adenoma.

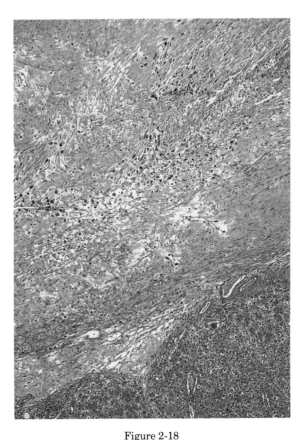

Figure 2-18
HEPATOCELLULAR ADENOMA
Segment of a large area of fibrosis containing hemosiderin-laden macrophages.

hyperchromatism, the history should be taken into account. If the patient had been taking oral contraceptives or other sex steroids, then the tumor is best regarded as an atypical HCA; but if it is certain that there is no such history, it is probably a well-differentiated hepatocellular carcinoma. It has been suggested that the expression of CD34 (detected with antibody Q Bend 10) may be helpful in the differentiation of hepatocellular carcinoma from HCA. In one study, this immunostain was reported to produce diffuse staining of a large number of sinusoids in hepatocellular carcinoma in contrast to HCA (and macroregenerative nodules) where the staining was focal or identified only marginal sinusoids (18). Similarly, it has been suggested that fluorescence in situ hybridization (FISH) may also help differentiate benign from malignant neoplasms of the liver; Nasarek et al. (52a) found that trisomy 1 and 8 occur frequently in hepatocellular carcinoma but not in HCA and focal nodular hyperplasia.

More recently, Wilkens et al. (123a) found multiple chromosomal aberrations, including gains or losses in one or more of six chromosomes (1q, 4q, 8p, 8q, 16p, and 17p) in six well-developed hepatocellular carcinomas, but not in any of 10 hepatocellular adenomas. They felt that the detection of frequent aberrations supports a diagnosis of carcinoma and makes HCA unlikely.

Treatment and Prognosis. Surgical excision is usually advised for HCA to prevent the possibility of rupture and hemorrhage, and because of the risk of malignant transformation. As already noted, pregnancy is reported to cause unresected HCA to grow, become symptomatic, and sometimes rupture (37,75), but women who have had their tumors resected do not have further problems during subsequent pregnancies (66). Contraceptive steroid–related tumors usually (but not always) regress if the patient stops taking the exogenous hormones (6,21,41,45), as do adenomas complicating anabolic steroid therapy

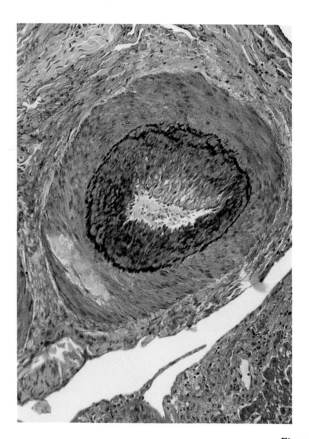
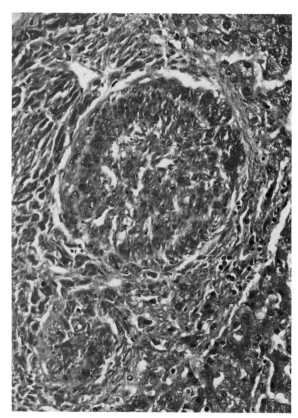

Figure 2-19
HEPATOCELLULAR ADENOMA

Left: The artery in the portal area adjacent to the tumor shows intimal hyperplasia and an abnormal elastica (Musto pentachrome stain).

Right: The portal vein branch from the same case shows total occlusion due to marked smooth muscle hypertrophy (Masson trichrome stain).

Figure 2-20
HEPATOCELLULAR
ADENOMA

The non-neoplastic parenchyma of an anabolic steroid-related tumor shows peliosis hepatis.

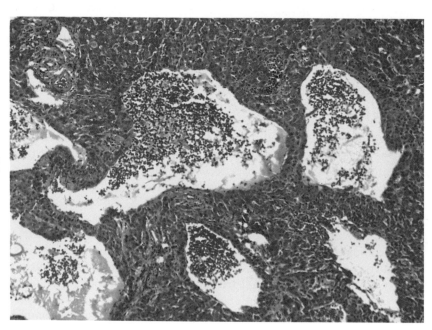

(11,22,48,51). Adenomas in type I glycogen storage disease may or may not regress with dietary therapy (55,67). Too few other cases have been followed to know whether this is generally true for spontaneous HCA, but there are some unresected tumors that have remained stable for up to 26 years (79). Recurrences of resected oral contraceptive–related tumors are rare unless the patient continues to use those agents. We have seen one case in which a recurrence (presumably an implant) of HCA was discovered in the omentum 11 years after the original tumor was removed. Alternative therapeutic modalities for HCAs that cannot be resected include arterial embolization (17,42,49) and orthotopic liver transplantation (52).

Malignant transformation is rare, since most HCAs are resected when discovered. However, there are a few well-documented cases of hepatocellular carcinoma arising in unresected solitary as well multiple adenomas (22,25,32,68). A case on file at the Armed Forces Institute of Pathology (AFIP) is illustrated in figures 2-21 through 2-23. There is one report of development of hepatocellular carcinoma at the site of an HCA that had regressed 5 years after discontinuation of oral contraceptive use (28): this may represent an adenoma-carcinoma sequence in hepatocellular neoplasia, similar to that seen in colonic neoplasms. It is advisable, therefore, to reserve the diagnosis of HCA for tumors that are well sampled histologically, have no microscopic evidence of malignancy, and have an association with a known etiologic factor. Whether all hepatocellular carcinomas reported in women who had used contraceptive steroids develop in a preexisting HCA is not established. There is, however, evidence from case control studies suggesting an etiologic relationship between hepatocellular carcinoma and the use of contraceptive steroids, particularly for more than 8 years (71,73); thus some cases must develop through that sequence.

A diagnostic problem arises when a hepatocellular tumor has features of both adenoma and carcinoma. In the past, we have usually maintained that if a tumor appears to be predominantly HCA but also has areas of unequivocal hepatocellular carcinoma, then the entire tumor is really hepatocellular carcinoma. The adenoma-like area is regarded as grade 1 carcinoma, while the more malignant areas are grade 2 or higher. It is pos-

sible that all hepatocellular carcinomas arising in noncirrhotic livers are adenoma-like when small and only later develop more frankly malignant features, a concept that is better established in cirrhosis, where small benign lesions called dysplastic nodules may develop atypical features (low- and high-grade dysplasia) and finally hepatocellular carcinoma (see chapter 7).

Hepatocellular carcinomas, at least some of which are presumed to have arisen in adenomas, have also been reported in patients on anabolic steroids and with the glycogenoses. In reference to the anabolic steroids, acceptable cases of hepatocellular carcinoma have to meet rigid criteria that include an elevated serum alpha-fetoprotein level, unequivocal histopathology, and/or distant metastases. Of the 10 acceptable cases (22,30,33, 41,50,53,54,63,76,78,80), one had documented postnecrotic cirrhosis (63) that could have been the underlying etiologic condition for the malignancy. Another tumor was the fibrolamellar variant of hepatocellular carcinoma (41). In reference to glycogenosis type Ia, there are at least seven cases of hepatocellular carcinoma reported in the literature; two unpublished examples are on file at AFIP. None of those patients had an underlying cirrhosis.

Liver Adenomatosis. There is no question that HCA can be multiple (fig. 2-3). Most patients have one, but some have two, three, or many tumors that are histologically similar. The term *adenomatosis,* although used previously by others, was defined by Flejou et al. (24) as more than three (but often more than 10) adenomas (fig. 2-3). According to these authors, the distinctive characteristics of this entity are: 1) it affects both men and women, as opposed to HCA that mainly occurs in women. However, HCA does occur in men, albeit much less frequently than in women (56,62). Furthermore, in a recently reported series of patients with liver adenomatosis by Ribeiro et al. (65) all were women; 2) the condition is unrelated to oral contraceptives, although 37 percent of the patients reviewed had used these agents, as was the case with some of the subsequently reported examples (40,65); and 3) increases in serum alkaline phosphatase and gamma-glutamyl transpeptidase are more frequent in adenomatosis than in HCA, a statement that is not corroborated by our experience when all causes of multiple adenomas are considered. None of the

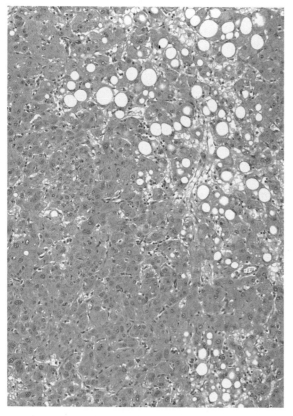

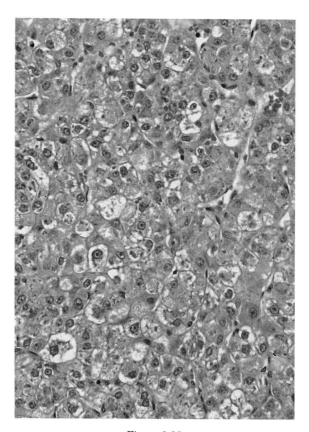

Figure 2-21
HEPATOCELLULAR ADENOMA
Cellular atypia and steatosis in an oral contraceptive-related tumor. (Figures 2-21 through 2-23 are from the same patient.)

Figure 2-22
HEPATOCELLULAR ADENOMA
This figure shows an area of well-differentiated hepatocellular carcinoma.

Figure 2-23
HEPATOCELLULAR
ADENOMA
Ki-67 is expressed in the nuclei of cells of hepatocellular carcinoma (right), but not in cells of the adenoma (left).

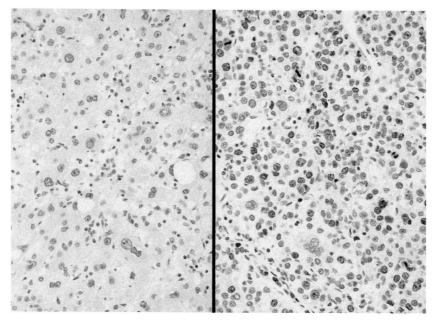

aforementioned characteristics are distinctive for multiple, as opposed to single HCA. Additionally, both Flejou et al. (24) and Ribeiro et al. (65) arbitrarily excluded the two most important causes of multiple HCA, viz, the glycogenoses and anabolic steroid therapy. In fact, almost all of the etiologic factors listed in Table 2-2 are associated with multiple as well as single adenomas. They include the contraceptive and anabolic steroids; other drugs such as danazol (34), clomiphene (9) or norethisterone (35), and carbamazepine (72a); glycogenoses Ia and III (14,42,70); Hurler's syndrome (64); and diabetes mellitus (26). As already mentioned, malignant transformation has occurred in some HCAs due to oral contraceptive use as well as use of anabolic steroids, glycogenesis Ia, and idiopathic hepatocellular adenomatosis, although all of these lesions may regress or remain unchanged for many years. There is a recent report of an 11-year follow-up of a patient with idiopathic adenomatosis with no complications (60). However, the development of hepatocellular carcinoma has been reported rarely (23,40).

The importance of liver adenomatosis is its morbidity. In the Mayo Clinic series (65), tumor bleeding occurred in 62.5 percent of patients. A conservative surgical approach is recommended by Ribeiro et al. (65); they suggest resection of large (greater than 5 cm) or symptomatic lesions, with observation of smaller (less than 3 cm) lesions.

NODULAR REGENERATIVE HYPERPLASIA

Definition. This condition is characterized by generally small regenerative nodules dispersed throughout the liver, associated with acinar atrophy and variably occluded portal vessels (particularly veins). Synonyms include *nodular transformation* (106,111), *noncirrhotic nodulation* (108), *micronodular transformation* (120), *partial nodular transformation* (85,88,94,107,114), *diffuse nodular hyperplasia without fibrous septa* (95), *adenomatous hyperplasia* (92), *miliary hepatocellular adenomatosis* (103), and *hepatocellular adenomatosis* (112).

Clinical Features. The autopsy incidence of NRH varies between 0.1 and 0.34 percent (110). It has been associated with a bewildering array of diseases that include hereditary hemorrhagic telangiectasia, persistent ductus venosus, Down's

syndrome, Krabbe's disease, tuberculosis, toxic oil syndrome, rheumatoid arthritis, Felty's syndrome, scleroderma, CRST syndrome (calcinosis cutis, Raynaud's phenomenon, sclerodactyly, telangiectasia), systemic lupus erythematosus, polyarteritis nodosa, Hashimoto's thyroiditis, hyperthyroidism, diabetes mellitus, myasthenia gravis, idiopathic thrombocytopenic purpura, celiac disease, primary biliary cirrhosis, primary sclerosing cholangitis, chronic hepatitis, extrahepatic portal vein obstruction, glomerulonephritis (chronic, membranous, or membranoproliferative), following renal dialysis or renal transplantation for end-stage renal disease, post-bone marrow transplantation, subacute bacterial endocarditis, cardiac valvulopathies, congestive heart failure, Budd-Chiari syndrome, primary pulmonary hypertension, Behcet's disease, monoclonal gammopathies, myeloproliferative disorders, lymphoproliferative disorders, and malignant neoplasms other than leukemia and lymphoma (including hepatocellular carcinoma). The interested reader is referred to several reviews of the topic for these and other disease associations (83,86, 96,105,110,111). It is worth noting that no clear-cut disease associations were evident in some of the reported cases of NRH.

NRH occurs in patients of all ages, with a mean age of 52 years (111). It is infrequently reported in childhood (99). No sex predilection has been observed in two large series of NRH in adults (86,111).

Patients with NRH may be completely asymptomatic. Symptoms and signs, when present, can be divided into the following broad categories: 1) those of the underlying disease, e.g., Felty's syndrome, myeloproliferative disorder; 2) manifestations of portal hypertension such as esophageal varices with or without gastrointestinal hemorrhage, splenomegaly, and ascites. Portal hypertension was recorded in 37.5 percent and 56.7 percent of patients with NRH in two series (86,111). However, as noted by Wanless (117), there is a bias toward symptomatic cases of NRH reported from research centers; in his review of 64 patients with NRH culled from 2,500 autopsies, only 4.7 percent had evidence of portal hypertension; 3) hepatic failure, usually in conjunction with portal hypertension; 4) an acute abdominal crisis from rupture of a large nodule, with hemoperitoneum. This rare complication occurred in 2 of the 30

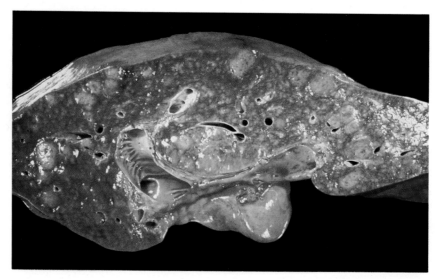

Figure 2-24
NODULAR REGENERATIVE
HYPERPLASIA
Pale nodules of varied size are
dispersed throughout this liver.

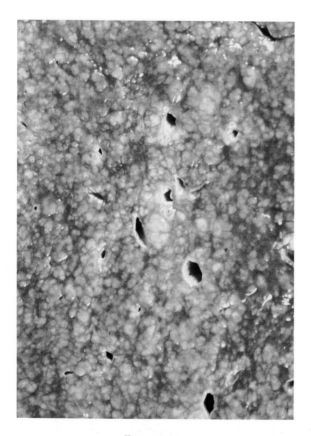

Figure 2-25
NODULAR REGENERATIVE HYPERPLASIA
Close-up of a section of liver showing multiple, small,
light tan nodules with no associated fibrosis.

patients studied by Stromeyer and Ishak (111); and 5) symptoms and signs of hypersplenism, a very rare mode of presentation (96). Liver tests are usually either normal or mildly abnormal, the most common abnormalities being elevations of the alkaline phosphatase and gamma-glutamyl transpeptidase. If elevated, the serum bilirubin value is generally below 2 mg/dl.

Radiologic Findings. These have been characterized in a series of 21 cases reported from the AFIP (87). The nodules take up technetium sulfur colloid, and have variable echogenicity on ultrasonography. They are often hypodense on computerized tomography (CT) without significant enhancement. Evidence of central hemorrhage may be noted in large nodules. Angiographically, the nodules fill from the periphery and are vascular, but they may display hypovascular areas due to hemorrhage. Liver biopsy is necessary for definitive diagnosis in the majority of cases.

Gross Findings. Typically, the liver is atrophic and riddled diffusely with multiple, light tan to yellowish white nodules; the majority vary from a millimeter to a centimeter in size, but occasionally measure up to 4 cm (figs. 2-24, 2-25). In cases of *partial nodular transformation*, a variant of NRH, even larger adenoma-like nodules (up to 8 cm in diameter) may be present (85,88,101,106,107,116). The larger nodules may be clustered at the hilum or may be intermingled with small lesions throughout the liver. Gross evidence of hemorrhage or infarction may be observed occasionally in the larger nodules. The

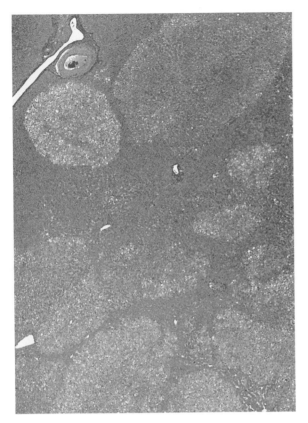

Figure 2-26
NODULAR REGENERATIVE HYPERPLASIA
The nodules are sharply defined and of varied size.

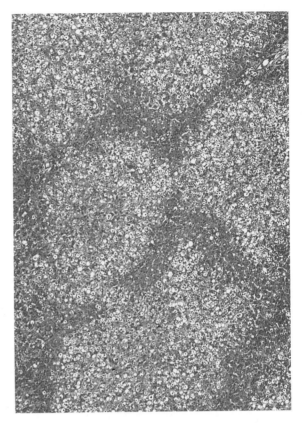

Figure 2-27
NODULAR REGENERATIVE HYPERPLASIA
Pale nodules are outlined by more darkly stained intervening parenchyma.

nodules are not encapsulated, and there is no associated fibrosis.

Microscopic Findings. Small nodules are often difficult to recognize microscopically, particularly in a needle biopsy specimen; they are usually periportal in location. As they continue to grow, they impinge on other nodules, and compress and distort terminal hepatic venules and portal tracts (figs. 2-26–2-29). The larger the nodules the easier they are to recognize because of compression atrophy of the intervening hepatic parenchyma (fig. 2-28). A reticulin stain is especially useful in outlining the nodules because of condensation of fibers at the periphery (fig. 2-30). Often, there is a different orientation of liver plates in the nodules compared to those in the surrounding parenchyma (fig. 2-30). The plates within the nodules are two cells thick. Internodular sinusoidal dilatation, often patchy, also helps to delineate the nodules. The hyperplastic liver cells, particularly in the smaller nodules,

often closely resemble those in the surrounding parenchyma. As the nodules grow, their cells tend to be larger than normal hepatocytes, and may have a pale or even vacuolated cytoplasm due to an increased content of glycogen or fat (fig. 2-29). Larger nodules also sometimes show pseudogland formation, and evidence of chronic cholestasis with cholate stasis (*pseudoxanthomatous transformation*) and copper storage (111). Liver cell dysplasia (large cell change) has been observed in NRH (fig. 2-31) (86,110). There is less lipofuscin in cells of NRH than in the normal hepatocytes; many of the cells contain no pigment (fig. 2-32). If hemosiderin is present in the internodular parenchyma none is detected in the cells of NRH. Immunoreactive alpha-1-antitrypsin but not alpha-fetoprotein is expressed (91,100). Endothelial and Kupffer cells are present in the nodules; the latter can be demonstrated by an immunostain for lysozyme.

25

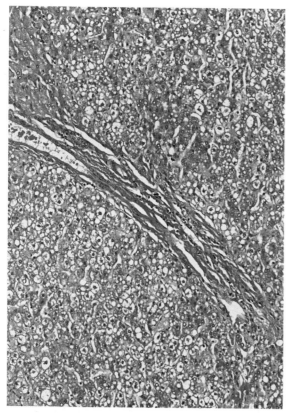

Figure 2-28
NODULAR REGENERATIVE HYPERPLASIA
Segments of two large nodules are separated by a non-collagenous "passive" septum.

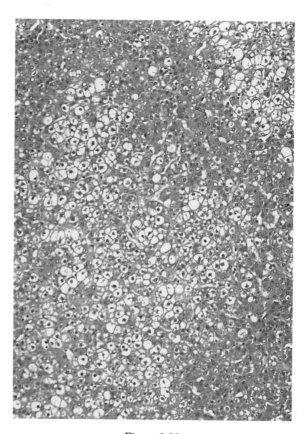

Figure 2-29
NODULAR REGENERATIVE HYPERPLASIA
The cells of a nodule are larger and paler than the nearby normal liver cells.

Figure 2-30
NODULAR
REGENERATIVE
HYPERPLASIA

Plates of a nodule (left) are thick, and there is compression of reticulin fibers of the adjacent parenchyma (right) (Manuel reticulin stain).

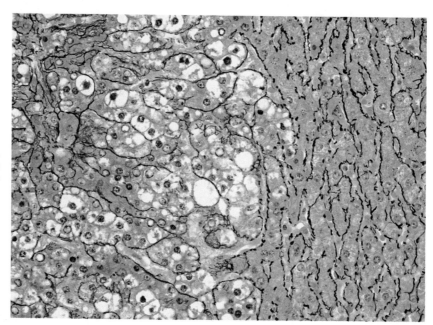

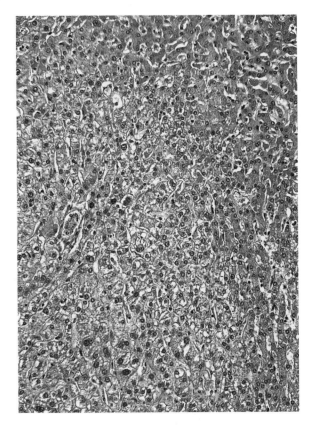

Figure 2-31
NODULAR REGENERATIVE HYPERPLASIA
Liver cell dysplasia in a nodule.

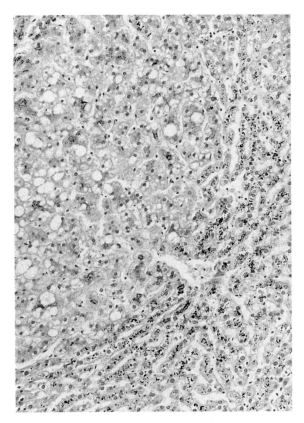

Figure 2-32
NODULAR REGENERATIVE HYPERPLASIA
The segment of a nodule contains little lipofuscin compared to the adjacent parenchyma (right and bottom) (Fontana stain).

Large nodules in NRH appear to form by the confluence of multiple smaller nodules. Portal areas and terminal hepatic venules incorporated into these larger nodules may be difficult to recognize since the interlobular bile ducts can atrophy and disappear. Eventually, these large nodules may resemble hepatocellular adenoma. In rare instances the large nodules rupture and lead to hemoperitoneum. Areas of multiacinar atrophy usually alternate with the nodules of NRH (fig. 2-33). They are recognized by the small size of the acini and the approximation of portal areas to each other and to terminal hepatic venules.

The portal areas in NRH may reveal no obvious light microscopic changes, but morphologic and morphometric studies by Wanless and collaborators (117–120) have furnished evidence of an underlying intrahepatic portal venopathy or, less commonly, an arteriopathy. When present, the vascular lesions include recent or old thrombi, or eccentric or concentric sclerosis of portal vein branches (figs. 2-34–2-36). Portal vein thrombi involving major vessels lead to larger areas of atrophy with big nodules (*partial nodular transformation*) (120). Occlusive lesions of large portal vein branches and the portal vein trunk have been reported in several cases of partial nodular transformation (107,120).

Pathogenesis. According to Wanless et al. (118–120), the common pathogenetic pathway for NRH is a nonuniform blood supply, in which the well-perfused acini become hyperplastic while the ischemic acini become atrophic. There is a possibility that in some instances NRH may be a neoplastic process, akin to the neoplastic foci and nodules induced in experimental animals by a wide variety of carcinogens (111). Many of the reported patients had been taking therapeutic drugs prior to discovery of their NRH. Of note are corticosteroids, contraceptive and anabolic steroids, and immunosuppressive and cancer

27

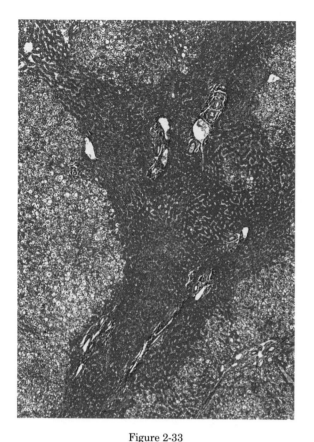

Figure 2-33
NODULAR REGENERATIVE HYPERPLASIA
Acinar atrophy, with approximation of portal areas, between several nodules (Masson trichrome stain).

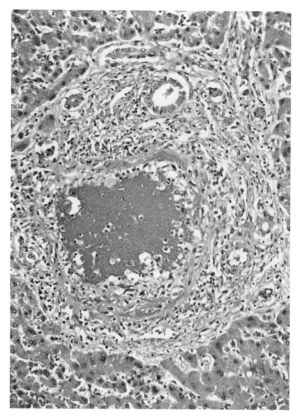

Figure 2-34
NODULAR REGENERATIVE HYPERPLASIA
Thrombophlebitis of an intrahepatic portal vein branch. (Figures 2-34 and 2-35 are from the same patient.)

chemotherapeutic agents (86,97,106,109,121). A third possible pathogenetic mechanism has been demonstrated in a rat model of selenium-induced NRH (81,89). In that model there is capillarization of sinusoids with deposition of laminin and type IV collagen, and transformation of perisinusoidal lipocytes into myofibroblasts, leading to an altered microcirculation and nodule formation. A recent study of hepatic hemodynamics in a patient with NRH supports the experimental evidence that the portal hypertension is primarily sinusoidal, as is the case in cirrhosis (115).

The relationship between NRH and other multiple benign hepatocellular tumors remains conjectural. Several authorities limit the size of nodules in NRH to 3 mm or less (83,110,118). Partial nodular transformation, a condition pathogenetically related to NRH, however, is characterized by large nodules (up to several centimeters in diameter) located in the hilum, though not exclusively so (85). Patients with this condition usually have portal hypertension. By contrast, most reported patients with multiple adenomas do not develop portal hypertension. Obliterative portal arterial and venous lesions and atrophy have not been observed in the livers of patients with hepatocellular adenomas due to oral contraceptives or anabolic steroids, whether single or multiple. NRH has, however, been reported in patients taking contraceptive or anabolic steroids (82,104,111). It is our experience that small lesions of "classic" NRH can continue to grow and coalesce to form larger nodules. Some years ago Sweeney and Evans (113) described generalized hyperplasia, hyperplastic nodules, and hepatocellular adenoma in patients treated with anabolic steroids. These authors and Stromeyer and Ishak (111) suggested that such lesions are analogous to those induced experimentally by a variety of carcinogenic compounds.

It is conceivable that most multiple, benign hepatocellular nodules arise as a result of vascular

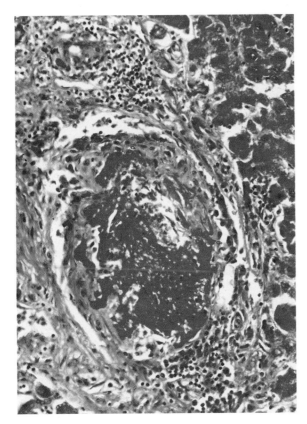

Figure 2-35
NODULAR REGENERATIVE HYPERPLASIA
Thrombosed intrahepatic portal vein branch (Masson trichrome stain).

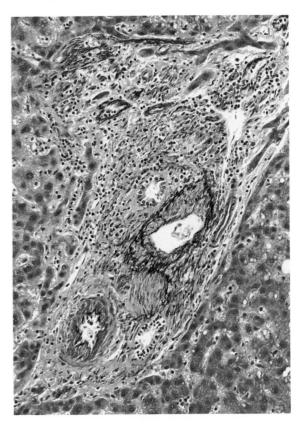

Figure 2-36
NODULAR REGENERATIVE HYPERPLASIA
Partially occluded portal vein branch in the portal area between nodules (Musto pentachrome stain).

lesions (venous and/or arterial) with resultant microcirculatory disturbances, as originally proposed for NRH (118). In support of a vascular basis for NRH is the experimental induction of a similar condition in portacaval-shunted rats (90, 122,123), and in rats with a congenital portacaval shunt (89). In another study, Haese et al. (93) found that mice infected with *Schistosoma mansoni* developed hepatic hyperplasia, presumably related to egg-induced obliterative lesions of small intrahepatic portal vein branches. Such hyperplasia was enhanced by the administration of hycanthone, resulting in the development of hepatocellular carcinoma in some animals.

Natural History and Prognosis. The majority of cases of "vasculopathy-induced" NRH seemingly do not progress any further. In one long-term follow-up study, 10 patients with NRH with portal hypertension treated by portal diversion had a favorable outcome, with survival from 1 to 6 years (83). On the other hand, the lesions of NRH could continue to grow under the influence of drugs (oral contraceptives, anabolic/androgenic steroids, corticosteroids) or hepatotrophic substances (glucagon, insulin, epidermal growth factor). Growth and coalescence of small nodules could eventually lead to formation of adenomatous or adenoma-like nodules which, with their precarious blood supply, may undergo infarction, hemorrhage, and even rupture, or become malignant. Resolution of benign hepatocellular tumors, whether single or multiple, has been repeatedly documented after cessation of use of the causative agent, for example anabolic steroid therapy (84,98), or after the lowering of glucagon levels in patients with liver cell adenomas associated with glycogen storage disease.

Liver cell dysplasia (large cell change) has been observed in 24 percent of patients with NRH in one series (111) and 42 percent in another series (86). Of 804 cases of hepatocellular carcinoma in North America studied by Nzeako et al. (102), 342 arose in a noncirrhotic liver; 13 (6.7 percent) of those livers had NRH. Seventeen of the patients (73.9 percent) with NRH had liver cell dysplasia and 16 (69.6 percent) had portal venous invasion by the carcinoma. Liver cell dysplasia occurred in a significantly greater proportion of patients with NRH than in those without (P<0.01), but there were no significant differences between both groups with regard to portal venous invasion. Nzeako et al. concluded that the temporal relationship between hepatocellular carcinoma and NRH is probably determined in each case by the interaction of multiple pathogenetic factors. Among patients with hepatocellular carcinoma, factors other than portal vein obstruction by tumor invasion, for example, chemotherapy and/or radiotherapy, could play a role in the pathogenesis of NRH.

FOCAL NODULAR HYPERPLASIA

Definition. Focal nodular hyperplasia (FNH) is a lesion composed of hyperplastic hepatocytes in two cell–thick plates, subdivided into nodules by fibrous septa, which may form stellate scars. Thick-walled arteries are present in the scars and septa, and ductules (but not ducts) are typically located between the scars and the parenchymal component.

Clinical Features. FNH occurs in both sexes and all ages, but more often in females than males. The percentages of females in three series of more than 20 cases were 86, 88, and 91 (127, 149,161). Most of the tumors occur in adults, but cases have been reported in children (171). Some FNHs in pediatric patients have not been recognized as such and have, instead, been referred to as mixed hamartoma (164).

In a series of 130 patients with FNH from the AFIP (146), only 20 percent had symptoms and signs related to their neoplasm; in the remainder, the FNH was discovered incidentally at surgery (58 patients), usually for diseases of the gallbladder, or at necropsy (46 patients). The majority (15 of 20) of the patients with symptoms and signs had a mass (either discovered by the patient or palpated during a routine physical check-up). Pain or discomfort was associated with the mass in 5 patients. In 1 patient the mass

was tender and pulsatile, and a loud bruit was heard over it. Two of the patients with negative physical findings had symptoms mimicking those of peptic ulcer or cholelithiasis; subsequent laparotomy in both patients showed pressure of the FNH on the stomach and gallbladder, respectively. Another patient had pain on pressure over the FNH, although no mass was palpated. One female patient had an acute abdominal crisis due to rupture of her lesion.

Three patients in the AFIP series had manifestations of portal hypertension associated with multiple FNH (146). One of the patients with this very rare complication, an 8-year-old child, had left hemihypertrophy; that patient was reported by Everson et al. (134). Another patient with multiple FNH, anomalous vascular supply to the liver, and hemihypertrophy, was reported by Haber et al. (142). Wanless et al. (176) described 13 patients with multiple FNH and vascular malformations of the liver (hemangiomas) and other organs (telangiectasia of the brain, berry aneurysm, and dysplastic systemic arteries), as well as neoplasms of the brain (meningioma, astrocytoma); they proposed the combination of lesions as a new syndrome. However, hemangiomas of the liver, as well as berry aneurysms and vascular malformations of the brain, have been reported with single FNH (136,140,163).

The majority of patients with FNH have normal results of liver tests. The serum alpha-fetoprotein value is always in the normal range. The tumor(s) may or may not show up as a filling defect(s) by hepatic scan. Indentation of, and pressure on, adjacent hollow viscera may be demonstrated by upper and lower gastrointestinal radiographic studies, intravenous pyelography, or cholecystography. The appearance of FNH in radionuclear scans was described by Kerlin et al. (149). Angiographic studies have been described by several groups of investigators (141,158,159). Comparative studies using various imaging modalities (angiography, computed tomography [CT], ultrasound, and scintigraphy) in two series of patients with FNH were reported by Kerlin et al. (149) and Welch et al. (179). The magnetic resonance imaging (MRI) appearance of FNH has been studied by several groups of investigators (153,154,175). Shamsi et al. (170) used a multimodality approach (ultrasound, CT, and MRI) in their radiologic evaluation of FNH.

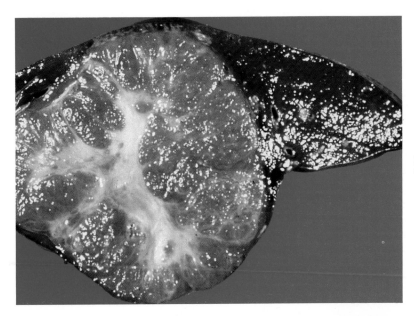

Figure 2-37
FOCAL NODULAR HYPERPLASIA
This well-circumscribed tumor displays a branching central scar and a tan-colored parenchyma.

Color doppler sonography has been found useful in diagnosis (131,152). However, in the latter study the best imaging procedure for FNH was enhanced MRI, which had a sensitivity of 70 percent and a specificity of 98 percent. On the basis of that study, Cherqui et al. (131) have proposed that histologic diagnosis is only necessary in the 30 percent of cases in which the clinical, biochemical, or imaging data are atypical for FNH. Calcification has been reported rarely in FNH by various imaging modalities; it may pose problems in differentiating this lesion from fibrolamellar carcinoma (130).

Gross Findings. The tumors in the AFIP series were most frequently found in the right lobe of the liver (63 of the 130 cases), followed by the left lobe (40 cases), both lobes (15 cases), caudate lobe (1 case), and Riedel's lobe (1 case); in 8 cases the location was not known (143). There was a single lesion in 78.5 percent of the patients, 12.3 percent had two nodules, 6.9 percent had multiple nodules, and 2.3 percent had left lobar FNH. This uncommon lobar form of FNH is only reported in one other patient (172). The majority of patients (84.6 percent) had single nodules which measured 5 cm or less in diameter, 16 patients (12.3 percent) had nodules of 5 to 10 cm, and only 4 patients (3.1 percent) had an FNH with a diameter greater than 10 cm.

The gross appearance of FNH is highly characteristic (figs. 2-37, 2-38). The lesions are usu-

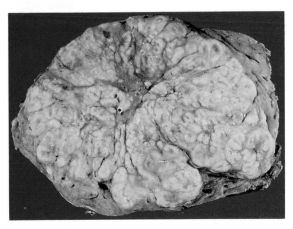

Figure 2-38
FOCAL NODULAR HYPERPLASIA
The section of this tumor has a cirrhosis-like appearance. Note the light color of the lesion in comparison to the adjacent liver.

ally globular, lobulated, and often bulge from one of the surfaces of the liver. Less than 5 percent of the tumors have a pedicle. Prominent vessels are often seen coursing over the surface. The consistency is firm to rubbery and, when transected, the tumor often bulges above the plane of the rest of the liver. FNH is usually well circumscribed but nonencapsulated. The color is invariably lighter than that of the adjacent, typically normal liver, being light brown, tan, or yellow-tan. Areas of hemorrhagic necrosis or infarction are very rare (128). The highly typical gross feature of FNH is

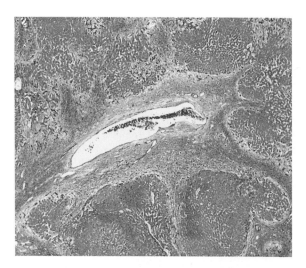

Figure 2-39
FOCAL NODULAR HYPERPLASIA
Low-power view of the architecture of the lesion.

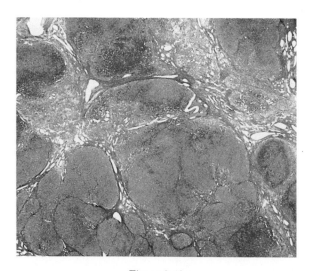

Figure 2-40
FOCAL NODULAR HYPERPLASIA
The tumor is subdivided into smaller nodules by fibrous
septa (Masson trichrome stain).

its subdivision into smaller nodules by fibrous septa that often run into retracted stellate scars; the latter may be central or eccentric and there may be several of them, particularly in large lesions. The resemblance of FNH to a localized cirrhotic process led Benz and Baggenstoss (126) to call it "focal cirrhosis." It should be emphasized, however, that FNH is not associated with cirrhosis or other intrinsic diseases of the liver.

In 3 of the 130 AFIP cases, cavernous hemangiomas (single in two and multiple in one) were found in the same liver (146). A much higher association with hemangiomas (20.6 percent and 23 percent) was reported in two other series of FNH: one was an autopsy series (126) while the other was a series of surgically resected FNH (157). In one case report FNH was associated with an intrahepatic portosystemic venous shunt (151). Two of the AFIP patients, both children, had stenosed portal veins. The simultaneous occurrence of FNH and hepatocellular adenoma is well documented but rare (137). A number of the patients with FNH had benign or malignant neoplasms of other organs, either synchronous or metachronous. One interesting association is with glioblastoma multiforme which was found in four of the AFIP patients, and has also been reported in other patients (133,176). Forty (30.8 percent) of the patients in the AFIP series had cholelithiasis and/or chronic cholecystitis or cholesterolosis; 33 of those patients were female.

Microscopic Findings. The earliest observations of the pathology of FNH were made by Begg and Berry (125) and Benz and Baggenstoss (126). FNH has a hepatocellular component, as well as bile ductules proliferating in a fibrous base (figs. 2-39–2-41). It is typically nonencapsulated. The hepatic parenchymal component of the tumor lacks an acinar architecture; thus, no terminal hepatic veins or portal areas are visible. The plates are generally two cells in thickness and are supported by a well-developed reticulin framework (fig. 2-42). They are separated by sinusoidal spaces lined by inconspicuous endothelial cells. The hyperplastic cells resemble the normal hepatocytes in the adjacent non-neoplastic parenchyma, but they may be slightly larger and paler (fig. 2-43). Variable steatosis may be seen. The nuclei occupy a relatively small part of the total cell volume and show little variation in size, with rare exceptions (180). They are normochromatic, and have fine chromatin granules and inconspicuous amphophilic nucleoli. Most of the cells contain one nucleus, and no mitoses are seen. Definite canaliculi are identifiable between the cells but none contain bile.

In our experience, the sinusoids (particularly those close to the septa) are capillarized, as shown by deposition of collagen IV, laminin, and even smooth muscle actin in the perisinusoidal spaces (figs. 2-44, 2-45). Recently, Scoazec et al. (169)

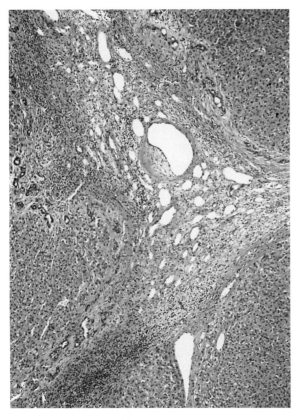

Figure 2-41
FOCAL NODULAR HYPERPLASIA
The scar in the center shows an eccentrically thickened artery and numerous smaller vessels. Note the periseptal ductular proliferation and the inflammatory cells. No interlobular bile ducts are present.

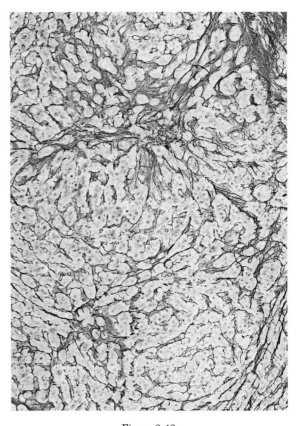

Figure 2-42
FOCAL NODULAR HYPERPLASIA
A well-developed reticulin network is typical of this tumor (Reticulin stain).

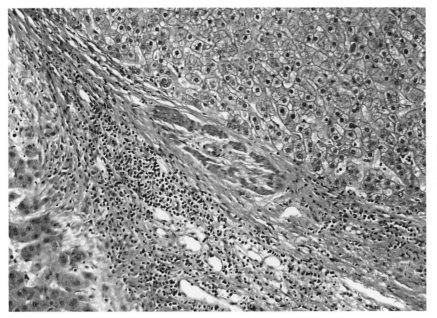

Figure 2-43
FOCAL NODULAR
HYPERPLASIA
The hepatocellular component resembles normal liver. Note the thick-walled artery in a septum that is infiltrated by numerous lymphocytes.

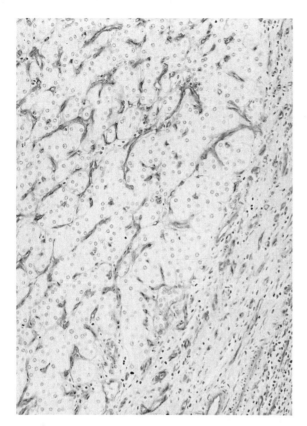

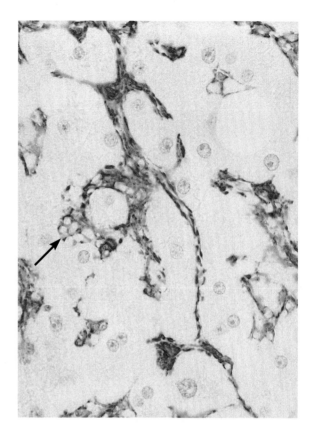

Figure 2-44
FOCAL NODULAR HYPERPLASIA
The sinusoids of the tumor are "capillarized," as demonstrated by the linear expression of CD34 by endothelial cells (CD34 immunostain).

Figure 2-45
FOCAL NODULAR HYPERPLASIA
Perisinusoidal myofibroblasts (modified stellate cells) are present in the hepatocellular component of this tumor. At least one vacuolated stellate cell is recognizable (arrow) (smooth muscle actin immunostain).

noted the presence of large amounts of laminin, von Willebrand factor, and thrombospondin in the zone surrounding the central scar, suggesting the development of perisinusoidal fibrosis accompanied by the induction of integrin receptors on hepatocytes and sinusoidal endothelial cells. Cells adjacent to the fibrous septa often show cholate stasis (pseudoxanthomatous transformation) (fig. 2-46), and may contain copper (demonstrable with the rhodanine stain) (fig. 2-47) and copper binding protein (demonstrable with orcein or Victoria blue stain). These features of chronic cholestasis are seen in almost all cases of FNH (129); in addition, some tumors may display "cholestatic" Mallory bodies in periseptal hepatocytes. The absence of bile ducts and a connection to the biliary outflow tract in part explains the cholestatic features.

Numerous ductules (but not interlobular bile ducts) are present at the junction of the fibrous septa with the hepatocellular component, with which they merge imperceptibly (fig. 2-48). The ductules stain intensely with cytokeratin stains 7, 8, 18, and 19 (fig. 2-49). Additionally, there is variable staining of the liver cells near the septa with cytokeratins 7 and 19 (specific in the normal liver for bile duct epithelium), indicating a change in phenotype of these cells (fig. 2-50). The ductules have a very fine lumen, though some may be slightly dilated. They have a thin basement membrane, and may be surrounded and infiltrated by neutrophils. Roskams and colleagues (165) found undifferentiated progenitor ("stem") cells in FNH and suggested that the ductules, at least in part, are derived by activation of these cells.

The fibrous septa of FNH are often infiltrated by varying numbers of inflammatory cells (lymphocytes, plasma cells, mast cells, and neutrophils); lymphoid aggregates are also observed

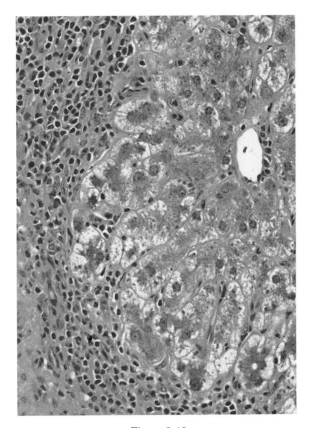

Figure 2-46
FOCAL NODULAR HYPERPLASIA
Cholate stasis of liver cells adjacent to a septum. The septum is infiltrated by many lymphoplasmacytic cells.

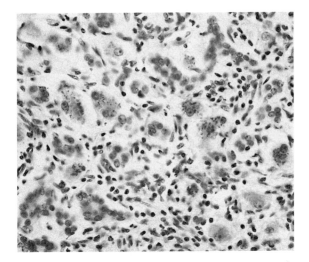

Figure 2-47
FOCAL NODULAR HYPERPLASIA
Copper accumulation (red granules) in liver cells adjacent to a septum (Rhodanine stain).

(figs. 2-41, 2-46). Interface hepatitis (piecemeal necrosis), including the presence of apoptotic bodies, may be observed. Numerous vessels, both arteries and to a lesser extent veins, course through the septa and the large scars. The large arteries often show eccentric thickening due to subintimal fibrosis, fibromuscular hyperplasia, and disruption or reduplication of the elastica (fig. 2-51). The veins show no histologic changes. The hepatic parenchyma immediately adjacent to FNH can show some compression atrophy but is architecturally normal.

Variants of FNH, all rare in our experience, have been described by Nguyen et al. (160a). These, referred to as "nonclassical" FNH, include a *telangiectatic form* (showing sinusoidal dilatation or marked ectasia and lacking a central scar), a *mixed hyperplastic and adenomatous form* (with transitional morphology between FNH and hepatocellular adenoma), and *FNH with cytologic atypia* (FNH with areas of large cell change).

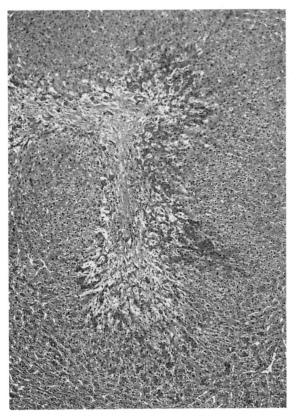

Figure 2-48
FOCAL NODULAR HYPERPLASIA
Numerous ductules are interposed between the liver cells and a septum. Note the absence of interlobular bile ducts.

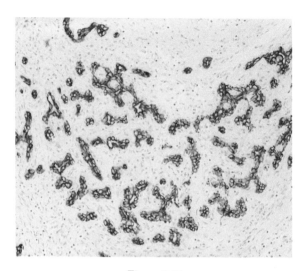

Figure 2-49
FOCAL NODULAR HYPERPLASIA
The ductules along a septum express cytokeratin (pancyto-keratin immunostain).

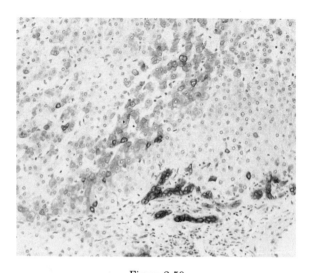

Figure 2-50
FOCAL NODULAR HYPERPLASIA
Liver cells adjacent to a septum show a phenotypic change characterized by aberrant expression of bile duct cytokeratin 19.

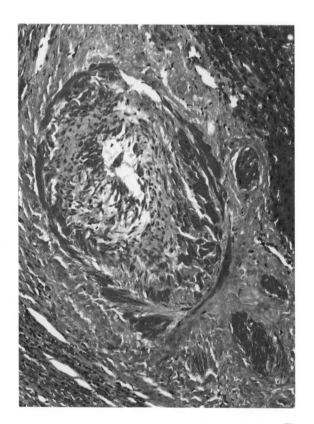

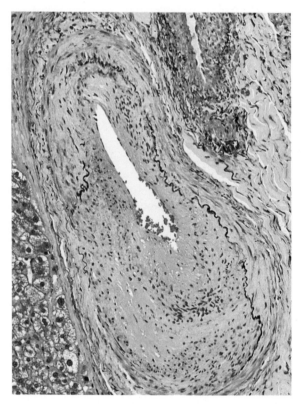

Figure 2-51
FOCAL NODULAR HYPERPLASIA
Left: Marked smooth muscle hypertrophy of an artery (Masson trichrome stain).
Right: Markedly occluded artery with mucopolysaccharide accumulation (green), smooth muscle hypertrophy, and a disrupted elastica (Musto pentachrome stain).

Differential Diagnosis. When FNH is seen in its entirety or with some adjacent parenchyma, pathologists usually have no trouble distinguishing it from cirrhosis. A needle or wedge biopsy specimen, however (when obtained at the time of laparotomy or at laparoscopy), may cause difficulties in differential diagnosis, particularly if the pathologist is not informed that the biopsy material is from a mass lesion. As pointed out by Knowles and Wolff (150), two histologic features permit differentiation of FNH from cirrhosis. The first is the complete lack of a normal acinar architecture and the second is the presence of areas of bile ductular proliferation in the nodules of FNH. To these may be added the characteristic vascular lesions of FNH, well described in an elegant study by Travers and D'Amato (173), the absence of lipofuscin, and the already enumerated chronic cholestatic features (cholate stasis, the accumulation of copper and copper-binding protein, and sometimes the presence of Mallory bodies).

The benign tumors and tumor-like lesions that may on occasion have to be distinguished microscopically from FNH include hepatocellular adenoma and nodular regenerative hyperplasia. Hepatocellular adenoma, which occurs mostly in females on birth control pills, lacks the substructure (fibrous septa and bile ductules) of FNH. Nodular regenerative hyperplasia occurs in adults of both sexes, is multiple, and may be accompanied by portal hypertension. It has been reported in association with many conditions, in particular myeloproliferative disorders, Felty's syndrome, rheumatoid arthritis, and the CRST syndrome. Microscopically, the nodules are typically small and scattered throughout the liver, are ill-defined, and contain plates two cells thick. A reticulin stain is invaluable, particularly in needle biopsy specimens, in defining the nodules because of condensation of fibers around them, and in demonstrating the thick liver cell plates within the nodules. Occlusive vascular (usually portal venous) lesions may be identified, and the parenchyma between the nodules is atrophic. Elastic stains (Musto or Movat pentachrome stains, orcein or Victoria blue) are very helpful in identifying occluded vessels in portal areas in NRH.

Pathogenesis. Various theories have been propounded to explain the pathogenesis of FNH, including a hamartomatous malformation or a reparative process in an area or areas of focal injury (e.g., amebic abscess). In 1973 Whelan et al. (181), on the basis of arteriographic studies of four cases, hypothesized that FNH may result from arterialization of a localized region of liver by an anomalous arterial supply. Their astute observations were subsequently confirmed by a study of 51 cases of FNH by Wanless and colleagues (177). These investigators proposed that FNH is a hyperplastic response of the hepatic parenchyma to a preexisting arterial, spider-like malformation. They found that the lesions were supplied by an anomalous artery larger than expected for their locale in the liver. The frequent association of FNH with hemangiomas of the liver, and the report of two cases of localized nodular proliferation surrounding hemangiomas of the liver (160), and one case of arterial malformations (148), lend further support to a vascular basis for such lesions. However, FNH has never been reported in a newborn or stillborn, unlike other malformations, and so we suspect that another factor may also play a role. In general, arteries throughout the body are accompanied by relatively equal-sized veins that provide drainage of the tissue supplied by the artery. In FNH, there are usually many small veins in the septa and central scar, but large veins are generally not seen. Fukukura et al. (138) showed that arterial blood perfuses the sinusoids of FNH and that most of the blood eventually drains into small hepatic veins surrounding the lesions rather than returning through veins of the septa or central scar; they found no portal blood flow in FNH. We suspect that in fetal life, the large artery that will eventually be present in the central scar is accompanied by an equally large vein, but that at some point in development, the venous drainage is disrupted. A likely time for this event is at birth, when the fetal circulation closes. Part of the fetal circulation is the ductus venosus, which allows oxygenated blood returning from the placenta by the umbilical veins to bypass the liver. Some of the venous drainage of the liver, particularly from the central portion and left lobe, is carried by the ductus venosus during fetal life, but after this closes, drainage is into the tributaries of the hepatic veins. We suspect that, in the presence of an abnormally large artery, closure of the ductus venosus and partial blockage of venous drainage may be the event that leads to the development of FNH. At least some reported cases of "mixed hamartoma" of the liver probably represent developing FNH in a young infant, as these have some but not all of the features of FNH. At the present time, however, this pathogenetic sequence remains a hypothesis, since it has not been investigated and there is no direct evidence to support it.

Evidence against an etiologic relationship between FNH and contraceptive steroids has been cited by a number of authors (145,146,150). Briefly, this includes the occurrence of FNH in infants and children, in males as well as in females, and in many patients prior to the introduction of oral contraceptives into clinical practice. We have only seen one patient with FNH present with rupture and hemoperitoneum, a complication frequently occurring in hepatocellular adenoma. In a review of the literature up to 1977, Fechner (135) found that of the nine women with FNH who had taken oral contraceptives, two presented with intrahepatic or intraperitoneal bleeding. He suggested that this complication could be a direct consequence of oral contraceptives and could occur even if the underlying lesion itself were not caused by hormone therapy. It is also possible that FNH, a very slow growing lesion, could undergo accelerated growth under the influence of contraceptive steroids or other conjugated estrogens. Such a possibility receives support from the discovery of FNH in some patients on estrogen (127), the occasional report of "regression" of FNH after discontinuation of oral contraceptive or estrogen therapy (124,166), and the demonstration of estrogen receptors in tumor cells (144). Two recent studies, however, have shown that neither pregnancy nor oral contraceptive use are risk factors in women with FNH (157,173). Weimann et al. (178) found no increase in size of FNH in 10 of 82 (12.2 percent) women who became pregnant; Mathieu et al. (156,157) found no relationship between the intake and type of oral contraceptive and the size and number of lesions of FNH, and no increase in size of FNH in 12 women who become pregnant.

As discussed earlier, the vascular pathogenesis of FNH is now firmly established. Recently, however, Gaffey et al. (139) suggested, on the basis of a study of X-chromosome inactivation, that FNH is clonal. That study was refuted by Paradis and colleagues (162) who found a random pattern of X-chromosome inactivation consistent with a polyclonal lesion.

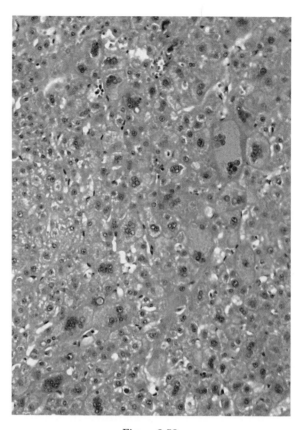

Figure 2-52
FOCAL NODULAR HYPERPLASIA
Large cell change (dysplasia) in the hepatocellular component. (Figures 2-52 through 2-54 are from the same patient.)

Treatment. Small lesions may require no treatment, but otherwise the treatment of choice for FNH is simple or segmental resection (147, 149). When this is not feasible, arterial embolization or ligation has been advocated (161). According to one experienced hepatobiliary surgeon, deep-seated lesions need not be resected (155).

Prognosis. The risk of hemorrhage and rupture is rare, as is malignant transformation. There are only 2 cases of malignant transformation in over 800 patients with FNH on file at the AFIP (figs. 2-52–2-54). The suggestion of Vecchio et al. (174) that the fibrolamellar variant of hepatocellular carcinoma arises from FNH has not been corroborated by other investigators. As already noted, FNH may be associated with other hepatic neoplasms; in the case of cavernous hemangioma the two tumors may be in close proximity. An FNH adjacent to a fibrolamellar carcinoma was reported by Saul et al. (167) and Saxena et al. (168). In both

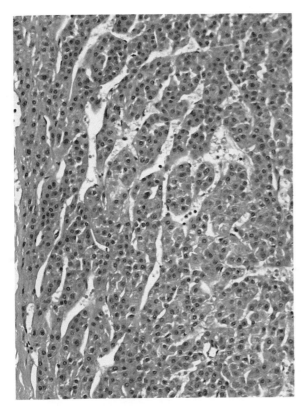

Figure 2-53
FOCAL NODULAR HYPERPLASIA
Trabecular hepatocellular carcinoma that arose in the tumor depicted in figure 2-52.

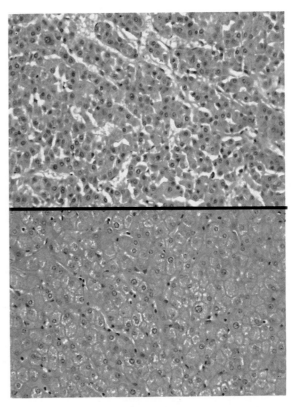

Figure 2-54
FOCAL NODULAR HYPERPLASIA
Cells of the carcinoma (top) shown in figure 2-53 are compared to the benign cells of the tumor (bottom).

case reports the authors suggested that the hyperplastic foci in the vicinity of the fibrolamellar carcinoma may be an epiphenomenon due to an abnormal blood supply, possibly derived from the tumor vasculature. The expression of the neurotensin gene by fibrolamellar carcinoma but not by FNH is considered further evidence against the suggestion that the latter lesion is the precursor of the former (132).

The salient features of hepatocellular adenoma, focal nodular hyperplasia, and nodular transformation are compared in Table 2-3.

COMPENSATORY HYPERTROPHY ASSOCIATED WITH LOBAR ATROPHY

Atrophy of a lobe of the liver may result in compensatory hypertrophy of the remaining lobes (fig. 2-55). The atrophy may be due to obstruction of the bile duct draining the lobe (stricture, cholangiocarcinoma) or blockage (thrombotic occlusion) of the portal or hepatic veins (182–184). The atro-

phy/hypertrophy complex has been reproduced in a rat model by selective portal vein ligation, but not by biliary ligation (185). The hypertrophied lobe may present as a palpable mass (186). The affected atrophic lobe (or segment) of the liver is markedly shrunken, firm, and pink, and is well demarcated from the rest of the liver. Microscopically, there are usually no hepatocellular elements; instead, the atrophic tissue consists of collapsed portal areas with intervening fibrosis and elasticization (figs. 2-56, 2-57). In cases related to vascular occlusion there may be recanalized thrombi in veins. The hypertrophied lobe has a normal acinar architecture, but the liver plates may be two cells thick.

POSTNECROTIC REGENERATIVE NODULES

Regenerative nodules may be visible grossly in livers from patients who sustained submassive injury from viral hepatitis, drugs, or toxins several

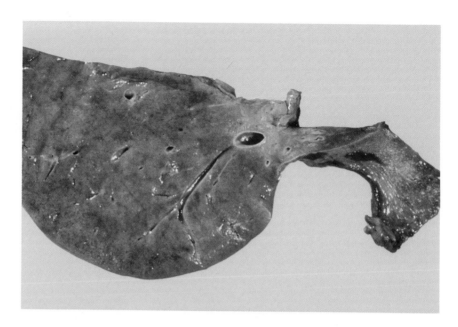

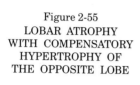

Figure 2-55
LOBAR ATROPHY
WITH COMPENSATORY
HYPERTROPHY OF
THE OPPOSITE LOBE

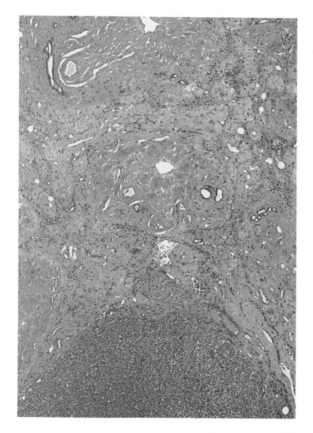
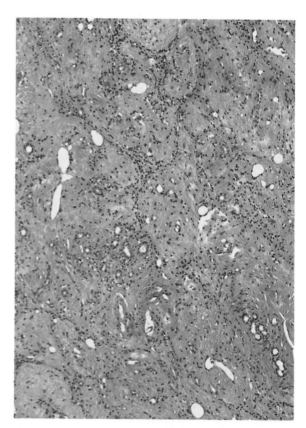

Figure 2-56
LOBAR ATROPHY
Left: The atrophic lobe (top) is sharply demarcated from the adjacent normal parenchyma.
Right: Higher magnification of the atrophic lobe shows residual portal areas and fibrosis.

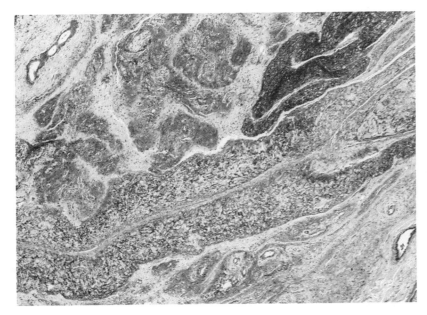

Figure 2-57
LOBAR ATROPHY
There is marked elasticization of the fibrous tissue of the atrophic lobe (Victoria blue stain).

Figure 2-58
NODULAR REGENERATION
Gross photograph of the inferior surface of the liver showing tumor-like nodules of regenerating parenchyma. (AFIP MIS #76094.)

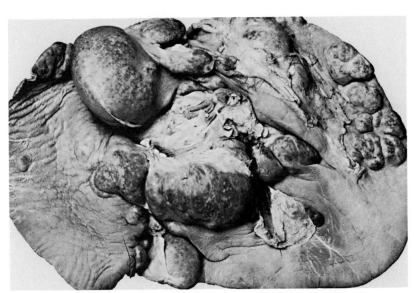

weeks previously (187–189). These lesions may present as large, tumor-like masses, several centimeters in diameter, that are pale yellow or green in color and separated from each other by deep indentations or broad areas of red-brown atrophy (figs. 2-58, 2-59). Edmondson (188) referred to these nodules as *adenomatous hyperplasia*. Baggenstoss (187) distinguished the large nodules ("lobar"), from smaller ones ("nodular" and "granular"). Microscopically, the re-

generative nodules can have an acinar architecture although portal tracts are small and have tiny bile ducts and a scanty stroma. The liver cells are arranged in two cell–thick plates, often have large hyperchromatic nuclei, and may be bi-, tri-, or multinucleated (fig. 2-60). The cells lack the "wear and tear" pigment lipofuscin. Bilirubinostasis, both cytoplasmic and canalicular, is often prominent.

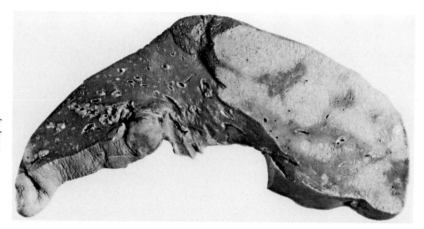

Figure 2-59
NODULAR REGENERATION
AFTER SUBMASSIVE
HEPATIC NECROSIS
Cut surface shows pale areas of regenerated parenchyma. The rest of the liver shows massive necrosis and collapse. (AFIP MIS #73602.)

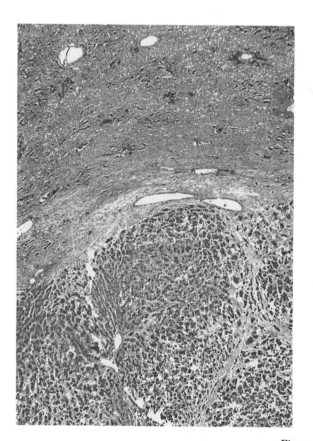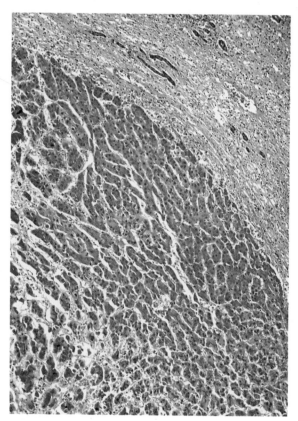

Figure 2-60
NODULAR REGENERATION
Left: Regenerative nodule (bottom) is sharply demarcated from collapsed, congested parenchyma (top).
Right: Segment of regenerative nodule (bottom), composed of two cell-thick plates, is sharply demarcated from the collapsed parenchyma (upper right).

REFERENCES

Hepatocellular Adenoma

1. Alshak NS, Cocjin J, Podesta L, et al. Hepatocellular adenoma in glycogen storage disease type IV. Arch Pathol Lab Med 1994;118:88–91.

2. Balazs M. Comparative electron-microscopic studies of benign hepatoma and icterus in patients on oral contraceptives. Virchows Arch [A] 1978;381:97–109.

3. Beuers U, Richter WO, Ritter MM, et al. Klinefelter's syndrome and liver adenoma. J Clin Gastroenterol 1991;13:214–6.

4. Bianchi L. Glycogen storage disease I and hepatocellular tumours. Eur J Pediatr 1993;152(Suppl 1):S63–70.

5. Bioulac-Sage P, Lamouliatte H, Saric J, et al. Ultrastructure of sinusoidal cells in a benign liver cell adenoma. Ultrastr Pathol 1986;10:49–54.

6. Buhler H, Pirovino M, Akovbiantz A, et al. Regression of liver cell adenoma. A follow-up study of three consecutive patients after discontinuation of oral contraceptive use. Gastroenterology 1982;82:775–82.

7. Cannon RO III, Dusheiko GM, Long JA Jr, et al. Hepatocellular adenoma in a young woman with beta-thalassemia and secondary iron overload. Gastroenterology 1981;81:352–5.

8. Carbone A, Vecchio FM. Presence of cytoplasmic progesterone receptors in hepatic adenomas. A report of two cases. Am J Clin Pathol 1986;85:325–9.

9. Carrasco D, Barrachina M, Prieto M, et al. Clomiphene citrate and liver cell adenoma [Letter]. N Engl J Med 1984;310:1120–1.

10. Carrasco D, Prieto M, Pallardo L, et al. Multiple hepatic adenomas after long-term therapy with testosterone enanthate: review of the literature. J Hepatol 1985;1:533–78.

11. Chandra RS, Kapur SP, Kelleher J, et al. Benign hepatocellular tumors in the young: a clinicopathologic spectrum. Arch Pathol Lab Med 1984;108:168–71.

12. Christopherson WM, Mays ET, Barrows GH. Liver tumors in young women: a clinical pathologic study of 201 cases in the Louisville Registry. In: Fenoglio CM, Wolff M, eds., Progress in surgical pathology, vol II. New York: Masson Publishing, 1980:187–205.

13. Cohen C, Lawson D, DeRose PB. Sex and androgenic steroid receptor expression in hepatic adenomas. Hum Pathol 1998;29:1428–32.

14. Coire CI, Qizilbash AH, Castelli MF. Hepatic adenomata in type Ia glycogen storage disease. Arch Pathol Lab Med 1987;111:166–9.

15. Cosme A, Horrajada JP, Vidaur F, et al. Systemic amyloidosis induced by oral contraceptive-associated hepatocellular adenoma: a 13-year follow up. Liver 1995;15:164–7.

16. Creagh TM, Rubin A, Evans DJ. Hepatic tumours induced by anabolic steroids in an athlete. J Clin Pathol 1988;41:441–3.

17. Derhy S, Soyer P, Roche A, et al. Adénomes hépatiques non résécable: Place de l'embolisation artérielle dans la conduite thérapeutique. Gastroenterol Clin Biol 1991;15:424–7.

18. Dhillon AP, Colombari R, Savage K, Scheuer PJ. An immunohistochemical study of the blood vessels with primary hepatocellular tumours. Liver 1992;12:311–8.

19. Edmonds AM, Hennegar GR, Crooks R. Galactosemia: report of a case with autopsy. Pediatrics 1952;10:40–7.

20. Edmondson HA, Henderson B, Benton B. Liver-cell adenomas associated with use of oral contraceptives. N Engl J Med 1976;294:470–2.

21. Edmondson HA, Reynolds TB, Henderson B, Benton B. Regression of liver cell adenomas associated with oral contraceptives. Ann Intern Med 1977;86:180–2.

22. Farrell GC, Joshua DE, Uren RF. Androgen-induced hepatoma. Lancet 1975;1:430–2.

23. Ferrell LD. Hepatocellular carcinoma arising in a focus of multilobular adenoma: a case report. Am J Surg Pathol 1993;17:524–9.

24. Flejou JF, Barge J, Menu Y, et al. Liver adenomatosis. An entity distinct from liver adenoma? Gastroenterology 1985;89:1132–8.

25. Foster JH, Berman MM. The malignant transformation of liver cell adenomas. Arch Surg 1994;129:712–7.

26. Foster JH, Donohue TA, Berman MM. Familial liver-cell adenomas and diabetes mellitus. N Engl J Med 1978;299:239–41.

27. Galassi A, Pasquinelli G, Guerini A. Benign myxoid hepatocellular tumor: a variant of liver cell adenoma. Liver 1995;15:233–5.

28. Gordon SC, Reddy KR, Livingstone S, Jeffers LJ, Schiff ER. Resolution of a contraceptive-steroid-induced hepatic adenoma with subsequent evolution into hepatocellular carcinoma. Ann Intern Med 1986;105:547–9.

28a. Hasan A, Coutts M, Portmann B. Pigmented liver cell adenoma in two male patients. Am J Surg Pathol 2000 24:1429–32.

29. Heffelfinger S, Irani DR, Finegold MJ. "Alcoholic hepatitis" in a hepatic adenoma. Hum Pathol 1987;18:751–4.

30. Henderson JT, Richmond J. Androgenic-anabolic steroid therapy and hepatocellular carcinoma [Letter]. Lancet 1973;1:434.

31. Ishak KG. Hepatic neoplasms associated with contraceptive and anabolic steroids. In: Lingeman CH, ed. Carcinogenic hormones. Berlin: Springer-Verlag, 1979:73–128.

32. Janes CH, McGill DB, Ludwig J, Krom RA. Liver cell adenoma at the age of 3 years and transplantation 19 years later after development of carcinoma: a case report. Hepatology 1993;17:583–5.

33. Johnson FL, Lerner KG, Siegel M, et al. Association of anabolic steroid therapy with development of hepatocellular carcinoma. Lancet 1972;2:1273–6.

34. Kahn H, Manzarbeitia C, Theise N, Schwartz M, Miller C, Thung SN. Danazol-induced hepatocellular adenomas. A case report and review of the literature. Arch Pathol Lab Med 1991;115:1054–7.

35. Kalra PA, Guthrie JA, Dibble JB, Turney JH, Brownjohn AM. Hepatic adenomas induced by norethisterone in patients receiving renal dialysis. Br Med J 1987;294:808.

36. Kay S, Schatzki PF. Ultrastructure of a benign liver cell adenoma. Cancer 1971;28:755–72.

37. Kent DR, Nissen ED, Nissen SE, Ziehm DJ. Effect of pregnancy on liver tumor associated with oral contraceptives. Obstet Gynecol 1978;51:148–51.

38. Kerlin P, Davis GL, McGill DB, et al. Hepatic adenoma and focal nodular hyperplasia: clinical, pathologic, and radiologic features. Gastroenterology 1983;84:994–1002.

39. Khoo US, Nicholls JM, Lee JS, Saing H, Ng IO. Cholestatic liver cell adenoma in a child with hirsutism and elevated serum levels of cortisol and ACTH. Histopathology 1994;25:586–8.

40. LeBail B, Jouhanole H, Deugnier Y, et al. Liver adenomatosis with granulomas in two patients on long-term oral contraceptives. Am J Surg Pathol 1992;16:982–7.

41. LeBrun DP, Silver MM, Freedman MH, Phillips MJ. Fibrolamellar carcinoma of the liver in a patient with Fanconi anemia. Hum Pathol 1991;22:396–8.

42. Leese T, Farges O, Bismuth H. Liver cell adenomas. A 12-year experience from a specialist hepatobiliary unit. Ann Surg 1988;208:558–64.

43. Lubbers PR, Ros PR, Goodman ZD, Ishak KG. Accumulation of technetium-99m sulfur colloid by hepatocellular adenoma: scintigraphic-pathologic correlation. AJR Am J Roentgenol 1987;148:1005–8.

44. Mariani AF, Livingston AS, Pereiras RV Jr, et al. Progressive enlargement of an hepatic cell adenoma. Gastroenterology 1979;77:1319–25.

45. Marks WH, Thompson N, Appleman H. Failure of hepatic adenomas (HCA) to regress after discontinuance of oral contraceptives: an association with focal nodular hyperplasia and leiomyoma. Ann Surg 1988;208:190–5.

46. Masood S, West AB, Barwick KW. Expression of steroid hormone receptors in benign hepatic tumors: an immunocytochemical study. Arch Pathol Lab Med 1992;116:1355–9.

47. Mathieu d, Kobeiter H, Cherqui D, et al. Oral contraceptive intake in women with focal nodular hyperplasia of the liver. Lancet 1998;352:1679–80.

48. McCaughan GW, Bilous MJ, Gallagher ND. Long-term survival with tumor regression in androgen-induced liver tumors. Cancer 1985;56:2622–6.

49. Meirowitz RF, Tobin KD, Elias EG, Iseri O, Pais SO, Knodell RG. Resolution of inferior vena cava syndrome after embolization of a hepatic adenoma. Gastroenterology 1990;99:1502–6.

50. Mokrohisky ST, Ambruso DR, Hathaway WE. Fulminant hepatic neoplasia after androgen therapy [Letter]. Lancet 1977;296:1411–2.

51. Montgomery RR, Ducore JM, Githens JH, August CS, Johnson ML. Regression of oxymetholone-induced hepatic tumors after bone marrow transplantation in aplastic anemia. Transplantation 1980;30:90–6.

52. Mueller J, Keeffe EB, Esquivel CO. Liver transplantation for treatment of giant hepatocellular adenomas. Liv Transpl Surg 1995;1:99–102.

52a. Nasarek A, Werner M, Nolte M, Klemphauer J, Georgii A. Trisomy 1 and 8 occur frequently in hepatocellular carcinoma but not in liver cell adenoma and focal nodular hyperplasia. Virchows Arch 1995;427:373–8.

53. Overly WL, Dankoff JA, Wang BK, Singh UD. Androgens and hepatocellular carcinoma in an athlete [Letter]. Ann Intern Med 1984;100:158–9.

54. Paradinas FJ, Bull TB, Westaby D, Murray-Lyon IM. Hyperplasia and prolapse of hepatocytes during longterm methyltestosterone therapy: possible relationships of these changes to the development of peliosis hepatis and liver tumours. Histopathology 1977;1:225–46.

55. Parker P, Burr I, Slonim A, Grishan FK, Greene H. Regression of hepatic adenomas in type Ia glycogen storage disease with dietary therapy. Gastroenterology 1981;81:534–6.

56. Pelletier G, Frija J, Szekely AM, Clauvel JP. L'adénome du foie chez l'homme. Gastroenterol Clin Biol 1984;8:269–72.

57. Peters RL. Neoplastic diseases. In: Peters RL, Craig JR, eds. Liver pathology. New York: Churchill Livingstone, 1986:337–64.

58. Poe R, Snover DC. Adenomas in glycogen storage disease type I. Two cases with unusual histologic features. Am J Surg Pathol 1988;12:477–83.

59. Porter LE, Van Thiel D, Eagon PK. Estrogens and progestins as tumor inducers. Semin Liver Dis 1987;7:24–31.

60. Propst A, Propst T, Waldenberger P, Vogel W, Judmaier G. A case of hepatocellular adenomatosis with a follow up of 11 years. Am J Gastroenterol 1995;90:1345–6.

61. Rabe T, Feldmann K, Grunwald K, Runnebaum B. Liver tumours in women on oral contraceptives [Letter]. Lancet 1994;344:1568–9.

62. Raoul JL, Darnault P, Deugnier Y, et al. L'adénome du foie chez lhomme: Étude d'un cas et revue de la littérature. Sem Hop Paris 1987;63:487–90.

63. Recant L, Lacy P. Fanconi's anemia and hepatic cirrhosis. Am J Med 1965;39:464–75.

64. Resnick MB, Kozakewich, HP, Perez-Atayde AR. Hepatic adenoma in the pediatric age group. Clinicopathologic observations with assessment of cell proliferative activity. Am J Surg Pathol 1995;19:1181–90.

65. Ribeiro A, Burgart LJ, Nagorney DM, Gores GJ. Management of liver adenomatosis: results with a conservative approach. Liver Transpl Surg 1998;4:388–98.

66. Rooks JB, Ory HW, Ishak KG, et al. Epidemiology of hepatocellular adenoma. The role of oral contraceptive use. JAMA 1979;242:644–8.

67. Rosh JR, Collins J, Groisman GM, et al. Management of hepatic adenoma in glycogen storage disease Ia. J Pediatr Gastroenterol Nutr 1995;20:225–8.

68. Scott FR, El-Refaie A, More L, Scheuer PJ, Dhillon AP. Hepatocellular carcinoma in an adenoma: value of Q Bend 10 immunostaining in diagnosis of liver cell carcinoma. Histopathology 1996;28:472–4.

69. Soe KL, Soe M, Gluud C. Liver pathology associated with the use of the anabolic-androgenic steroids. Liver 1992;12:73–9.

70. Smit GP, Fernandes J, Leonard JV, et al. The long-term outcome of patients with glycogen storage diseases. J Inher Metab Dis 1990;13;411–8.

71. Tavani A, Negri E, Parazzini F, Franceschi S, La-Vecchia C. Female hormone utilization and risk of hepatocellular carcinoma. Br J Cancer 1993;67:635–7.

72. Taylor W, Snowball S, Lesna M. The effects of long-term administration of methyl testosterone on the development of liver lesions in BALB/c mice. J Pathol 1984;143:211–8.

72a. Tazawa K, Yasuda M, Ohtani Y, Makuurchi H, Osamura RY. Multiple hepatocellular adenomas associated with long-term carbamazepine. Histopathology 1999;35:86–95.

73. Thomas DB. Exogenous steroid hormones and hepatocellular carcinoma. In: Tabor E, DiBisceglie AM, Purcell RH, eds. Etiology, pathology, and treatment of hepatocellular carcinoma in North America. Houston: Gulf Publishing Co, 1991:77–89.

74. Thysell H, Ingvar C, Gustafson T, Holmin T. Systemic reactive amyloidosis caused by hepatocellular adenoma. A case report. J Hepatol 1986;2:450–7.

75. Tsang V, Halliday AW, Collier N, et al. Hepatic cell adenoma: spontaneous rupture during pregnancy. Dig Surg 1989;6:86–7.

76. Turani H, Levi J, Zevin D, Kessler D. Hepatic lesions in patients on anabolic androgenic therapy. Isr J Med Sci 1983;19:332–7.

77. Wanless IR, Medline A. Role of estrogens as promoters of hepatic neoplasia. Lab Invest 1982;46:313–20.

78. Westaby D, Portmann B, Williams R. Androgen related primary hepatic tumors in non-Fanconi patients. Cancer 1983;51:1947–83.

79. Wheeler DA, Edmondson HA, Reynolds TB. Spontaneous liver cell adenoma in children. Am J Clin Pathol 1986;85:6–12.

80. Zevin D, Turani H, Cohen A, Levi J. Androgen-associated hepatoma in a hemodialysis patient. Nephron 1981;29:274–6.

Nodular Regenerative Hyperplasia

81. Bioulac-Sage P, Dubuisson L, Bedin C, et al. Nodular regenerative hyperplasia in the rat induced by a selenium-enriched diet: study of a model. Hepatology 1992;16:418–25.

82. Bretagne JF, Deugnier Y, Launois B, Gosselin M, Ferrand B, Gastard J. Hyperplasie nodulaire regenerative, carcinomes hepatocellulaire et contraceptifs oraux. Gastroenterol Clin Biol 1994;8:768–9.

83. Capron JP, Degott C, Bernuau J, et al. L'hyperplasie nodulaire regenerative du foie. Etude de 15 cas et revue de la litterature. Gastroenterol Clin Biol 1993;7:761–9.

84. Carrasco D, Prieto M, Pallardo L, et al. Multiple hepatic adenomas after long-term therapy with testosterone enanthate. Review of the literature. J Hepatol 1985;1:573–8.

85. Classen M, Elster K, Pesch HJ, Demling L. Portal hypertension caused by partial nodular transformation of the liver. Gut 1970;11:245–9.

86. Colina F, Alberti N, Solis JA, Martinez-Tello FJ. Diffuse nodular regenerative hyperplasia of the liver (DNRH). A clinicopathologic study of 24 cases. Liver 1989;9:253–65.

87. Dachman AH, Ros PR, Goodman ZD, Olmsted WW, Ishak KG. Nodular regenerative hyperplasia of the liver: clinical and radiographic observations. AJR Am J Roentgenol 1987;148:717–22.

88. Dick AP, Gresham GA. Partial nodular transformation of the liver presenting with ascites. Gut 1972;13:289–92.

89. Dubuisson L, Boussarie L, Bedin CA, Balabaud C, Bioulac-Sage P. Transformation of sinusoids into capillaries in a rat model of selenium-induced nodular regenerative hyperplasia: an immunolight and immunoelectron microscopic study. Hepatology 1995;21:805–14.

90. Dubuisson L, Vonnahme FJ, Stzark F, et al. Hyperplastic foci in the atrophic liver of rats after portacaval anastomosis. Liver 1985;5:21–8.

91. Gerber MA, Thung SN, Shen S, Stromeyer FW, Ishak KG. Phenotypic characterization of hepatic proliferations. Am J Pathol 1983;110:70–4.

92. Gindhart TD, Cimis RJ, Mosenthal WT, Longnecker DS. Adenomatous hyperplasia of the liver. Arch Pathol Lab Med 1979;103:34–7.

93. Haese WH, Smith L, Bueding E. Hycanthone-induced hepatic changes in mice infected with Schistosoma mansoni. J Pharmacol Exp Ther 1973;186:430–40.

94. Hoso M, Terada T, Nakanuma Y. Partial nodular transformation of liver developing around intrahepatic portal venous emboli of hepatocellular carcinoma. Histopathology 1996;29:580–2.

95. International Working Party. Terminology of nodular hepatocellular lesions. Hepatology 1995;22:983–93.

96. Ishak KG. Nodular regenerative hyperplasia of the liver and other rare disorders associated with intrahepatic portal hypertension. In: Okuda K, Benhamou JP, eds. Portal hypertension. Tokyo: Springer-Verlag, 1991:325–42.

97. Key NS, Kelly PM, Emerson PM, Chapman RW, Allan NC, McGee JO. Oesophageal varices associated with busulphan-thioguanine combination therapy for chronic myeloid leukaemia. Lancet 1987;2:1050–2.

98. Montgomery RR, Ducore JM, Githens JH. Regression of oxymetholone-induced hepatic tumors after bone marrow transplantation in aplastic anemia. Transplantation 1980;30:90–6.

99. Moran CA, Mullick FG, Ishak KG. Nodular regenerative hyperplasia in children. Am J Surg Pathol 1991;15:449–54.

100. Nakhleh RE, Snover DC. Use of alpha-1-antitrypsin in the diagnosis of nodular regenerative hyperplasia of the liver. Hum Pathol 1988;19:1048–52.

101. Nguyen TD, Oakes D, Fogel MR, Williams L, Sherck JP, Kozar M. Hepatocellular adenoma and nodular regenerative hyperplasia of the liver in a young man. J Clin Gastroenterol 1986;8:478–82.

102. Nzeako UC, Goodman ZD, Ishak KG. Hepatocellular carcinoma and nodular regenerative hyperplasia: possible pathogenetic relationship. Am J Gastroenterol 1996;91:879–84.

103. Ranstrom S. Miliary hepatocellular adenomatosis. Acta Pathol Microbiol Scand 1953;33:225–9.

104. Roschlau VG. Nodulare hyperplasie der Leber bei kontrazeptive Behandlung. Zbl Allg Pathol Anat 1977;121:517–21.

105. Rougier P, Degott C, Rueff B, Benhamou JP. Nodular regenerative hyperplasia of the liver. Report of six cases and review of the literature. Gastroenterology 1978;75:169–72.

106. Shedlofsky S, Koehler RE, De Schryver-Kecskemeti K, Alpers DH. Noncirrhotic nodular transformation of the liver with portal hypertension: clinical, angiographic, and pathological correlation. Gastroenterology 1980;79:938–94.

107. Sherlock S, Feldman CA, Moran B, Scheuer PJ. Partial nodular transformation of the liver with portal hypertension. Am J Med 1966;40:195–203.

108. Smith JC. Noncirrhotic nodulation of the liver. Arch Pathol Lab Med 1978;102:398–401.

109. Snover DC, Weisdorf S, Bloomer J, McClave P, Weisdorf D. Nodular regenerative hyperplasia of the liver following bone marrow transplantation. Hepatology 1989;9:443–8.

110. Solis-Herruzo JA, Colina-Ruizdelgado FA. Nodular regenerative hyperplasia of the liver. Hepatogastroenterology 1983;30:171–3.

111. Stromeyer FW, Ishak KG. Nodular transformation (nodular regenerative hyperplasia) of the liver. A clinicopathologic study of 30 cases. Hum Pathol 1981;12:60–71.

112. Stumpf HH, Liber AF. Hepatocellular adenomatosis. Report of a case with liver function tests. Am J Med 1954;17:887–90.

113. Sweeney EC, Evans DJ. Hepatic lesions in patients treated with synthetic anabolic steroids. J Clin Pathol 1976;29:626–33.

114. Tsui WM, So KT. Partial nodular transformation of liver in a child. Histopathology 1993;22:594–6.

115. Ueno S, Tanabe G, Sueyoshi K, et al. Hepatic hemodynamics in a patient with nodular regenerative hyperplasia. Am J Gastroenterol 1996;91:1012–15.

116. Variend S. An unusual nodular lesion of the liver: probable partial nodular transformation. Histopathology 1978;2:363–71.

117. Wanless IR. Micronodular transformation (nodular regenerative hyperplasia) of the liver: a report of 64 cases among 2,500 autopsies and a new classification of benign hepatocellular nodules. Hepatology 1990;11:787–97.

118. Wanless IR, Godwin TA, Allen F, Feder A. Nodular regenerative hyperplasia of the liver in hematologic disorders: a possible response to obliterative portal venopathy. A morphometric study of nine cases with an hypothesis on the pathogenesis. Medicine 1980;59:367–79.

119. Wanless IR, Gryfe A. Nodular transformation of the liver in hereditary hemorrhagic telangiectasia. Arch Pathol Lab Med 1986;110:331–5.

120. Wanless IR, Lentz JS, Roberts EA. Partial nodular transformation of liver in an adult with persistent ductus venosus: review with hypothesis on pathogenesis. Arch Pathol Lab Med 1985;109:427–32.

121. Washington K, Lane KL, Meyers WC. Nodular regenerative hyperplasia in partial hepatectomy specimens. Am J Surg Pathol 1993;17:1151–8.

122. Weinbren K. Experimental diffuse nodular hepatic hyperplasia. Toxicol Pathol 1982;10:81–94.

123. Weinbren K, Mutum SS. Pathological aspects of diffuse nodular hyperplasia of the liver. J Pathol 1984;143:81–92.

123a. Wilkens L, Bredt M, Flemming P, Becker T, Klempnauer J, Kreipe HH. Differentiation of liver cell adenoma from well-differentiated hepatocellular carcinoma by comparative genomic hybridization. J Pathol 2001;193:476–82.

Focal Nodular Hyperplasia

124. Aldinger K, Ben-Menachem Y, Whalen G. Focal nodular hyperplasia of the liver associated with high-dosage estrogens. Arch Intern Med 1977;137:357–9.

125. Begg CF, Berry WH. Isolated nodules of regenerative hyperplasia of the liver. Am J Clin Pathol 1953;27:447–53.

126. Benz EJ, Baggenstoss AH. Focal cirrhosis of the liver. Its relation to the so called hamartoma (adenoma, benign hepatoma). Cancer 1953;6:743–55.

127. Brady MS, Coit DG. Focal nodular hyperplasia of the liver. Surg Gynecol Obst 1990;171:377–81.

128. Brunt EM, Flye MW. Infarction in focal nodular hyperplasia of the liver. A case report. Am J Clin Pathol 1991;95:503–6.

129. Butron Vila MM, Haot J, Desmet VJ. Cholestatic features in focal nodular hyperplasia of the liver. Liver 1984;4:387–95.

130. Caseiro-Alves F, Zins M, Mahfouz AE, et al. Calcification in focal nodular hyperplasia: a new problem for differentiation from fibrolamellar hepatocellular carcinoma. Radiology 1996;198:889–92.

131. Cherqui D, Rahmouni A, Charlotte F, et al. Management of focal nodular hyperplasia and hepatocellular adenoma in young women: a series of 41 patients with clinical, radiological, and pathological correlations. Hepatology 1995;22:1674–81.

132. Ehrenfried JA, Zhou Z, Thompson JC, Evers BM. Expression of the neurotensin gene in fetal human liver and fibrolamellar carcinoma. Ann Surg 1994;220:484–91.

133. Everson RB, Fraumeni JF Jr. Familial glioblastoma with hepatic focal nodular hyperplasia. Cancer 1976;38:310–3.

134. Everson RB, Museles M, Henson DE, Grundy GW. Focal nodular hyperplasia of the liver in a child with hemihypertrophy. J Pediatr 1976;88:985–7.

135. Fechner RE. Benign hepatic lesions and orally administered contraceptives. A report of seven cases and a critical analysis of the literature. Hum Pathol 1977;8:255–68.

136. Forns X, Castells A, Bruix J, et al. Hiperplasia nodular focal asociada a malformaciones vasculares cerebrales. Gastroenterol Hepatol 1992;15:405–7.

137. Friedman LS, Gang DL, Hedberg SE, Isselbacher KJ. Simultaneous occurrence of hepatic adenoma and focal nodular hyperplasia: report of a case and review of the literature. Hepatology 1984;4:536–40.

138. Fukukura Y, Nakashima O, Kusaba A, et al. Angioarchitecture and blood circulation in focal nodular hyperplasia of the liver. J Hepatol 1998;29:470–5.

139. Gaffey MJ, Iezzoni JC, Weiss LM. Clonal analysis of focal nodular hyperplasia of the liver. Am J Pathol 1996;148:1089–96.

140. Goldin RD, Rose DS. Focal nodular hyperplasia of the liver associated with intracranial vascular malformation. Gut 1990;31:554–5.

141. Goldstein HM, Neiman HL, Mena E, Bookstein JJ, Appelman HD. Angiographic findings in benign liver cell tumors. Radiology 1973;110:339–43.

142. Haber M, Reuben A, Burrell M, et al. Multiple focal nodular hyperplasia of the liver associated with hemihypertrophy and vascular malformations. Gastroenterology 1995;108:1256–62.

143. Holder LE, Gnarra DJ, Lampkin BC, Nishiyama H, Perkins P. Hepatoma associated with anabolic steroid therapy. AJR Am J Roentgenol Rad Ther Nucl Med 1975;124:638–42.

144. Hunt RF, Sali A, Kune GA. Oestrogen receptors in focal nodular hyperplasia of the liver. M J Aust 1985;143:519–20.

145. Ishak KG. Benign tumors and pseudotumors of the liver. Appl Pathol 1988;6:82–104.

146. Ishak KG, Rabin L. Benign tumors of the liver. Med Clin N Am 1975;59:995–1013.

147. Jenkins RL, Johnson LB, Lewis WD. Surgical approach to benign liver tumors. Semin Liver Dis 1994;14:178–89.

148. Kaji K, Kaneko S, Matsushita E, Kobayashi K, Matsui O, Nakanuma Y. A case of progressive multiple focal nodular hyperplasia with alteration of imaging studies. Am J Gastroenterol 1998;93:2568–72.

149. Kerlin P, Davis GL, McGill DL, Weiland LH, Adson MA, Sheedy PF. Hepatic adenoma and focal nodular hyperplasia: clinical, pathologic and radiologic features. Gastroenterology 1983;84:994–1002.

150. Knowles DM, Wolff M. Focal nodular hyperplasia of the liver. A clinicopathologic study and review of the literature. Hum Pathol 1976;7:533–45.

151. Lalonde L, Van Beers B, Trigaux JP, Delos M, Melange M, Pringot J. Focal nodular hyperplasia in association with spontaneous portosystemic intrahepatic venous shunt. Gastrointest Radiol 1992;17:154–6.

152. Learch TJ, Ralls PW, Johnson MB, et al. Hepatic focal nodular hyperplasia: findings with color doppler sonography. J Ultrasound Med 1993;12:541–4.

153. Lee MJ, Saini S, Hamm B, et al. Focal nodular hyperplasia of the liver: MR findings in 35 proved cases. AJR Am J Roentgenol 1991;156:317–20.

154. Mahfouz AE, Hamm B, Taupitz M, Wolf KJ. Hypervascular liver lesions: differentiation of focal nodular hyperplasia form malignant tumors with dynamic Gadolinium-enhanced MR imaging. Radiology 1993;186:133–8.

155. Malt RA. Current concepts: surgery for hepatic neoplasms. N Engl J Med 1985;313:1591–6.

156. Mathieu D, Kobeiter H, Cherqui D, Rahmouni A, Dhumeaux D. Oral contraceptive intake in women with focal nodular hyperplasia of the liver [Letter]. Lancet 1998;352:1679–80.

157. Mathieu D, Zafrani ES, Anglade MC, Dhumeaux D. Association of focal nodular hyperplasia and hepatic hemangioma. Gastroenterology 1989;97:154–7.

158. McLoughlin MJ, Colapinto RF, Gilday DL, et al. Focal nodular hyperplasia of the liver. Angiography and radioisotope scanning. Radiology 1973;107:257–63.

159. McLoughlin MJ, Gilday DL. Angiography and colloid scanning of benign mass lesions of the liver. Clin Radiol 1973;23:377–91.

160. Ndimbie OK, Goodman ZD, Chase RL, Mack L, Lee MW. Hemangiomas with localized nodular proliferation of the liver. A suggestion on the pathogenesis of focal nodular hyperplasia. Am J Surg Pathol 1990;14:142–50.

160a. Nguyen BN, Flejou JF, Terris B, Belghiti J, Degott C. Focal nodular hyperplasia of the liver: a comprehensive pathologic study of 305 lesions and recognition of new histologic forms. Am J Surg Pathol 1999;23:1441–54.

161. Pain JA, Gimson AE, Williams R, Howard ER. Focal nodular hyperplasia of the liver: results of treatment and options on management. Gut 1991;32:524–7.

162. Paradis V, Laurent A, Flejou JF, Vidaud M, Bedossa P. Evidence for the polyclonal nature of focal nodular hyperplasia of the liver by the study of X-chromosome inactivation. Hepatology 1997;26:891–5.

163. Portmann B, Stewart S, Higenbottam TW, et al. Nodular transformation of the liver associated with portal pulmonary arterial hypertension. Gastroenterology 1993;104:616–21.

164. Rhodes RH, Marchildon MB, Luebke DC, et al. A mixed hamartoma of the liver: light and electron microscopy. Hum Pathol 1978;9:211–21.

165. Roskams T, De Vos R, Desmet V. Undifferentiated progenitor cells in focal nodular hyperplasia of the liver. Histopathology 1996;28:291–9.

166. Ross D, Pina J, Mirza M, Gavalan A, Ponce L. Regression of focal nodular hyperplasia after discontinuation of oral contraceptives [Letter]. Ann Intern Med 1976;85:203–4.

167. Saul SH, Titelbaum DS, Gansler TS, et al. The fibrolamellar variant of hepatocellular carcinoma. Its association with focal nodular hyperplasia. Cancer 1987;60:3049–55.

168. Saxena R, Humphreys S, Williams R, Portmann B. Nodular hyperplasia surrounding fibrolamellar carcinoma: a zone of arterialized hepatic parenchyma. Histopathology 1994;25 275–8.

169. Scoazec JY, Flejou JF, D'Errico A, et al. Focal nodular hyperplasia of the liver: composition of the extracellular matrix and expression of cell-cell and adhesion molecules. Hum Pathol 1995;26:1114–25.

170. Shamsi K, De Schepper A, Degyse H, Deckers F. Focal nodular hyperplasia of the liver: radiologic findings. Abdom Imaging 1993;18:32–8.

171. Stocker JT, Ishak KG. Focal nodular hyperplasia of the liver: a study of 21 pediatric patients. Cancer 1981;48:336–45.

172. Thomas PA, McCusker JJ, Merrigan EH, Conte NF. Lobar cirrhosis with nodular hyperplasia (hamartoma) of the liver treated by left hepatic lobectomy. Am J Surg 1966;112:831–4.

173. Travers H, D'Amato NA. Vascular alterations in focal nodular hyperplasia of the liver. Mil Med 1978;143:96–101.

174. Vecchio FM, Fabiano A, Ghirlanda G, Manna R, Massi G. Fibrolamellar carcinoma of the liver: the malignant counterpart of focal nodular hyperplasia with oncocytic change. Am J Clin Pathol 1984;81:521–6.

175. Vilgrain V, Flejou JF, Arrive L, et al. Focal nodular hyperplasia of the liver: MR imaging and pathologic correlation in 37 patients. Radiology 1992;184:699–703.

176. Wanless IR, Albrecht S, Belbao J, et al. Multiple focal nodular hyperplasia of the liver associated with vascular malformations of various organs and neoplasia of the brain: a new syndrome. Mod Pathol 1989;2:456–62.

177. Wanless IR, Mössinger M, Fronhoff K, Nadalin S, Raab R. Pregnancy in woman with observed focal nodular hyperplasia of the liver. Lancet 1998;351:1251–2.

178. Weimann A, Mawdsley C, Adams R. On the pathogenesis of focal nodular hyperplasia of the liver. Hepatology 1985;5:1194–200.

179. Welch TJ, Sheedy II PF, Johnson CM, et al. Focal nodular hyperplasia and hepatic adenoma: comparison of angiography, CT, US, and scintigraphy. Radiology 1985;156:593–5.

180. Wetzel WJ, Alexander RW. Focal nodular hyperplasia with alcoholic hyalin bodies and cytologic atypia. Cancer 1979;44:1322–6.

181. Whelan TJ, Baugh JH, Chandor S. Focal nodular hyperplasia of the liver. Ann Surg 1973;177:150–8.

Compensatory Hypertrophy Associated with Lobar Atrophy

182. Benz HH, Baggenstoss. AH, Wollaeger EE. Atrophy of the left lobe of the liver. Arch Pathol 1952;53:315–462.

183. Hadjis NS, Blenkharn JI, Hatzis G, Demianiuk C, Guzail M. Pathologic and hemodynamic sequelae of unilobar biliary obstruction and associated liver atrophy. Surgery 1999;109:671–6.

184. Ham JM. Lobar and segmental atrophy of the liver. World J Surg 1990;14:457–62.

185. Schweizer W, Duda P, Tanner S, et al. Experimenteller Atrophied/Hypertrophie-Komplex der Leber nach portale und/oder biliärrer bei der Ratte. Helv Chir Acta 1992;59:389–98.

186. Tsuzaki T, Hoshino Y, Uchiyama T, et al. Compensatory hypertrophy of the lateral quadrant of the left hepatic lobe due to atrophy of the rest of the liver, appearing as a mass in the left upper quadrant of the abdomen: report of a case. Ann Surg 1973;177:406–10.

Postnecrotic Regenerative Nodules

187. Baggenstoss AH. Pathological anatomy of hepatitis. JAMA 1957;165:1099–1107.

188. Edmondson HA. Benign epithelial tumors and tumor-like lesions of the liver. In: Okuda K, Peters RL, eds. Hepatocellular carcinoma. New York: John Wiley & Sons, 1976:309–30.

189. Ishak KG. Viral hepatitis. In: Binford CH, Connor DH, eds. Pathology of tropical and extraordinary diseases. An Atlas. Vol. 1. Washington, D.C., Armed Forces Institute of Pathology, 1976:13–36.

✧✧✧

3

BENIGN CHOLANGIOCELLULAR TUMORS

SOLITARY BILE DUCT CYST

Definition. This is a unilocular cyst lined by a single layer of columnar or low cuboidal epithelium, which rests on a basement membrane and a layer of fibrous tissue.

Clinical Features. Bile duct cysts occur at all ages, although the majority present in the fourth to the sixth decades. They are rare in the pediatric age group; at the Boston Children's Hospital, 31 solitary nonparasitic cysts (26 unilocular and 5 multilocular) were diagnosed in 63 years (12). The female to male ratio in two adult series was 4 to 1 (18) and 5.25 to 1 (16). Cysts smaller than 8 to 10 cm rarely cause symptoms. When present, symptoms include fullness or an upper abdominal mass, nausea, and occasional vomiting. Rapid enlargement has been reported in infancy (7). Jaundice is an infrequent complication (8,16,23). An acute abdominal crisis may result from torsion, strangulation, hemorrhage into the cyst, or rupture (2,3,10,25,28). Diagnosis is usually established by ultrasonography, computed tomography (CT), or other imaging modalities.

Gross Findings. Solitary bile duct cysts involve the right lobe twice as often as the left.

Rarely, they can arise in the falciform ligament (6,13). They are usually round, and some have a pedicle; the lining is typically smooth (fig. 3-1). The larger ones may contain one to several liters of fluid which is usually clear, but may be mucoid, purulent (if the cyst is infected), bile stained (if the cyst communicates with a bile duct), or hemorrhagic.

Microscopic Findings. The cyst lining usually consists of a single layer of columnar, cuboidal, or flat epithelium (fig. 3-2). The epithelium rests on a basement membrane that in turn is supported by a layer of fibrous issue. Malignant tumors, usually adenocarcinomas (20,21), may arise in the cyst. Other malignancies reported to arise in solitary cysts include carcinosarcoma (29), squamous cell carcinoma (fig. 3-3) (5,26), and carcinoid tumor (31).

Differential Diagnosis. *Autosomal dominant polycystic disease* of the kidney and liver usually does not pose a problem in the differential diagnosis since the imaging studies show multiple cysts in the liver (as well as renal cysts). The cysts may also be accompanied by *von Meyenburg complexes (biliary microhamartomas)* that are the precursor lesions of the larger cysts. Caroli's disease (segmental dilatation of the intrahepatic

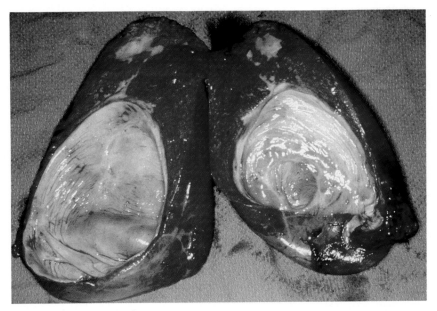

Figure 3-1
SOLITARY BILE DUCT CYST
Sectioned cyst has a smooth inner lining.

bile ducts) is unlikely to be confused with solitary bile duct cyst since the cyst-like dilatations are part of a generally dilated biliary tree. Moreover, these patients typically present with recurrent cholangitis with or without obstructive jaundice. *Alimentary (intestinal) duplications,* which can present as cysts in the liver, are very rare; two such cases have been reported: one was a duodenal duplication (19) and the other an ileal duplication (27). These duplications are recognized by

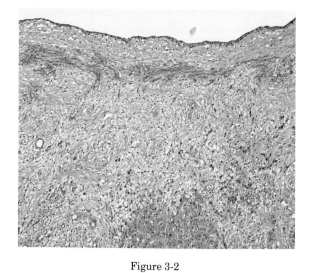

Figure 3-2
SOLITARY BILE DUCT CYST
The cyst epithelium consists of a single layer of cuboidal to low columnar cells.

the presence of the usual layers of the bowel wall, although they are not as well organized as normal. Mesothelial cysts are rare; they are usually small and subcapsular, and are lined by a single layer of flat mesothelial cells. *Pancreatic pseudocysts* of the liver may complicate both acute and chronic pancreatitis. They have been described in the left or caudate lobes and more recently, in both hepatic lobes (1). They are fluid collections rich in pancreatic secretions, and can be appropriately managed by percutaneous aspiration and biopsy. The cysts lack an endothelial lining but have a wall of fibrous tissue with chronic inflammation. Three examples of an *endometrial cyst* of the liver or hepatic endometriosis have been reported (15,32). In our opinion the possibility that these cysts represent biliary cystadenomas with mesenchymal stroma has not been ruled out. *Echinococcal (hydatid) cysts* have a characteristic imaging appearance, often with calcification. Grossly, they have a thick wall, an inner laminated membrane, brood capsules, and daughter cysts. The characteristic scoleces or hooklets are diagnostic.

Pathogenesis. A congenital origin is supported by the occurrence of the solitary bile duct cyst in fetuses and newborns (18), by a case presenting as a congenital diaphragmatic hernia (9), and the association of another case with the Peutz-Jeghers syndrome (30). Kida et al. (22) have suggested an origin of some solitary cysts

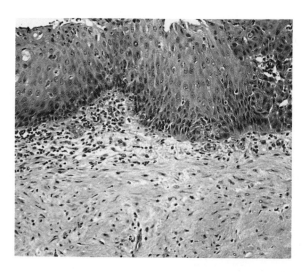 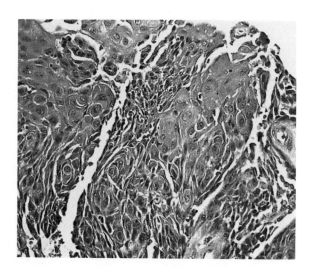

Figure 3-3
SQUAMOUS CELL CARCINOMA ARISING IN SOLITARY BILE DUCT CYST
The cyst lining shows squamous metaplasia (left). Well-differentiated squamous cell carcinoma is present in another area (right).

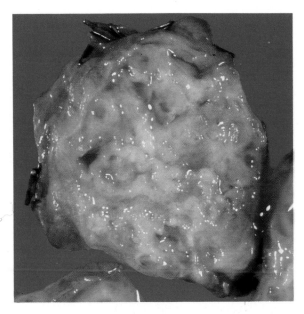

Figure 3-4
CILIATED FOREGUT CYST
Section of resected tumor shows multiple cysts.

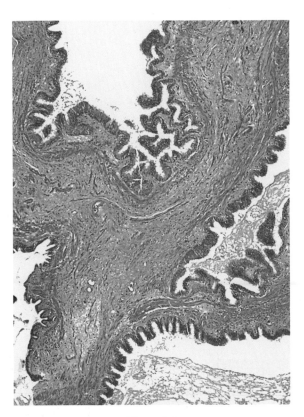

Figure 3-5
CILIATED FOREGUT CYST
Several cyst locules are lined by pseudostratified columnar epithelium. Note the smooth muscle bundles surrounding the cysts.

from dilatation of peribiliary glands, probably related to congenital or genetic factors.

Treatment. In the past, the treatment of choice of solitary cysts was excision (11), but this has been supplanted by aspiration and sclerotherapy (4,17), or laparoscopic fenestration (14,24).

CILIATED HEPATIC FOREGUT CYST

Clinical Features. Vick et al. (35) recently reviewed 49 reported ciliated hepatic foregut cysts and studied 6 previously unpublished cases on file at the Armed Forces Institute of Pathology (AFIP). The average age of the AFIP patients was 48 years (range, 14 to 61 years), with an equal incidence in males and females. The majority of the cysts were small and asymptomatic. Wu et al. (37) reported a high serum level of CA19-9 in a patient with a relatively large (5 cm) bilocular cyst. Imaging characteristics are described by Kadoya et al. (33). The case reported by Wu et al. revealed calcification radiographically.

Gross and Microscopic Findings. The cysts are typically subcapsular, small (less than 4 cm in diameter), and unilocular, except for one of the AFIP cases that was multicystic (fig. 3-4). Since publication of the AFIP series we have seen another multilocular cyst that measured 9 x 4.5

x 1.5 cm. The cysts contain clear fluid and rarely, viscid mucus. The histopathologic features include a lining of ciliated, pseudostratified, columnar epithelium resting on a basement membrane and supported by a loose lamina propria (figs. 3-5, 3-6). Mucin production can be demonstrated by special stains (fig. 3-7). The epithelium is in turn surrounded by bundles of smooth muscle and an outer fibrous capsule (figs. 3-8, 3-9) (35). The cilia are immunoreactive to actin and tubulin, and have a characteristic 9+2 ultrastructural pattern (34).

Malignant Transformation. This is exceptionally rare. We have seen one case of a squamous cell carcinoma arising in a ciliated foregut cyst in a 51-year-old male (36).

Pathogenesis. Ciliated foregut cysts are believed to arise from the embryonic foregut and to differentiate toward bronchial structures in the liver (34).

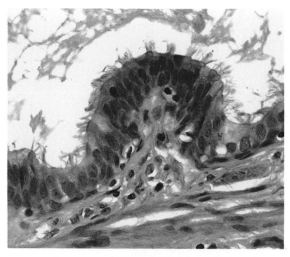

Figure 3-6
CILIATED FOREGUT CYST
High-power view of epithelium with cilia.

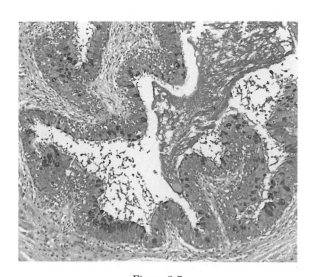

Figure 3-7
CILIATED FOREGUT CYST
Mucin is present in the cytoplasm of the lining cells and in the lumen (Alcian blue stain).

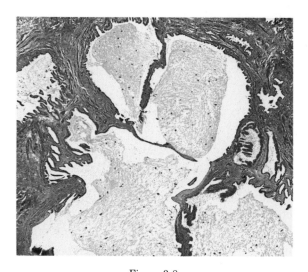

Figure 3-8
CILIATED FOREGUT CYST
Cysts are surrounded by collagen (blue) and smooth muscle bundles (red) (Masson trichrome stain).

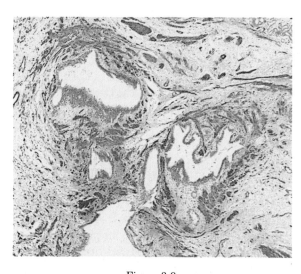

Figure 3-9
CILIATED FOREGUT CYST
Smooth muscle fibers are demonstrated immunohistochemically by antismooth muscle antibody.

PERIBILIARY GLAND HAMARTOMA (BILE DUCT ADENOMA)

Definition. This is a well-circumscribed lesion composed of acini and tubules that express the antigens of peribiliary glands, set in a fibrous stroma. This entity was formerly regarded as a bile duct adenoma, but the studies of Bhathal et al. (39) have shown convincingly that its cells actually have the phenotype of normal peribiliary glands rather than bile ducts, and so we now recognize this as peribiliary gland hamartoma.

Clinical Features. These are based on a series of 152 cases studied at the AFIP (38). There were 89 (58.6 percent) males and 63 (41.4 percent) females ranging in age from 1 to 99 years (mean, 55 years). Only two patients (1.3 percent) were under 20 years of age (1 1/2 and 12 years), while

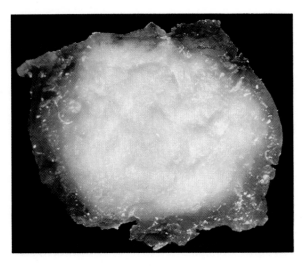

Figure 3-10
PERIBILIARY GLAND HAMARTOMA
Section shows a sharply circumscribed, white nodule that was firm in consistency.

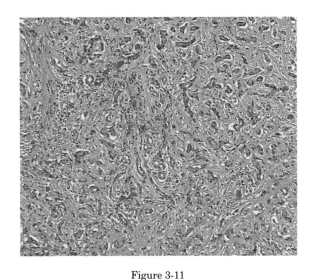

Figure 3-11
PERIBILIARY GLAND HAMARTOMA
The lesion is composed of small tubules lined by a single layer of cuboidal cells. Note the portal area in center.

24 (15.8 percent) were older than 70 years. No clinical signs or symptoms were attributable to the lesion. The lesion was always discovered incidentally: during intra-abdominal surgery in 103 patients (67.8 percent) and at autopsy in 49 (32.2 percent). There was no history of polycystic disease of the liver and kidneys in any case.

Peribiliary gland hamartomas encountered incidentally at surgery are excised locally (wedge resection) because of concern about the possibility of a malignant tumor, especially in patients with known malignant neoplasms of extrahepatic origin. Of the 38 patients in the AFIP series who were followed, 30 were alive and well 4 to 154 months (mean, 54.6) after surgery (38). Eight patients died of an unrelated condition 9 to 156 months (mean, 58.6) after surgery; autopsies in three cases did not show residual or recurrent tumor in the liver.

Gross Findings. In the AFIP series, 82.9 percent of the patients had solitary lesions, 6.6 percent had two lesions, and 10.5 percent had multiple lesions (38). The size was 10 mm or less in 92.8 percent of cases. Grossly, the lesions are round or ovoid, and well-demarcated but nonencapsulated (fig. 3-10); a few appear as small, flat, subcapsular scars. The color can be gray, grayish white, white, yellow, or tan. The consistency is typically firm.

Microscopic Findings. Peribiliary gland hamartoma is composed of tubules and acini that may show slight branching and tortuosity (figs. 3-11–3-14); some may exhibit minimal dilatation of the lumen. The lumen does not contain bile, and may be compressed or slightly dilated (figs. 3-11, 3-12). The tubules and acini are lined by a single layer of cuboidal to columnar cells resting on a basement membrane; nuclei are basally placed and show no hyperchromasia, atypia, or mitoses. Mucin production can be demonstrated with special stains (fig. 3-13). Normal portal tracts are often identified in the lesion. The stroma of the peribiliary gland hamartoma is fibrous and may be loose and scanty, or dense and hyalinized (fig. 3-14); microcalcification is rare.

The stroma often shows mild to marked inflammation. The inflammatory cells are predominantly lymphocytes; at the periphery of the nodule, they tend to be grouped in small clusters, sometimes forming lymphoid aggregates or follicles. In addition, polymorphonuclear leukocytes may be present occasionally; these cells may infiltrate the wall or lumen of the tubules. Rarely, small noncaseating granulomas may be present at the periphery of the nodule.

In a study of 30 cases, Bhathal et al. (39) found a spatial relationship between the lesions and a histologically normal bile duct; the ducts were either within or alongside the peribiliary gland hamartoma, although some were not be evident until serial sections were performed. The liver

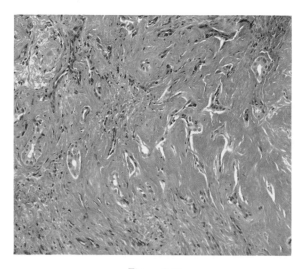

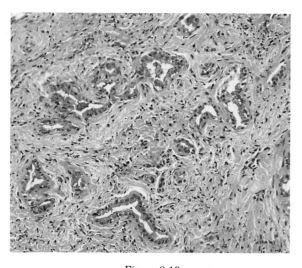

Figure 3-12
PERIBILIARY GLAND HAMARTOMA
Tubules are compressed and distorted due to the abundant, hyalinized stroma.

Figure 3-13
PERIBILIARY GLAND HAMARTOMA
Mucin production is highlighted by the Alcian blue stain.

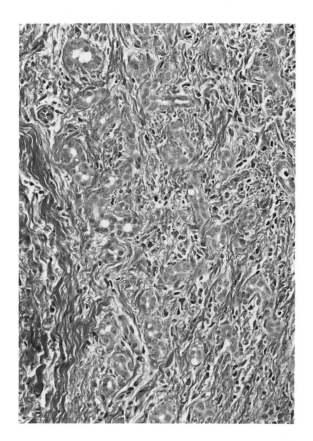

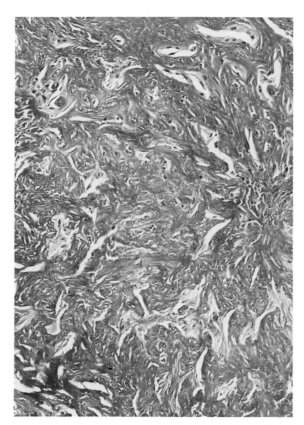

Figure 3-14
PERIBILIARY GLAND HAMARTOMA
Left: The trichrome stain shows the collagenous nature of the stroma.
Right: A densely hyalinized stroma surrounds the tubules (Masson trichrome stain).

surrounding a peribiliary gland hamartoma is either normal or shows nonspecific changes, but occasional lesions may be located in a background of cirrhosis.

Immunohistochemical Findings. The cells of the acini and tubules of peribiliary gland hamartoma express cytokeratin (pooled monoclonal antibodies [fig. 3-15]) as well as CK19; a basement membrane surrounds the tubules and glands. They also express the antigens D10 and 1F6, which are expressed by intrahepatic peribiliary glands but not by bile ducts of the normal liver (fig. 3-16) (39). Also expressed are polyclonal carcinoembryonic antigen and epithelial membrane antigen (39). Two tumors reported by O'Hara et al. (44) contained nests and clusters of uniform, round cells that stained for neuroendocrine markers.

Differential Diagnosis. The major importance of peribiliary gland hamartoma is its possible confusion with intrahepatic cholangiocarcinoma or metastatic adenocarcinoma (38). Helpful features distinguishing peribiliary gland hamartoma from adenocarcinoma are the presence of preexisting portal areas, the absence of cytologic features of malignancy (hyperchromasia, pleomorphism, loss of polarity, mitoses), and the absence of lymphatic or vascular invasion. The only benign lesion in the differential diagnosis that requires comment is the von Meyenburg complex. This lesion, also known as biliary microhamartoma, is a developmental anomaly consisting of multiple, small (less than 5 mm) nodules that are typically paraportal, and are composed of a variable number of ductal structures embedded in a hyalinized stroma. The ductal elements tend to be variably dilated and frequently exhibit microcystic dilatation; their lumen often contains bile (figs. 3-17, 3-18). These findings contrast with the morphologic features of peribiliary gland hamartoma, which is more frequently single and does not show cystic changes or contain bile (fig. 3-19). Von Meyenburg complexes are part of the spectrum of adult polycystic liver disease and can be associated with polycystic kidneys. A distinctive tumor, named *biliary adenofibroma,* was described recently by Tsui et al. (45). The histologic features include a complex tubulocystic biliary epithelial component set in an abundant fibroblastic stromal background. The glandular element is nonmucin secreting and contains bile concretions. Adenomatous neoplastic transformation

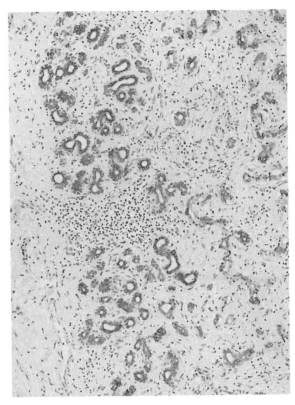

Figure 3-15
PERIBILIARY GLAND HAMARTOMA
Peribiliary gland hamartoma showing immunoreactivity of epithelial cells to pooled monoclonal cytokeratin antibodies.

of von Meyenburg complexes was considered but was ruled out by the authors. Histologically, this tumor is unlikely to be confused with peribiliary gland hamartoma.

Malignant Transformation. Follow-up studies of patients with peribiliary gland hamartoma have confirmed its benign nature (38,40, 42). There are, however, at least two documented cases that have developed malignancy (41,43), and we have seen three such cases at the AFIP.

Etiology and Pathogenesis. Allaire et al. (38) could not identify an etiologic factor in the 152 cases they studied. Based on the overall gross and microscopic findings, they suggested that the lesions were a reactive process to a focal injury, possibly postinflammatory or traumatic. Bhathal et al. (39) showed that these lesions actually represent disorganized, hamartomatous peribiliary glands, and that a more appropriate name for the lesion is peribiliary gland hamartoma, which is the preferred term.

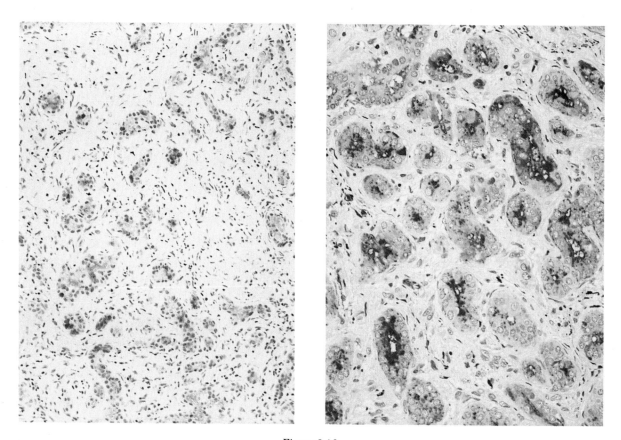

Figure 3-16
PERIBILIARY GLAND HAMARTOMA
Immunohistochemical expression of peribiliary gland antigen D10 (left) and 1F6 (right).

Figure 3-17
VON MEYENBURG
COMPLEX, SUBCAPSULAR

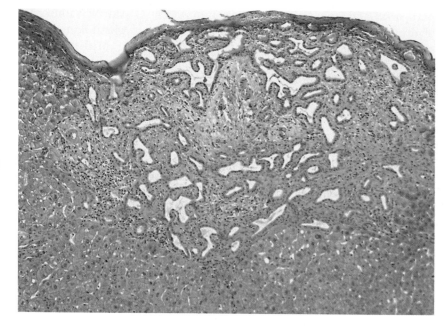

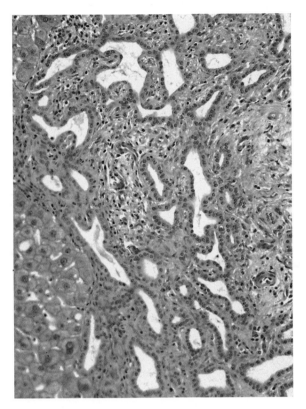

Figure 3-18
VON MEYENBURG COMPLEX
Von Meyenburg complex showing irregular bile ducts, some slightly dilated, embedded in a fibrous stroma.

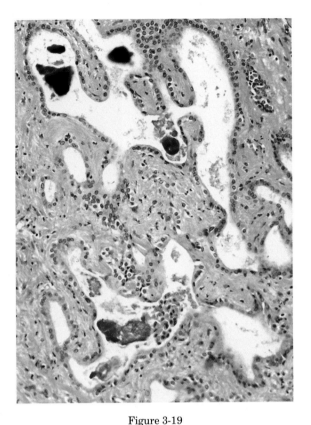

Figure 3-19
VON MEYENBURG COMPLEX
Von Meyenburg complex showing bile in the lumen of the ducts. Note the atypical configuration of the ducts.

PERIBILIARY CYSTS

Definition. Peribiliary cysts are retention cysts of peribiliary (periductal) glands located in the hilum of the liver and large portal areas. Synonyms include *hepatic cysts of periductal gland origin* and *hepatic hilar cysts.*

Clinical Features. The male to female ratio of reported cases is about 4 to 1 (46–48). The mean age in the largest series of 12 patients was 57 years, with a range of 38 to 69 years (46). To date, no cases have been reported in children. No symptoms or signs have been specifically attributed to the cysts, with the exception of the few cases with biliary obstruction (46,47,50,52). Associated hepatobiliary conditions (one or more) have included chronic cholecystitis/cholelithiasis (46,52), chronic hepatitis (51), cirrhosis (46, 49,50), portal vein thrombosis and/or portal hypertension (46,49,51,52), and hepatocellular carcinoma (46,49). The cysts can be detected by CT,

sonography, magnetic resonance imaging (MRI) (46,51,52), and endoscopic retrograde cholangiopancreatectomy (ERCP) (50,52). After studying 12 cases by various imaging modalities, Baron et al. (46) concluded that sonography was the most sensitive technique for detecting the thin septa between the cysts, thus allowing differentiation of a dilated bile duct from a linear collection of the peribiliary cysts.

Gross Findings. The cysts are located along the bile ducts in the hepatic hilum or in the large intrahepatic portal areas (fig. 3-20). They are round to ovoid and vary from 0.2 to 2.5 cm in diameter. They contain clear fluid. The larger cysts can compress and in some cases occlude the bile ducts. There is no communication between the cysts and the lumen of the bile ducts (49).

Microscopic Findings. The cysts are lined by a single layer of cuboidal to flat epithelial cells, depending on their size (fig. 3-21), which rest on a basement membrane. The cysts are

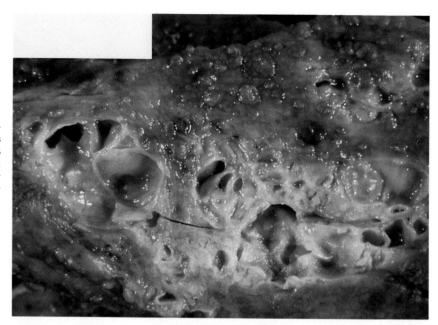

Figure 3-20
PERIBILIARY CYSTS
Section of liver showing a linear arrangement of multiple cysts of varied size. A bile duct is not clearly visualized in this section. The cysts have a smooth inner lining. Note the surrounding cirrhotic parenchyma.

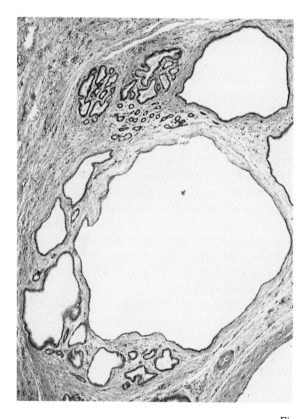 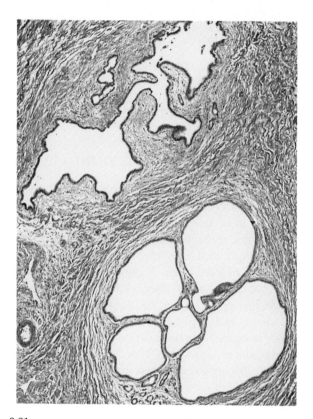

Figure 3-21
PERIBILIARY CYSTS
Left: The cysts are of varied size and are lined by a single layer of cuboidal or flattened epithelial cells. Clusters of typical, small peribiliary glands are intimately associated with the cysts.
Right: The peribiliary glands are surrounded by mature collagen. Note the cross section of a bile duct with a contorted lumen in the upper part of the figure (Masson trichrome stain).

surrounded by fibrous tissue in which are scattered periliary glands, some showing microcyst formation. There is a sprinkling of chronic inflammatory cells. Portal vein branches may show sclerosis or recanalized thrombi.

Pathogenesis. Nakanuma (49), who first described the cysts, concluded from the study of his autopsy cases that they were the result of dilatation of periliary glands. He suggested that disturbances of the portal venous flow could be the precipitating factor in their pathogenesis. Wanless et al. (52) postulated that periductal inflammation, fibrosis, and portal venous thrombosis could obliterate the necks of the periliary glands and result in the formation of retention cysts.

Treatment and Prognosis. Most of the reported cases have been found in autopsy livers or in total hepatectomy specimens (46,48,49). As already noted, the cysts have been associated with a variety of often severe hepatobiliary diseases. Only one of the patients who presented with obstructive jaundice was treated by dilatation of a strictured bile duct; he later died of pneumonia (52).

HEPATOBILIARY CYSTADENOMA

Definition. This is a solitary, multilocular cyst that can arise within the liver, extrahepatic bile ducts, or gallbladder. The cyst locules are lined by a layer of columnar to flattened epithelial cells that rests on a basement membrane, usually supported by a cellular mesenchymal stroma, which in turn is surrounded by a layer of collagenous tissue. Synonyms include *hepatobiliary cystadenoma with mesenchymal stroma* and *biliary cystadenoma.*

Clinical Features. These are based on an AFIP study of the largest series of cystadenomas published to date (59). The 52 patients ranged in age from 2 to 87 years at the time of initial presentation (mean age at presentation, 45 years; median age, 46 years). Cystadenomas were only rarely encountered in males: 96 percent of the patients were female; white patients predominated (89 percent).

Of the 52 patients, 22 (42.3 percent) complained of an upper abdominal mass; 15 (28.8 percent) complained of upper abdominal discomfort or pain. Four patients (7.7 percent) had a mass (associated with pain in two and nausea and vomiting in two). Five patients (9.6 percent)

had jaundice (that was painless in one and symptomatic in four). Only one patient (1.9 percent) had an abnormally elevated serum alkaline phosphatase value. Five of the tumors (9.6 percent) were discovered incidentally (two at autopsy and three at laparotomy for cholecystectomy or peptic ulcer surgery). The duration of illness prior to diagnosis varied considerably, from days to several months or, in six cases, from 1 to 7 years. The preoperative diagnosis of cystadenoma is largely based on imaging studies (see Radiologic Findings). Elevated levels (serum and cyst fluid) of CA19-9 have been helpful in distinguishing cystadenoma from other cystic lesions (63,68) although, as already noted, elevated serum levels were detected in a patient with a ciliated foregut cyst (37). It is also worth noting that a patient with a cystadenoma of the common hepatic duct had elevated serum CA19-9 levels (57).

The period of follow-up for the AFIP patients with cystadenoma ranged from 1 to 15 years (average, 7.6 years) (59). Of the 50 patients treated surgically, total excision was carried out in 43 (88 percent), while 12 percent were initially treated by some form of biopsy or subtotal resection (often accompanied by marsupialization of the remainder of the cyst to permit drainage of the contents). Of the patients treated by cyst excision in toto, recurrence of (benign) disease occurred in only one. Three of the six patients initially treated by biopsy/subtotal resection, later underwent definitive resections; two survived with persistent disease and one was lost to follow-up.

Radiologic Findings. These have been detailed in two relatively large series (55,58), as well as in individual case reports. The cystadenomas are solitary, multilocular, and cystic. Connections to the intrahepatic bile ducts and calcifications may be seen. Papillary excrescences, nodular thickening of internal septa, and mural nodules that show contrast enhancement are typical in cystadenocarcinoma.

Gross Findings. The majority of cystadenomas are located within the liver. Of the 52 cases studied by Devaney et al. (59), 22 arose in the left lobe of the liver, 18 in the right lobe, and 3 occupied both right and left lobes. An additional three cystadenomas were found in the common bile duct, while two arose in the hepatic duct, two in the cystic duct, and one was in the gallbladder. Gadzijev et al. (60) reported two cystadenomas

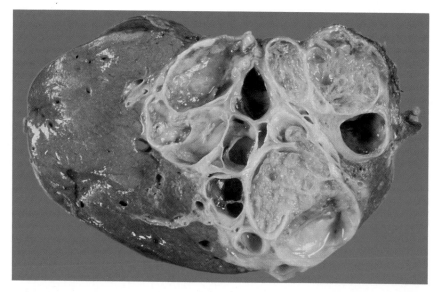

Figure 3-22
BILIARY CYSTADENOMA
This sectioned tumor is composed of multiple locules of varied size.

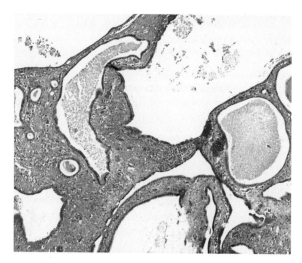

Figure 3-23
BILIARY CYSTADENOMA
The locules of varied size are lined by a single layer of cuboidal to columnar epithelium.

of the liver that protruded and grew into the extrahepatic bile ducts.

Hepatobiliary cystadenomas vary in size from 2.5 to 28 cm (mean, 15 cm). They are globular with a shiny, smooth, or bosselated surface through which stretched vessels course in different directions. Sections reveal multiple communicating locules of varied size that generally have a smooth and glistening lining (fig. 3-22). Roughened or elevated areas, or papillary excrescences, should arouse a suspicion of malignancy

(64). The fluid contents are often clear and thin but can be glairy or opalescent. Purulent material is present in infected locules. Blood-tinged or frankly bloody fluid may be found in cysts undergoing malignant degeneration (64).

Microscopic Findings. Cystadenomas are nearly always mucinous, but a serous variety is recognized (59). The locules of the *mucinous cystadenoma* are lined by columnar, cuboidal, or even flattened epithelium (fig. 3-23). Polypoid projections and papillary areas may be present (fig. 3-24). Mucin production is readily demonstrable by special stains (fig. 3-25). Focal intestinal metaplasia was observed in 11 of the 52 cystadenomas (21 percent) in the AFIP cases (fig. 3-26) (59). The epithelial cells rest on a basement membrane. Typically, the epithelium is surrounded by a layer of highly cellular mesenchymal tissue resembling ovarian stroma (fig. 3-27) (53, 59,64,70). This stroma is only found in females. Differentiation towards fibroblasts, smooth muscle, adipose tissue, and capillaries has been noted in the stroma (70). A layer of compact collagenous tissue in turn surrounds the mesenchymal stroma. A few cystadenomas, including some in women on file at the AFIP (fig. 3-28), and several in children (64), do not have the cellular mesenchymal stroma.

Inflammation may be noted in the wall, with infiltration by both acute and chronic inflammatory cells, and the epithelium may be ulcerated focally (fig. 3-29). The wall can be markedly

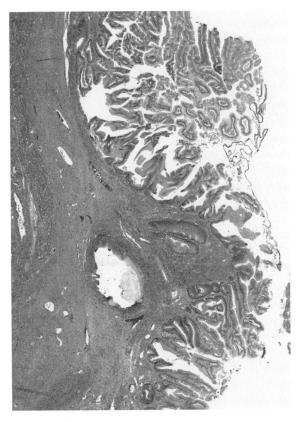

Figure 3-24
BILIARY CYSTADENOMA
The epithelium is hyperplastic and focally papillary, and shows low-grade dysplasia.

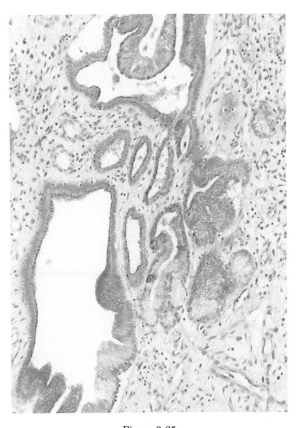

Figure 3-25
BILIARY CYSTADENOMA
Mucin production by the lining cells is highlighted by the Alcian blue stain.

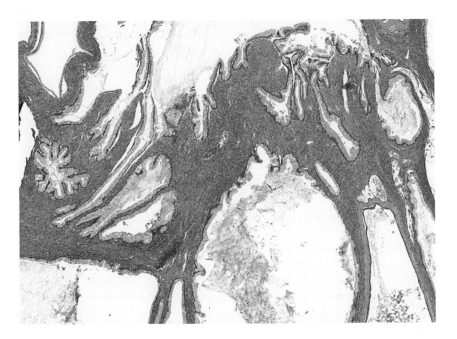

Figure 3-26
BILIARY CYSTADENOMA
Intestinal metaplasia.

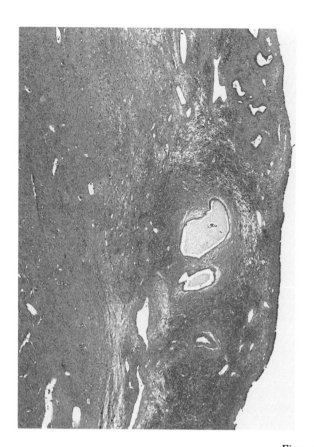
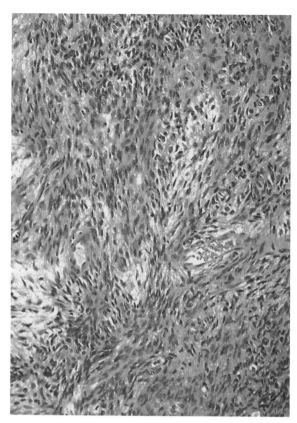

Figure 3-27
BILIARY CYSTADENOMA
Left: The epithelium is supported by a very cellular stroma.
Right: High magnification shows the cellular, mesenchymal stroma.

Figure 3-28
BILIARY CYSTADENOMA
This tumor lacks the cellular mesenchymal stroma.

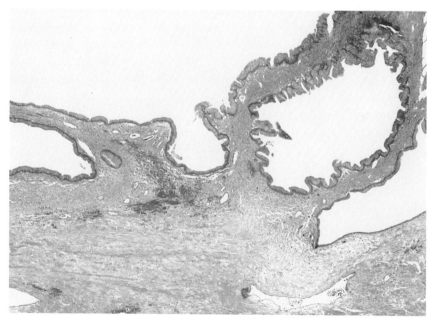

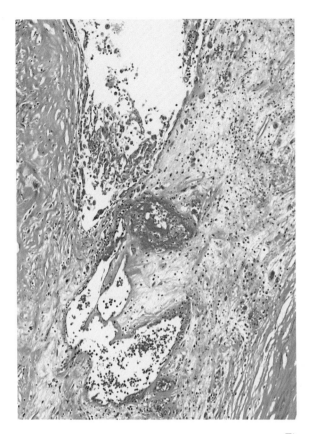
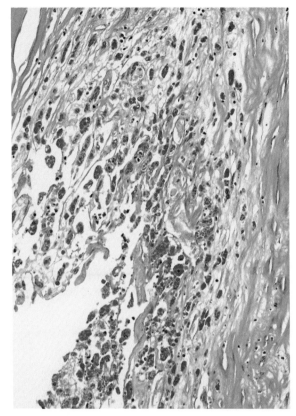

Figure 3-29
BILIARY CYSTADENOMA
Left: The wall of a locule shows epithelial ulceration and inflammation.
Right: Numerous macrophages containing ceroid are present in the ulcerated wall (PAS stain).

thickened by a xanthogranulomatous inflammation, with cholesterol accumulation and numerous ceroid-laden macrophages (fig. 3-29) (64). Calcification is rare (fig. 3-30).

The *serous ("microcystic") cystadenoma* is identical to the lesion more commonly described in the pancreas. It is composed of multiple small cysts lined by a single layer of cuboidal epithelial cells that are rich in glycogen (figs. 3-31–3-33). These cells rest on a basement membrane that in turn is supported by a coat of collagenous tissue. The cellular mesenchymal stroma, typical of the mucinous variety, is not seen in the serous cystadenoma.

Foci of dysplasia (enlargement of cells, multilayering, hyperchromasia, and loss of polarity) were reported in 7 of the 52 cases (13.5 percent) studied at the AFIP (59). The development of malignancy is a recognized complication of mucinous cystadenoma (53,59,64,69–71). In such

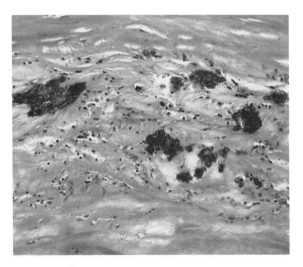

Figure 3-30
BILIARY CYSTADENOMA
Focal calcification is seen.

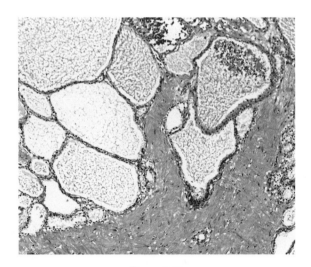

Figure 3-31
BILIARY CYSTADENOMA, SEROUS TYPE
The locules are small and the stroma is collagenous and acellular.

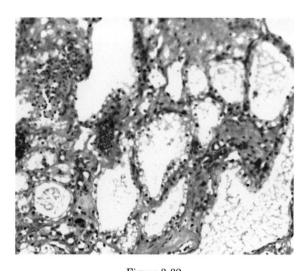

Figure 3-32
BILIARY CYSTADENOMA, SEROUS TYPE
Higher magnification shows the lining of a single layer of cuboidal clear cells.

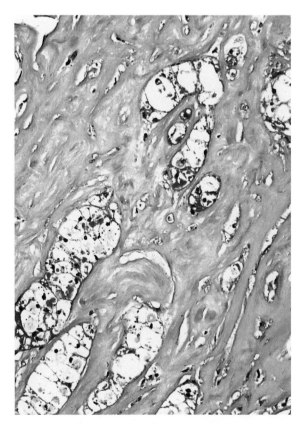

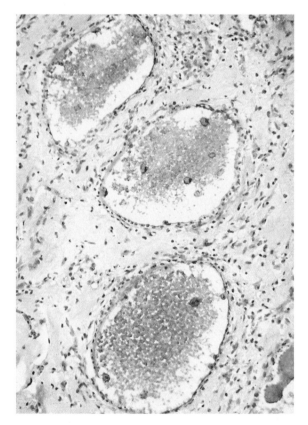

Figure 3-33
BILIARY CYSTADENOMA, SEROUS TYPE
Left: The lining cells focally contain glycogen (PAS stain).
Right: The lumen of the locules contains mucin (Alcian blue stain).

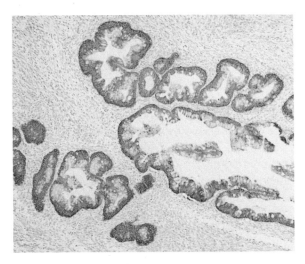

Figure 3-34
BILIARY CYSTADENOMA
Cytokeratin immunostain decorates the epithelial lining.

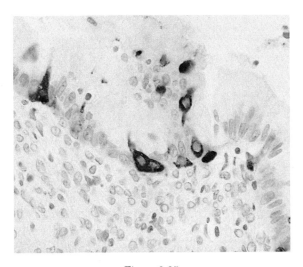

Figure 3-35
BILIARY CYSTADENOMA
There is focal expression of chromogranin antigen.

an event the basement membrane is breached and there is invasion of the underlying stroma. Other features of malignancy, such as loss of polarity, back-to-back glands, nuclear pleomorphism and hyperchromasia, and increased mitotic activity, are all helpful in distinguishing cystadenocarcinoma from cystadenoma (see chapter 10).

Immunohistochemical Findings. These are based on the study of the 52 cases from the AFIP (59). The epithelial lining of 20 of the cystadenomas was positive with antibodies to cytokeratin and carcinoembryonic antigen (fig. 3-34). Six (11.5 percent) had focal positive chromogranin staining (fig. 3-35); each of these cases arose in a female and showed foci of ovarian-like stroma. Intestinal metaplasia had been identified on light microscopy in four of these six patients. Diffuse to focal staining with antibody to lysozyme (a cytoplasmic pattern in all cases, with apical accentuation in one) appeared in the epithelium of 11 cystadenomas.

The stromal cells of the 20 cystadenomas studied by immunohistochemistry were negative with antibodies to cytokeratin, epithelial membrane antigen, carcinoembryonic antigen, chromogranin, and synaptophysin (59); vimentin positivity appeared in the stromal components of all 20 cystadenomas (fig. 3-36). Diffuse positivity with antibody to muscle-specific actin appeared in 17 of the 20 cases; focal desmin positivity was noted 8 of

these. Fifteen of the 17 actin-positive cases and 8 of the 8 desmin-positive cases had ovarian-like stroma identified on light microscopy. Positive staining with antibody to type IV collagen was found in each of the stromal regions studied; this positivity followed a basement membrane–like linear pattern (adjacent to the epithelial component) in 13 cases, while staining in the remaining 7 cases was focal throughout the cyst wall and not localized to a discrete basement membrane–like region.

Differential Diagnosis. Although of rare occurrence, metastases from mucinous cystic neoplasms of other organs (e.g., pancreas, ovary, appendix) must be ruled out by appropriate clinical and imaging studies. Several lesions, mesenchymal hamartoma, rare lobar forms of adult polycystic disease and Caroli's disease (54,62), and the alveolar type of echinococcal cyst, require differentiation from biliary cystadenoma. Mesenchymal hamartoma is diagnosed mainly in early infancy and childhood. Microscopically, although cystically dilated bile ducts may be present, most of the cystic areas of the tumor typically represent fluid accumulation in the primitive mesenchyme. Moreover, the bile ductal component of mesenchymal hamartoma has a very intricate branching pattern, and the tumor contains hepatocellular elements as well as an abundance of immature mesenchyme and many blood vessels.

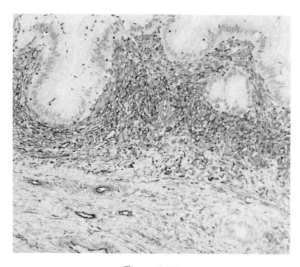

Figure 3-36
BILIARY CYSTADENOMA
Vimentin is strongly expressed by the stromal cells.

The lobar form of adult polycystic disease is exceptionally rare. Its biliary cysts do not intercommunicate (as they do in biliary cystadenoma), there is no mesenchymal stroma, and stretches of normal hepatic parenchyma are interposed between the cysts. Unilobar Caroli's disease shows segmental dilatation of intrahepatic bile ducts that are thickened by inflammation, both acute and chronic. Soft bilirubin calculi may be found in the dilated ducts. The parenchyma between the dilated ducts may be green from cholestasis.

Alveolar echinococcal cyst consists of multiple small cysts that are lined by the typical laminated (strongly periodic acid–Schiff [PAS]-positive) membrane of the parasite; the cyst is usually sterile. In one case report a cystadenoma protruding into the common bile duct mimicked a hydatid cyst in imaging studies (62). Calcification in another case also led to a mistaken radiologic diagnosis of hydatid cyst (66).

Histogenesis. This remains speculative. The occurrence of most of these tumors in adults raises the possibility that some environmental factor plays a role in their genesis (59). However, the presence of the mesenchymal stroma that resembles the primitive mesenchyme of the embryonic gallbladder and large bile ducts has suggested the possibility of origin from embryonic foregut rests (61,67,70).

Treatment. The treatment of choice of cystadenoma is complete surgical resection or enucleation (53,56,59,64,65). Incomplete resection, curettage, or internal surgical drainage procedures are likely to be followed by recurrence.

BILIARY PAPILLOMATOSIS

Definition. Biliary papillomatosis is a disease characterized by multiple, benign papillary tumors that are typically located in the intrahepatic and extrahepatic bile ducts, with involvement of the gallbladder or pancreatic duct in some cases. The lesions can be unilobar, usually involving the ducts of the left lobe.

Clinical Features. The following account is based on the comprehensive reviews of Rambaud et al. (84) and Gigot et al. (76); they reviewed 33 cases up to 1989, and collectively added 4 new cases. Since then other case reports have been published (72,73,75,81,86,87). The average age of patients with biliary papillomatosis is 56.3 years (range, 19 to 82 years) (76), but occasional cases have been reported in children. More males are affected than females: 21 of the 33 cases (63.6 percent) reviewed by Rambaud et al. were males. Jaundice, often recurrent, may be accompanied by fever and/or pain, and occurs in over 90 percent of patients; pain (epigastric or right hypochondrial) occurs in 70 percent; and hepatomegaly in 38 percent. Other signs and symptoms include fever (72 percent), weight loss (23.5 percent), and nausea, diarrhea, and vomiting in a small number (6 percent) of patients. Uncommon complications include acute pancreatitis, hemobilia, and anemia. The prognosis is poor because of recurrence, spread along the bile ducts, and malignant transformation, but metastases have only been reported in one instance (78). The mortality rate is estimated to be 65 percent.

Radiologic Findings. The intrahepatic and/or extrahepatic bile ducts are dilated in abdominal sonograms or CT scans, with some ducts containing polypoid masses (79,82). Endoscopic retrograde cholangiopancreatography shows the dilatation of the ducts as well as filling defects; "floating" defects corresponding to mucus secretion may also be seen (82).

Gross Findings. The affected ducts are dilated and contain friable, papilliferous lesions and inspissated mucus (fig. 3-37). Rarely, the lesions involve one lobe only, typically the left (83,87). The liver may show a green discoloration and the fine nodularity of secondary biliary cirrhosis.

Microscopic Findings. The affected bile ducts are variably dilated and partially or completely filled with papillary excrescences, which are composed of columnar epithelial cells supported by delicate fibrovascular stalks (fig. 3-38). The epithelium of the ducts between the papillary lesions may be ulcerated and involved by acute and chronic inflammation. The lumen of the ducts often contains inspissated mucin, blood, or tumor debris. Malignant transformation (to a papillary adenocarcinoma) is characterized by marked dysplasia with loss of polarity, hyperchromasia, numerous mitoses, and invasion beyond the confines of the ducts (see chapter 8). Discontinuities of the epithelial basement membrane in the three cases of Padfield et al. (83) (evaluated by the use of antilaminin antibodies) led to the conclusion that biliary

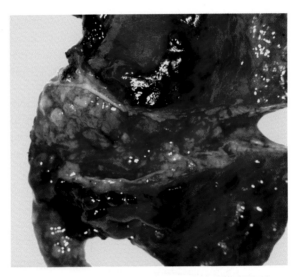

Figure 3-37
BILIARY PAPILLOMATOSIS
Section of a dilated duct showing an irregular lining with polypoid, tan excrescences.

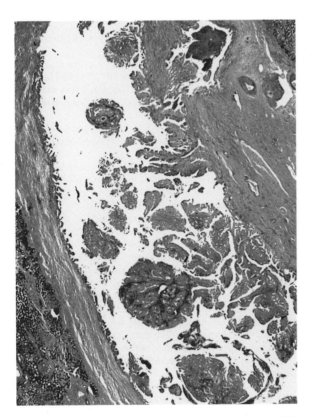
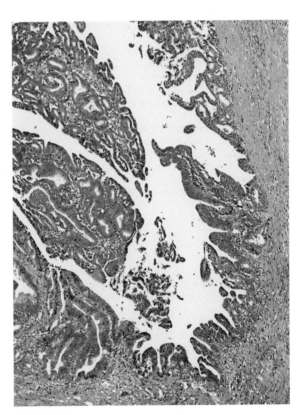

Figure 3-38
BILIARY PAPILLOMATOSIS

Left: Low-power appearance of the lesions.

Right: Higher magnification showing papillary excrescences in dilated intrahepatic bile ducts. The cells show high-grade dysplasia. There is no mural invasion.

papillomatosis should be considered a low-grade malignancy. In the review of Gigot et al. (76), 57 percent of cases of biliary papillomatosis were benign and 43 percent were malignant, either from first detection or secondarily.

Etiopathogenesis. No etiologic factors have been identified (76). A possible developmental error cannot be ruled out and, in this context, the occurrence of biliary papillomatosis in patients with Gardner's syndrome is worthy of note (74).

Treatment. Surgical treatment has included curettage of the bile ducts, excision of the bile duct by pancreaticoduodenectomy, hepaticoje-junostomy, and partial hepatectomy for the rare lobar form (77,80,84,85,88). Relapses and malignant transformation render the prognosis very poor. Liver transplantation has been recommended by Rambaud et al. (84,85).

REFERENCES

Solitary Bile Duct Cyst

1. Aiza I, Barkin JS, Casillas VJ, Molina EG. Pancreatic pseudocysts involving both hepatic lobes. Am J Gastroenterol 1993;88:1450–2.
2. Akriviadis EA, Steindel H, Ralls P, Redeker AG. Spontaneous rupture of a nonparasitic cyst of the liver. Gastroenterology 1989;97:312–5.
3. Ayyash K, Haddad J. Spontaneous rupture of solitary nonparasitic cyst of the liver. Acta Chir Scand 1988;154:241–3.
4. Bean WJ, Rodan BA. Hepatic cysts: treatment with alcohol. AJR Am J Roentgenol 1985;144:237–41.
5. Bloustein PA, Silverberg SG. Squamous cell carcinoma originating in a hepatic cyst. Case report with a review of the hepatic cyst-carcinoma association. Cancer 1976;38:2002–5.
6. Brock JS, Pachter HL, Schreiber J, Hofstetter SR. Surgical diseases of the falciform ligament. Am J Gastroenterol 1992;67:757–8.
7. Byrne WJ, Fonkalsrud EW. Congenital solitary nonparasitic cyst of the liver. A rare cause of a rapidly enlarging abdominal mass in infancy. J Pediatr Surg 1982;17:316–7.
8. Capell MS. Obstructive jaundice from benign nonparasitic hepatic cysts: identification of risk factors and percutaneous aspiration for diagnosis and treatment. Am J Gastroenterol 1988;83:93–6.
9. Chu DY, Olson AL, Mishalany HG. Congenital liver cyst presenting as congenital diaphragmatic hernia. J Pediatr Surg 1986;21:897–9.
10. Coustsoftides T, Hermann RE. Nonparasitic cysts of the liver. Surg Gynecol Obstet 1974;138:906–10.
11. Deziel DJ, Rossi RL, Munson JL, Brach JW, Silverman ML. Management of bile duct cysts in adults. Arch Surg 1986;121:410–5.
12. Donovan MJ, Kozakewich H, Perez-Atayde A. Solitary nonparasitic cysts of the liver. The Boston Children's Hospital experience. Pediatr Pathol Lab Med 1995;15:419–28.
13. Enterline DS, Rauch RE, Hayashi N, Silverman PM, Korobkin M, Akwari OE. Cyst of the falciform ligament of the liver. AJR Am J Roentgenol 1984;142:327–8.
14. Fabiani P, Mazza D, Toouli J, Bartels AM, Gugenheim J, Mouiel J. Laparoscopic fenestration of symptomatic nonparasitic cysts of the liver. Br J Surg 1997;84:321–2.
15. Finkel L, Marchersky A, Cohen B. Endometrial cyst of the liver. Am J Gastroenterol 1986;81:576–8.
16. Flagg RS, Robinson DW. Solitary nonparasitic hepatic cysts. Arch Surg 1967;95:964–73.
17. Furuta T, Yoshida Y, Saku M, et al. Treatment of symptomatic nonparasitic liver cyst—surgical treatment versus alcohol injection therapy. HPB Surgery 1990;2:269–79.
18. Geist DC. Solitary nonparasitic cyst of the liver. Arch Surg 1995;71:867–80.
19. Imamoglu KH, Walt AJ. Duplication of the duodenum extending into liver. Am J Surg 1977;133:628–32.
20. Kasai Y, Sasaki E, Tamaki A, Koshino I, Kawanishi N. Carcinoma arising in the cyst of the liver. Report of three cases. Jpn J Surg 1977;7:65–72.
21. Kashima S, Asanuma Y, Nwa M, Koyama K. A case of true hepatic cyst with malignant change. Acta Hepatol Jpn 1988;29:1265–8.
22. Kida T, Nakanuma Y, Terada T. Cystic dilatation of peribiliary glands in livers with adult polycystic disease and livers with solitary nonparasitic cysts: an autopsy study. Hepatology 1992;16:334–40.
23. Morin ME, Baker DA, Vanagunas A, et al. Solitary nonparasitic hepatic cyst causing obstructive jaundice. Am J Gastroenterol 1980;73:434–6.
24. Morino M, De Giuli M, Festa V, Garrone C. Laparoscopic management of symptomatic cysts of the liver. Indications and results. Ann Surg 1994;219:157–64.
25. Morgenstern L. Rupture of solitary nonparasitic cyst of the liver. Ann Surg 1959;150:167–71.
26. Pliskin A, Cualing H, Stenger RJ. Primary squamous cell carcinoma originating in congenital cysts of the liver. Report of a case and review of the literature. Arch Pathol Lab Med 1992;166:105–70.
27. Seidman JD, Yale-Loehr AJ, Beaver B, Sun CC. Alimentary duplication presenting as an hepatic cyst in a neonate. Am J Surg Pathol 1991;15:695–8.
28. Sood SC, Watson A. Solitary cyst of the liver presenting as an abdominal emergency. Postgrad Med J 1974;50:48–50.
29. Terada T, Notsumata K, Nakanuma Y. Biliary carcinosarcoma arising in nonparasitic cyst of the liver. Virchows Arch 1994;424:331–5.

30. Thrasher S, Adelman S, Chang CH. Hepatic cyst associated with Peutz-Jeghers syndrome. Arch Pathol Lab Med 1990;114:1278–80.
31. Ueyama T, Ding J, Hashimoto H, et al. Carcinoid tumor arising in the wall of a congenital bile duct cyst. Arch Pathol Lab Med 1992;116:291–3.

32. Verbeke C, Härle M, Sturm J. Cystic endometriosis of the upper abdominal organs. Report on three cases and review of the literature. Pathol Res Pract 1996;192:300–4.

Ciliated Foregut Cyst

33. Kadoya M, Matsui O, Nakanuma Y, et al. Ciliated hepatic foregut cyst: radiologic features. Radiology 1990;175:475–7.
34. Terada T, Nakanuma Y, Kono N, et al. Ciliated hepatic foregut cyst. A mucus histochemical, immunohistochemical, and ultrastructural study in three cases in comparison with normal bronchi and intrahepatic bile ducts. Am J Surg Pathol 1990;14:356–63.

35. Vick, DJ, Goodman ZD, Deavers MT, et al. Ciliated hepatic foregut cyst: a study of 6 cases and review of the literature. Am J Surg Pathol 1999;23:671–7.
36. Vick DJ, Goodman ZD, Ishak KG. Squamous cell carcinoma in a ciliated hepatic foregut cyst. Arch Pathol Lab Med 1999;123:1115–7.
37. Wu ML, Abecassis MM, Rao MS. Ciliated foregut cyst mimicking neoplasm. Am J Gastroenterol 1998;93:2212–4.

Peribiliary Gland Hamartoma (Bile Duct Adenoma)

38. Allaire GS, Rabin L, Ishak KG, Sesterhenn IA. Bile duct adenoma. A study of 152 cases. Am J Surg Pathol 1988;12:708–15.
39. Bhathal PS, Hughes NR, Goodman ZD. The so-called bile duct adenoma is a peribiliary gland hamartoma. Am J Surg Pathol 1996;20:858–64.
40. Colombari R, Tsui WM. Biliary tumors of the liver. Sem Liver Dis 1995;15:402–13.
41. Foucar E, Kaplan LR, Gold JH, Kiana DT, Sibley RK, Bosi G. Well-differentiated peripheral cholangiocarcinoma with an unusual clinical course. Gastroenterology 1979;77:347–53.

42. Govindarajan S, Peters RL. The bile duct adenoma. A lesion distinct from Meyenburg complex. Arch Pathol Lab Med 1984;108:922–4.
43. Hasebe T, Sakamoto M, Mukai K, et al. Cholangiocarcinoma arising in bile duct adenoma with focal area of bile duct hamartoma. Virchows Arch 1995;426:209–13.
44. O'Hara BJ, McCue PA, Miettinen M. Bile duct adenomas with endocrine component. Immunohistochemical study and comparison with conventional bile duct adenomas. Am J Surg Pathol 1992;16:21–5.
45. Tsui WM, Loo KT, Chow LT, Tse CC. Biliary adenofibroma. A heretofore unrecognized benign biliary tumor of the liver. Am J Surg Pathol 1993;17:186–92.

Peribiliary Cysts

46. Baron RL, Campbell WL, Dodd GD. Peribiliary cysts associated with severe liver disease: imaging-pathologic correlation. AJR Am J Roentgenol 1994;162:631–6.
47. Chin NW, Chapman I, Jimenez FA. Mucinous hamartoma of the biliary duct system causing obstructive jaundice. Hum Pathol 1988;19:1112–4.
48. Dumas A, Thung SN, Lin CS. Diffuse hyperplasia of the peribiliary glands. Arch Pathol Lab Med 1998;122:87–9.
49. Nakanuma Y, Kurumaya H, Ohta G. Multiple cysts in the hepatic hilum and their pathogenesis. A suggestion

of periductal gland origin. Virchows Arch [A] 1984;404:341–50.
50. Stevens W, Harford W, Lee E. Obstructive jaundice due to multiple hepatic peribiliary cysts. Am J Gastroenterol 1996;91:155–7.
51. Terada T, Minato H, Nakanuma Y, Shinozaki K, Kobayashi S, Matsui O. Ultrasound visualization of hepatic peribiliary cysts: a comparison with morphology. Am J Gastroenterol 1992;87:1499–502.
52. Wanless IR, Zahradnik J, Heathcote EJ. Hepatic cysts of periductal gland origin presenting as obstructive jaundice. Gastroenterology 1987;93:894–8.

Hepatobiliary Cystadenoma

53. Akwari OE, Tucker A, Seigler HF, Itani KM. Hepatobiliary cystadenoma with mesenchymal stroma. Ann Surg 1990;211:18–27.
54. Boyle MJ, Doyle GD, McNulty JG. Monolobular Caroli's disease. Am J Gastroenterol 1989;84:1437–44.
55. Buetow PC, Buck JL, Pantongrag Brown L, et al. Biliary cystadenoma and cystadenocarcinoma: clinical-imaging-pathologic correlation with emphasis on the importance of ovarian stroma. Radiology 1995;1996:805–10.
56. Cadranel JF, Vilgrain V, Flejou JF, et al. Cystadénome du foie. Etudes clinique, radiologique et anatomopathologique de 5 cas dont un associé a un cystédenocarcinome. Gastroenterol Clin Biol 1994;18:84–9.

57. Caturelli E, Bisceglia M, Villani MR, de Maio G, Siena DA. CA 19-9 production by a cystadenoma with mesenchymal stroma of the common hepatic duct: a case report. Liver 1998;18:221–4.
58. Choi BI, Lim JH, Han MC, et al. Biliary cystadenoma and cystadenocarcinoma: CT and sonographic findings. Radiology 1989;171:57–61.
59. Devaney K, Goodman ZD, Ishak KG. Hepatobiliary cystadenoma and cystadenocarcinoma. A light microscopic and immunohistochemical study of 70 patients. Am J Surg Pathol 1994;18:1078–91.

60. Gadzijev EM, Pleskovic A, Stanisavljevic D, et al. Hepatobiliary cystadenoma can protrude and grow into the bile ducts. Hepatogastroenterology 1998;45:1446–51.
61. Gourley WK, Kumar D, Bouton MS, Fish JC, Nealon W. Cystadenoma and cystadenocarcinoma with mesenchymal stroma of the liver. Immunohistochemical analysis. Arch Pathol Lab Med 1992;116:1047–50.
62. Guntz P, Coppo B, Lorimiert G, et al. La maladie de Caroli unilobaire. J Chir (Paris) 1991;128:167–81.
63. Horsmans Y, Laka A, Gigot JF, et al. Serum and cystic fluid CA 19-9 determinations as a diagnostic help in liver cysts of uncertain nature. Liver 1996;16:255–7.
64. Ishak KG, Willis GW, Cummins SD, Bullock AA. Biliary cystadenoma and cystadenocarcinoma: report of 14 cases and review of the literature. Cancer 1977;29:322–38.
65. Lewis WD, Jenkins RL, Rossi RL, et al. Surgical treatment of biliary cystadenoma. A report of 15 cases. Arch Surg 1988;123:563–8.
66. Rutledge JN, Pratt MC, Taupmann RE. Biliary cystadenoma mistaken for an echinococcal cyst. South Med J 1983;76:1575–7.

67. Subramony C, Herrera GA, Turbat-Herrera EA. Hepatobiliary cystadenoma. A study of 5 cases with reference to histogenesis. Arch Pathol Lab Med 1993;117:1036–42.
68. Thomas JA, Scriven MW, Puntis MC, Jasani B, Williams GT. Elevated serum CA 19-9 levels in hepatobiliary cystadenoma with mesenchymal stroma. Two case reports with immunohistochemical confirmation. Cancer 1992;70:1841–6.
69. Voigt JJ, Freligny E, Cassigneul J, Marty C, Monrozies X. Cystadenocarcinome primitif du foie associe a un cystadenome. Gastroenterol Clin Biol 1982;6:279–82.
70. Wheeler DA, Edmondson HA. Cystadenoma with mesenchymal stroma (CMS) in the liver and bile ducts. A clinicopathologic study of 17 cases, 4 with malignant change. Cancer 1985;56:1434–45.
71. Woods GL. Biliary cystadenocarcinoma. Case report of hepatic malignancy originating in benign cystadenoma. Cancer 1981;47:2936–40.

Biliary Papillomatosis

72. Bines JE, Shamberger RC, Perez-Atayde A, Rosenberg ST, Winter HS. Multiple biliary papillomatosis in a child. J Pediatr Gastroenterol Nutr 1992;14:309–13.
73. Bottger T, Sorger K, Junginger T. Progressive papillomatosis of the intrahepatic and extrahepatic bile ducts. Case report. Acta Chir Scand 1989;155:125–9.
74. Cougard P, Gelle LC, Collin P, Ferry C. La papillomatose des voies biliares dans le syndrome de Gardner. Med Chir Dig 1987;16:417–9.
75. Gertsch P, Thomas P, Baer H, Lerut J, Zimmermann A, Blumgart LH. Multiple tumors of the biliary tract. Am J Surg 1990;159:386–8.
76. Gigot JF, Geubel A, Haot J, et al. Papillomatose des voies biliares. Acta Endoscopica 1989;19:345–66.
77. Gouma DJ, Mutum SS, Benjamin IS, Blumgart LH. Intrahepatic biliary papillomatosis. Br J Surg 1984;71:72–4.
78. Griessen F. La papillomatose diffuse des voies biliares. Med Hyg 1979;32:227–7.
79. Harshfield DL, Teplick SK, Stanton M, Tunuguntla K, Diner WC, Read WC. Obstructing villous adenoma and papillary adenomatosis of the bile ducts. Am J Roentgenol 1990;154:1217–8.
80. Helpap B. Malignant papillomatosis of the intrahepatic bile ducts. Acta Hepatogastroenterol 1977;24:419–25.

81. Hubens G, Delvaux G, Williams G, et al. Papillomatosis of the intra- and extrahepatic bile ducts with involvement of the pancreatic duct. Hepatogastroenterology 1991;38:413–8.
82. Kawakatsu M, Vilgrain V, Zins M, et al. Radiologic features of papillary adenoma and papillomatosis of the biliary tract. Abdom Imaging 1997;22:87–90.
83. Padfield CJ, Ansell ID, Furness PN. Mucinous biliary papillomatosis: a tumour in need of wide recognition. Histopathology 1988;13:687–94.
84. Rambaud S, Nores JM, Meeus F, Paolaggi JH. Malignant papillomatosis of the bile ducts. Am J Gastroenterol 1989;84:448–9.
85. Rambaud S, Nores JM, Paolaggi JA. Papillomatose des voies biliares. Presse Med (Paris) 1989;18:1329–32.
86. Taguchi J, Yasunaga M, Kojiro M, Arita T, Nakayama T, Simokobe T. Intrahepatic and extrahepatic biliary papillomatosis. Arch Pathol Lab Med 1993;117:944–7.
87. Terada T, Mitsui T, Nakanuma Y, Miura S, Toya D. Intrahepatic biliary papillomatosis arising in nonobstructive intrahepatic biliary dilatations confined to the hepatic left lobe. Am J Gastroenterol 1991;86:1523–6.
88. Veloso FT, Ribeiro AT, Teixeira AA, Ramalhao J, Saleiro J, Serrao D. Biliary papillomatosis: report of a case with a 5-year follow-up. Am J Gastroenterol 1983;78:645–8.

❖❖❖

4

BENIGN MESENCHYMAL TUMORS AND PSEUDOTUMORS

MESENCHYMAL HAMARTOMA

Definition. Mesenchymal hamartoma is a benign lesion that occurs primarily in young children. It is composed of large, serous fluid–filled cysts surrounded by loose mesenchymal tissue containing small bile ducts.

Clinical Features. Mesenchymal hamartoma accounts for 7.9 percent of all liver tumors and pseudotumors in patients from birth to 21 years of age and 17.5 percent of the benign tumors and pseudotumors. During the first 2 years of life, however, mesenchymal hamartoma accounts for 12.4 percent of all tumors and pseudotumors and 22.2 percent of the benign ones (42); nearly 80 percent are detected in the first 2 years of life (Table 4-1) and another 17 percent in the next 3 years. Mesenchymal hamartoma has been reported in 15 patients 18 years and older; the oldest patients were a 62-year-old male and a 69-year-old female (6,12,13,19–21,29,33,45,48,50), but we suspect that many of these may be misdiagnoses. There is a slight male predominance but no apparent racial predilection.

Infants with mesenchymal hamartoma usually are noted by parents or physicians to have a nontender enlarging abdomen that may increase in size rapidly over a period of only a few days to weeks. These infants are rarely symptomatic. Respiratory distress, however, had been noted in a newborn infant with massive ascites from a ruptured lesion (3). Congestive heart failure has been described in two infants with highly vascular lesions, although this presentation is more often associated with infantile hemangioendothelioma (2,38). Other unusual presentations include jaundice in a newborn girl whose extrahepatic ducts were partially obstructed by the lesion (16), pyrexia in an 8-year-old girl whose lesion had become infected (36), and two patients with disseminated intravascular coagulation from intravascular thrombosis in the lesion (2,32). Mesenchymal hamartoma has also been found incidentally at autopsy (43).

Rarely, congenital anomalies and other diseases are seen in association with mesenchymal hamartoma. Alanen (1) noted the presence of mesenchymal stem villus hyperplasia in the placenta of an infant male who at age 6 months presented with a large mesenchymal hamartoma. Other associated anomalies have included adrenal cytomegaly, endocardial fibroelastosis, idiopathic thrombocytopenic purpura, and diffuse endocrinopathy (43).

Radiologic Findings. Ultrasound has been used to detect the presence of mesenchymal hamartoma in utero, during the neonatal period, in children, and in adults (1,3,5,11,13,17,20,22, 25,29,44,46,49). Tovbin and colleagues (44) observed a mesenchymal hamartoma by ultrasound in a 29-week fetus. Bartho and colleagues (4) described an abdominal mass in a female fetus in the 31st week of pregnancy that enclosed

Table 4-1

CLINICAL FINDINGS IN REPORTED PATIENTS WITH MESENCHYMAL HAMARTOMA*

Age	Cases	(%)
Birth to 1 month	16	(15)
1–12 months	42	(40)
1–2 years	25	(23)
2–5 years	18	(17)
5 years	5	(5)
	106	

Sex		
Male	72	(58)
Female	51	(42)
	123	

Race		
Caucasian	21	(55)
Black	10	(26)
Hispanic	3	(8)
Other	4	(11)
	38	

*Table 5.7 from Stocker J, Conran R, Selby D. Tumor and pseudotumors of the liver. In Stocker TJ, Askin F, eds. Pathology of solid tumors in children. London: Chapman & Hall, 1998:83–110.

the inferior vena cava. Hirata and colleagues (22) noted in utero, a complex, multicystic, well-circumscribed mass in a 38-week gestation male. The mass contained areas of echolucency surrounded by multiple echodense membranes. After delivery, the ultrasound was repeated, again demonstrating the mass which, by Doppler ultrasound, was negative for any pulsatile blood flow, an important feature in differentiating mesenchymal hamartoma from infantile hemangioendothelioma. In older children and adults, complex multicystic lesions are noted by ultrasound, although Alanen and colleagues (1) described a noncystic mass in a young woman. Computed tomography (CT) demonstrates the cystic or solid nature of the lesion, often showing considerable variation in size of the septa and cysts (1,9,11,18,21,25,35,37,46,48). Kaufman (23) noted that dynamic incremental contrast CT of a mesenchymal hamartoma in a 10-year-old male displayed peripheral and septal enhancement with centripetal fill, in a manner similar to that seen with infantile hemangioendothelioma and cavernous hemangioma. Magnetic resonance imaging (MRI) also demonstrates the multicystic nature of the lesion and can be helpful in delineating its extent (3,49). Roberts and colleagues (34) noted a multiseptate mass with fluid-filled compartments and some displacement of major intra-abdominal blood vessels in a 10-month-old male. By arteriography, mesenchymal hamartomas are generally hypovascular (9,17,47,48). Peripheral hypervascularity with a septated avascular center, however, has been described by Stanley and colleagues (40).

Gross Findings. Mesenchymal hamartomas involve the right lobe in 75 percent of cases, the left lobe in 22 percent, and both lobes in 3 percent (41). About 20 percent are pedunculated, extending from the surface of the liver as a mass attached by a thin to thick pedicle. The lesions vary in size from a few centimeters, when found incidentally at autopsy, to 30 cm or more in young children (43). The average weight is 1,300 to 1,900 g, but weights up to 6,810 g have been noted, as well as a 3,500 g lesion in a 1-month-old male whose birth weight had been 8,300 g (7,19).

Cysts are present in over 85 percent of cases, varying in size from a few millimeters to 14 cm (figs. 4-1, 4-2) (43). Average maximum cyst size is from 4 to 7 cm. The youngest infants may have

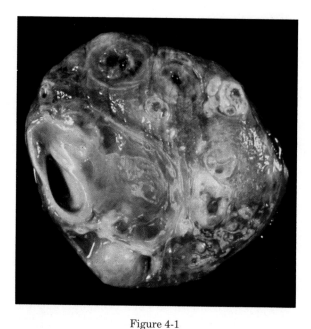

Figure 4-1
MESENCHYMAL HAMARTOMA
There are cysts of varied size with a smooth lining, as well as solid tan-brown tissue.

lesions without grossly visible cysts (fig. 4-3). The cysts are filled with clear amber to yellow fluid or gelatinous material; the fluid is similar in content to serum except for lower contents of total protein, albumin, immunoglobulin, cholesterol, and glucose (12). Rarely, the cysts have a smooth to ragged lining of gray-tan to yellow tissue, with older patients often displaying a lining similar to that of a bile duct.

Hemorrhage or necrosis is only infrequently seen and is more suggestive of an embryonal sarcoma or hepatoblastoma. Lennington and colleagues (26), however, noted the presence of a single vascular supply to a mesenchymal hamartoma in one case and recent vascular thrombi in two other cases, suggesting that mesenchymal hamartoma may represent a lesion with a solitary vascular supply and that the pattern of the stromal cysts may be a result of early ischemic changes.

Microscopic Findings. Mesenchymal hamartoma consists of a mixture of bile ducts, hepatocyte cords, clusters of vessels, and loose mesenchyme containing variably sized cysts, often with no discernible lining (figs. 4-4, 4-5). The mesenchyme consists of scattered stellate-shaped cells in a matrix rich in mucopolysaccharide (figs. 4-6, 4-7). Collagen may be present as

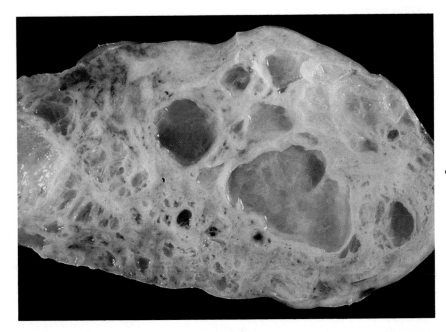

Figure 4-2
MESENCHYMAL
HAMARTOMA
The tumor is composed largely of cysts.

Figure 4-3
MESENCHYMAL
HAMARTOMA
Section shows solid, glistening, pink tissue in one area, and mottled pink and red-brown tissue in another area. Note the small separate ("satellite") nodules at the junction with the nontumor parenchyma.

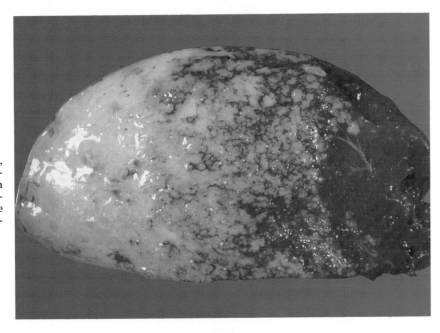

fibrils or small bundles associated with vessels and bile ducts within the mesenchyme (fig. 4-5). Extramedullary hematopoiesis (fig. 4-6) adjacent to the bile ducts or small vessels near the periphery of the lesion is noted within the mesenchyme in over 85 percent of cases (43). Plasma cells and lymphocytes, although rarely prominent, may also be seen within the mesenchyme.

Loose areas of fluid-rich mesenchyme may display fibrils of collagen separated into an alveolar pattern. These fibrils appear to expand to form the cysts characteristic of the lesion (fig. 4-8). The cyst walls are often composed only of denser mesenchymal tissue with no apparent epithelial lining. In older children and adults, however, a portion or the entire cyst wall may be

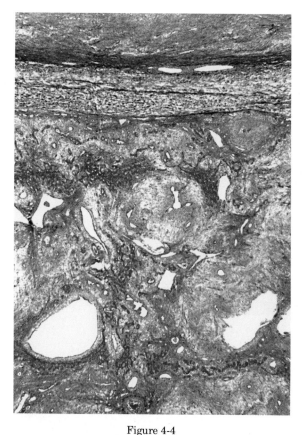

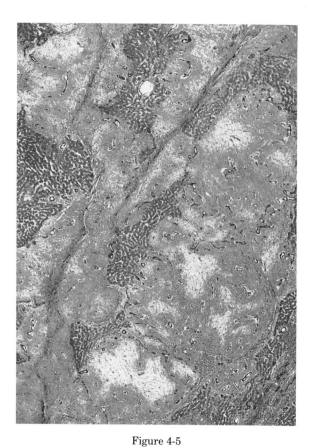

Figure 4-4
MESENCHYMAL HAMARTOMA
Low-power view shows the admixture of ducts, cysts, vessels, irregular liver cell plates, and mesenchymal stroma (Masson trichrome stain).

Figure 4-5
MESENCHYMAL HAMARTOMA
Low-power view shows numerous bile ducts surrounded by fibrous tissue, as well as liver plates lacking an acinar architecture.

Figure 4-6
MESENCHYMAL
HAMARTOMA
Extramedullary hematopoiesis. Note the loose mesenchyme and the hepatic parenchymal elements.

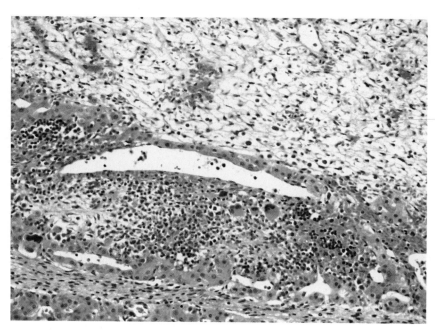

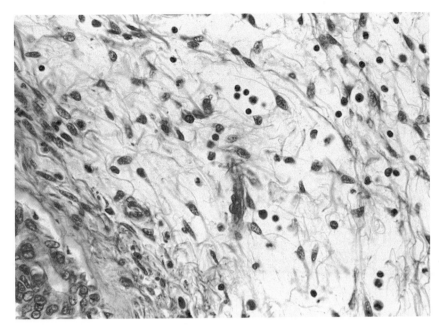

Figure 4-7
MESENCHYMAL
HAMARTOMA
At higher magnification the mesenchyme consists of stellate cells in a loose matrix.

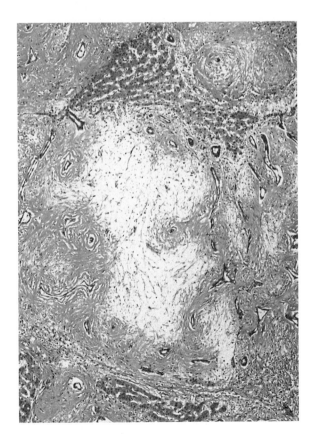
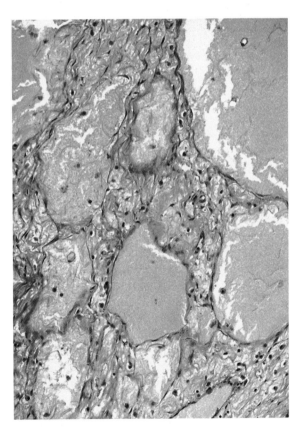

Figure 4-8
MESENCHYMAL HAMARTOMA
Left: Early cyst formation.
Right: Higher magnification of fully developed cysts. Note the absence of an endothelial lining.

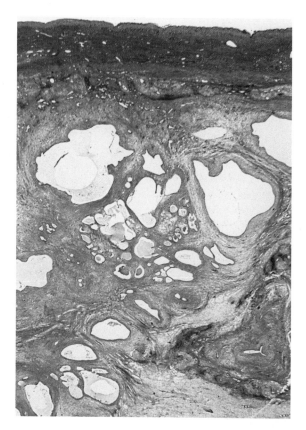
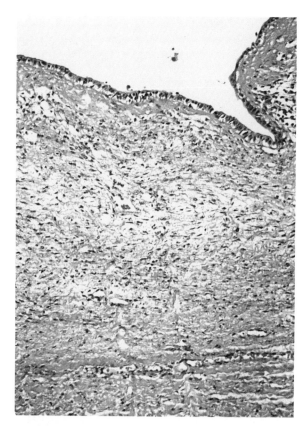

Figure 4-9
MESENCHYMAL HAMARTOMA
Left: The cysts in this low-power view are dilated ducts (Masson trichrome stain).
Right: On higher magnification, the ducts have an epithelial lining.

lined by cuboidal epithelium resembling that seen in the ducts of the normal liver (fig. 4-9).

Small bile ducts are usually present throughout the lesion. They may be single or intricately branching, and they appear to be an active or proliferating component of the lesion (fig. 4-10, left). The ducts often have the appearance of a ductal plate malformation (fig. 4-10, right). Bile is rarely present within the ducts. These ducts are surrounded by loose mesenchyme to dense collagen, which may distort the duct (figs. 4-10, 4-11). Hepatocyte cords may be present within the lesion but are usually confined to the periphery as thin compressed strips between expanding mesenchymal tissue (figs. 4-4–4-6) (43).

Areas of highly vascular connective tissue may be present as clusters of thin-walled vessels surrounded by loose collagen. Occasionally, the ducts disclose inflammatory or degenerative changes (fig. 4-12). This vascular tissue may extend to portal areas at the periphery of the lesion (satellite lesions) and be accompanied by mesenchymal tissue that appears to expand and compress intervening hepatic lobules, causing atrophy of the hepatocyte cords (fig. 4-13). Growth of the lesion may occur through this extension and expansion of mesenchymal tissue along portal tracts (42).

Immunohistochemical Findings. Immunohistochemical studies display vimentin positivity of the mesenchyme and "unlined" cysts while bile ducts stain for cytokeratin. Alpha-fetoprotein and alpha-1-antitrypsin stains are negative (13).

Differential Diagnosis. Rarely, myxoid change in the stroma of infantile hemangioendothelioma may lead to confusion with mesenchymal hamartoma. However, this tumor is composed predominantly of small vessels lined by plump endothelial cells, and the bile ducts in the tumor are small and lack the tortuosity of those

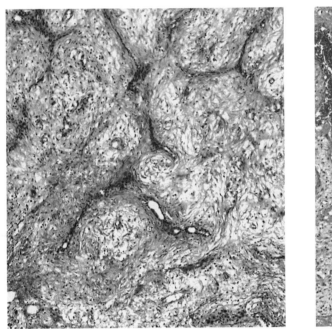
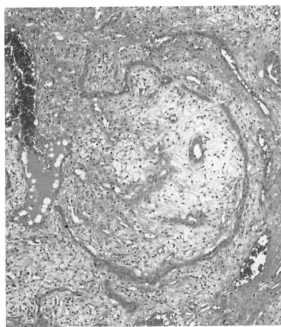

Figure 4-10
MESENCHYMAL HAMARTOMA
Left: The compressed, branching bile ducts are surrounded by a loose mesenchyme.
Right: The bile ducts, showing a ductal-plate malformation, are surrounded by a loose mesenchyme.

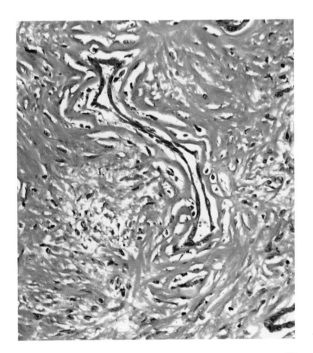
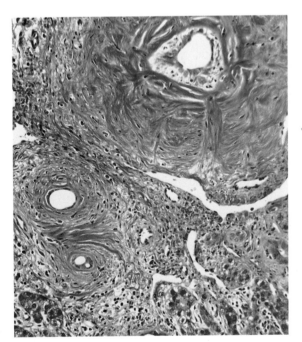

Figure 4-11
MESENCHYMAL HAMARTOMA
Left: The ducts are distorted by dense fibrous tissue.
Right: Ducts are surrounded by thick collars of collagen (Masson trichrome stain).

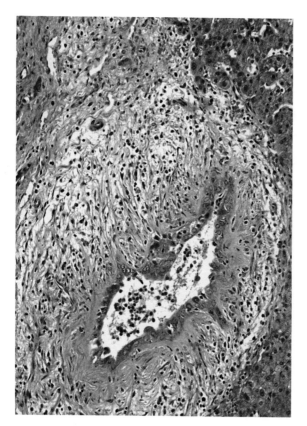

Figure 4-12
MESENCHYMAL HAMARTOMA
Bile duct inflammation and degeneration.

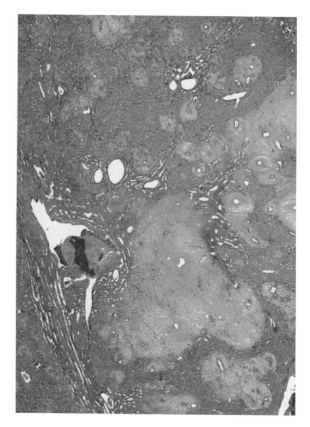

Figure 4-13
MESENCHYMAL HAMARTOMA
A satellite lesion is in the parenchyma adjacent to the tumor.

of mesenchymal hamartoma. Embryonal sarcoma (see chapter 12) should not pose difficulties in differential diagnosis since the stromal cells are clearly malignant. This tumor is compared with mesenchymal hamartoma in Table 4-2.

Pathogenesis. Maresch (27) in 1903 first described, as a "lymphangiomatous" lesion of the liver, what appears to have been a mesenchymal hamartoma in a 5-year-old female with an enlarged abdomen. Edmondson (14,15) coined the term "mesenchymal hamartoma" and suggested in 1958 that the lesion may result from a failure in the normal development of the embryonic and fetal liver resulting in a "congenital fibrodysplasia." Other authors have supported the concept of a developmental anomaly, while some suggest that the lesion is lymphangiomatous or the result of biliary obstruction (10,30). Based on a study of 30 cases (43), we suggested a developmental origin from primitive mesenchymal tissue late in embryogenesis. Noting the expansion

of portal areas at the periphery of the lesion, we postulated that the primitive mesenchymal tissue proliferates along portal tracts, compressing the hepatic parenchyma and eventually leading to atrophy of the hepatic lobule, resulting in the development of cysts as fluid accumulates in areas of mesenchymal degeneration.

A balanced translocation between chromosomes 11 and 19 with a breakpoint at 19q13.4 has been noted by Mascarello and Krous (28), similar to the balanced translocation between chromosomes 15 and 19 described by Speleman and colleagues (39). Otal et al. (31) performed flow cytometric analysis on paraffin-embedded tissue in 8 cases of mesenchymal hamartoma (4 male and 4 female) and noted that 6 cases were diploid and 2 were aneuploid, the latter with indices of 1.13 and 1.25. The presence of aneuploidy would seem to support the suggestion that mesenchymal hamartoma is a true neoplasm rather than a developmental anomaly.

Table 4-2

COMPARISON OF FEATURES OF MESENCHYMAL HAMARTOMA AND EMBRYONAL SARCOMA*

Feature	Mesenchymal Hamartoma	Embryonal Sarcoma
Sex	Twice as many males	Equal distribution
Age (median)	10 months	8 years
Presenting symptoms	Enlarging abdomen	Abdominal mass and/or pain
Physical examination	Nontender mass	Tender mass
Gross appearance	Mass with fluid-filled cysts	Mass with large areas of necrosis and hemorrhage
Pedunculation	17 to 30 percent	3 percent
Histologic features		
Bile ducts	Integral (proliferative) component of lesion	Entrapped (passive) component of lesion
Mesenchyme	Bland uniform tissue	Highly anaplastic tissue
Multinucleated tumor giant cells	Absent	Present
PAS-positive diastase-resistant globules	Absent	84 percent
Hematopoietic foci	87 percent	50 percent
Survival	90 percent	21 percent

*Table 5 from Stocker JT, Ishak KG. Mesenchymal hamartoma of the liver: report of 30 cases and review of the literature. Pediatr Pathol 1983;1:245–67.

Treatment and Prognosis. Surgical excision is the most frequent therapy, although the large size of the lesion and the involvement of vital structures, such as the inferior vena cava, the common bile duct, or the hepatic artery, may make complete excision difficult or impossible. Partial resection or excision and drainage of cysts may be all that is possible in some cases. Shuto and colleagues (37) described a 16-year-old girl who underwent bilateral lobectomy with preservation of the caudate lobe after having been previously treated at 7 months and 3 years of age with partial resection. In the Armed Forces Institute of Pathology (AFIP) series, there were six patients who, because of the size of the lesion, had only a biopsy and/or partial excision of the lesion initially. While one of the patients eventually required reoperation and excision, the others had no further treatment and survived without complications or recurrence. Alkalay and colleagues (2) reported on the successful use of cyclophosphamide to treat a newborn infant with a highly vascular mesenchymal hamartoma who presented with hydrops fetalis, congestive heart failure, and disseminated intra-vascular coagulation. The survival rate in patients with mesenchymal hamartoma is approximately 90 percent (43). Mortality and morbidity is largely related to intraoperative or postoperative complications. Almost all deaths associated with this lesion have occurred within the immediate postoperative period (9,24,35,43).

Relationship to Embryonal Sarcoma. The relationship between mesenchymal hamartoma and embryonal sarcoma (chapter 12) is unclear. De Chadarevian et al. (8) described a 12-year-old girl who developed an embryonal sarcoma in conjunction with a mesenchymal hamartoma. A second case was reported by Lauwers et al. (25a). This was a 15-year-old girl who had a typical mesenchymal hamartoma that transformed gradually into an embryonal sarcoma composed of anaplastic stromal cells; the former tumor was diploid and the latter aneuploid as determined by flow cytometry. Additionally, karyotypic analysis of the sarcoma showed structural alterations of chromosome 19, which have been implicated as a potential genetic marker of mesenchymal hamartoma. These two cases, however, are the only ones reported among over 200 cases of mesenchymal hamartoma.

INFANTILE HEMANGIOENDOTHELIOMA

Definition. This is a benign vascular tumor which occurs almost exclusively in the first year of life. It may be single or multicentric and is composed of vascular channels lined by a single layer of endothelial cells.

Clinical Features. Infantile hemangioendothelioma accounts for 17.7 percent of all liver tumors and pseudotumors in children (birth to 21 years) and 40 percent of the benign tumors and pseudotumors. During the first 2 years of life, infantile hemangioendothelioma accounts for 39.5 percent of all tumors and pseudotumors and 69.8 percent of the benign ones (94). Nearly 90 percent of infantile hemangioendotheliomas are seen in the first 6 months of life (Table 4-3), with 33 percent occurring in the first month. Almost all cases present by 2 years of age with only a rare report in older patients. Selby and colleagues (90) noted an infantile hemangioendothelioma in an 18-year-old. The lesion occurs more frequently in females (63 percent) and there appears to be no racial predilection (53,60,64,70,71,77,84,87,90–98).

Nearly 40 percent of infants are asymptomatic at the time the tumor is first noted by the mother or a physician as an abdominal mass. Symptoms and signs in the remaining cases include nausea, vomiting, gastrointestinal bleeding, respiratory compromise from upward compression of the diaphragm, fever, lethargy, jaundice, congestive heart failure, and liver failure (54,68,90). Congestive heart failure has been noted in 15 percent of patients in larger series and portends a poor prognosis (90). Samuel and Spitz (89), however, in a report of 16 cases, noted high-output cardiac failure in as many as 69 percent of the patients, along with consumptive coagulopathy and anemia in 75 percent. In 11 percent of cases from large series, hemangiomas are noted at other sites including skin, gastrointestinal tract, trachea, pleura, heart, adrenal gland, and dura and may be the first indication of an accompanying liver lesion (90). Rarely, acute abdominal pain from hemoperitoneum due to rupture of the tumor may be the initial symptom (58,84). Hepatomegaly and a diffusely enlarged abdomen are the most common physical findings (90). Infants with congestive heart failure may display difficulty in feeding, cough, dyspnea, or cyanosis (89,90).

Table 4-3

CLINICAL FEATURES OF INFANTILE HEMANGIOENDOTHELIOMA

Age	Cases	(%)
<1 month	42	(33)
1–6 months	69	(53)
6 months–3 years	16	(13)
>3 years	1	(1)
	128	
Sex		
Male	46	(37)
Female	79	(63)
	125	
Race		
Caucasian	74	(91)
Black	5	(6)
	79	

A variety of conditions have been noted in association with infantile hemangioendothelioma (Table 4-4). As noted earlier, hemangiomas at other sites are reported in 8 to 68 percent of cases, but larger series indicate the true incidence to be in the range of 10 to 15 percent (68,94). Marton and colleagues (74) described the presence of a multifocal hemangioendothelioma involving the placenta, liver, and left adrenal gland of a 29-week gestation, 1,460 g infant. The histology, with endothelial proliferation and atypia, however, suggests that the lesion may have been a chorangioma of the placenta or an angiosarcoma with metastases (74).

Sequestering of platelets occurs in some cases, leading to thrombocytopenia and hypofibrinogenemia (*the Kasabach-Merritt syndrome*) (92). Other findings may include anemia with hemoglobin of less than 10 mg/dl in 52 percent of cases, hyperbilirubinemia in 21 percent of cases, and elevated aspartate aminotransferase (AST) of greater than 100 U/L in 32 percent of cases (90). Alpha-fetoprotein (AFP) is rarely elevated beyond the expected levels for infants, recognizing that "adult" levels of AFP (less than 25 ng/ml) are not reached until 6 months of age. Since infants under 1 month of age may have AFP levels as high as 2,500 ng/dl, it is important to correlate the level of AFP with the age of the infant (80).

Table 4-4

CONDITIONS ASSOCIATED WITH INFANTILE HEMANGIOENDOTHELIOMA

Hydrocele (90)

Congenital heart disease (90), transposition of the great vessels (38)

Hydrocephalus (90)

Extranumerary digit (90)

Trisomy 21 (90)

Duplicate ureter (90)

Hemangiomas of skin, adrenal gland, trachea, pleura, heart, dura (90)

Deletion of chromosome 6q (66)

Cornelia de Lange syndrome and Wilms' tumor (75)

Heterotopic lobe of liver in left side of thorax (91)

Congenital hemihypertrophy (99)

Kasabach-Merritt syndrome (92)

Hepatic angiosarcoma (79,95)

Radiologic Findings. Plain films of the abdomen demonstrate hepatomegaly or an abdominal mass. Calcification as fine speckles may be seen in approximately 15 percent of cases (68). Tc-99m red blood cell single emission computed tomography (SPECT) produces an early "blush" as a diagnostic feature along with pooling of blood (78,82). Lesions with hemorrhage, necrosis, and fibrosis, however, may display decreased activity (68). Ultrasonography reveals a single nodule in one lobe in some cases or multiple nodules throughout the liver in others (86). The margins of the lesion may be well defined but irregular. Lesions are most frequently hypo-echoic or complex, with only a minority of cases displaying the hyperechoic features similar to those seen in adults (68). Ultrasonography may be used to follow the progression of the lesion (81). Doppler ultrasound studies may demonstrate enlargement of the hepatic artery and proximal aorta, with tapering of the aorta distal to the celiac artery (68). With nonenhanced CT, low-attenuation masses may be demonstrated (73). Calcification may be recognized in approximately 50 percent of cases by CT, ultrasound, or radiography; single lesions are most likely to calcify (68,72). Intravenous injection of a bolus of contrast material produces peripheral enhancement of the lesion in over 70 percent of cases, with delayed scans showing filling of the central low-attenuation areas. Infarction or hemorrhage, often present in large lesions, may result in failure of enhancement by CT, while multifocal lesions usually lack hemorrhage or necrosis and enhance completely (68). The presence or absence of hemorrhage and infarction results in a varied image with MRI. With T1-weighted images heterogeneity and low signal intensity is usually seen, although hemorrhagic areas may produce high signal intensity (68). With T2-weighted images, high signal intensity of the type seen in adult hemangiomas is usual (85). MRI may be helpful in determining the multicentricity of a lesion.

The vascular nature of infantile hemangioendothelioma is readily demonstrated with arteriography in all cases except those with extensive hemorrhage and infarction. Arteries feeding the tumor, both of hepatic and extrahepatic origin, are usually enlarged and tortuous (68). The lesion may also be supplied by the portal vein (55,63,76). Arteriovenous shunting may be demonstrated, along with pooling of contrast material within some or all of the lesion (68). Arteriography may be helpful in predicting the effectiveness of tumor embolization, with lesions with little collateral circulation responding better than those with extensive collateral circulation (63).

Gross Findings. Infantile hemangioendothelioma occurs as a single tumor in 55 percent of patients and as a multifocal tumor in the rest (figs. 4-14–4-16) (90). Single tumors are present equally in the right and left lobes; about 6 percent extend across the midline to involve both lobes. Single tumors may vary from 0.5 cm to as large as 13 cm in maximum dimension. Multifocal lesions may number from 2 to as many as 25 to 30 and may be localized to one lobe of the liver, but frequently involve large portions of the liver (fig. 4-16). When near the surface of the liver, the lesions may protrude slightly above the capsule, with smaller multifocal lesions displaying central umbilication. The lesions vary from well-demarcated, soft, spongy, red-tan masses to firm, tan-white to dark brown lesions with central areas of hemorrhage, necrosis, and gritty calcification (figs. 4-14, 4-15). The amount of hemorrhage and

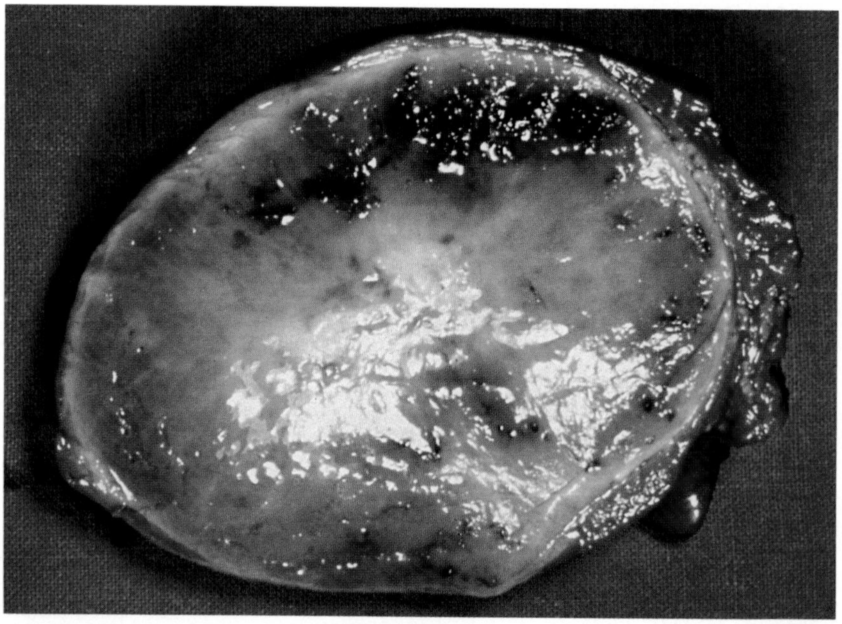

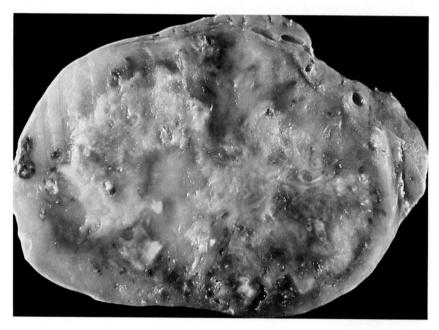

Figure 4-14
INFANTILE
HEMANGIOENDOTHELIOMA
This section of a single tumor shows a red to pink-brown periphery and a light tan-white center.

Figure 4-15
INFANTILE
HEMANGIOENDOTHELIOMA
The section of this tumor reveals mottled yellow, tan, and brown tissue.

necrosis is often influenced by preoperative or intraoperative hepatic artery ligation or transarterial embolization, with some lesions displaying nearly complete infarction.

Microscopic Findings. Infantile hemangioendotheliomas are composed of thin vascular channels lined by a single layer of bland-appearing endothelial cells (fig. 4-17). These flattened to plump endothelial cells contain a single round to oval nucleus with finely granular nuclear chromatin and a single nucleolus. The cytoplasm is usually scant and spread over the surface of the vascular channel in a thin layer. The vascular channels vary from small and capillary-like to slightly dilated and tortuous, the "type 1" lesion described by Dehner and Ishak (61). We now consider their "type 2" lesion an angiosarcoma (see chapter 12).

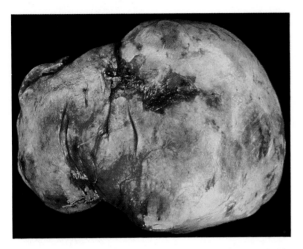 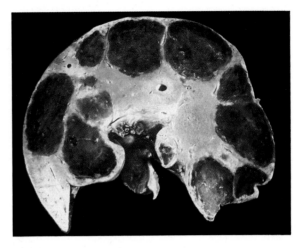

Figure 4-16
INFANTILE HEMANGIOENDOTHELIOMA
Left: Multiple, bluish subcapsular nodules.
Right: On sectioning, the nodules consist of large cavities filled with blood.

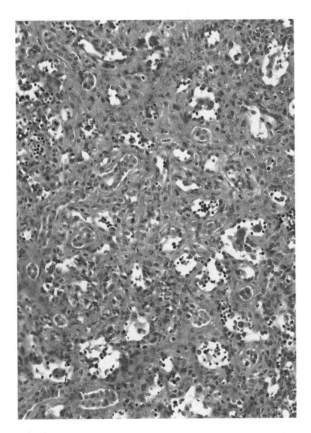 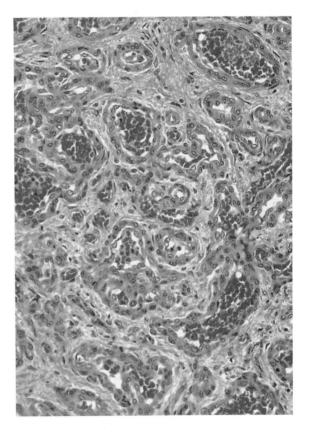

Figure 4-17
INFANTILE HEMANGIOENDOTHELIOMA
Left: The tumor consists of multiple vascular channels lined by a single layer of endothelial cells, surrounded by a scanty fibrous stroma. Note the small, scattered bile ducts.
Right: Higher magnification shows the endothelial lining of the vessels.

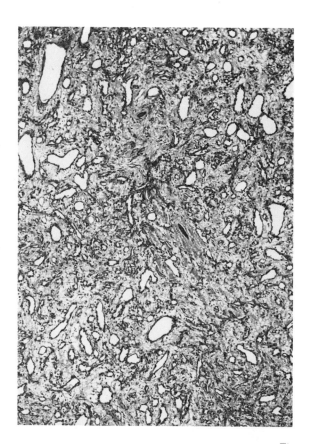 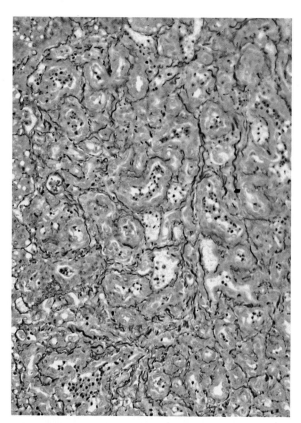

Figure 4-18
INFANTILE HEMANGIOENDOTHELIOMA
Left: The stroma contains collagen bundles (Masson trichrome stain).
Right: Reticulin fibers surround the vascular channels (Manuel reticulin stain).

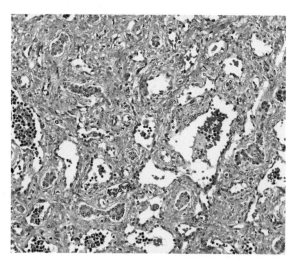

Figure 4-19
INFANTILE HEMANGIOENDOTHELIOMA
Bile ducts are noted throughout the lesion.

The walls of the vascular channels vary considerably in thickness and are composed of a central myxoid to dense fibrous stroma (fig. 4-18, left) with reticulin fibers (fig. 4-18, right), which may contain small bile ducts; these are particularly prominent near the margin of the lesion (fig. 4-19). Tumor margins in single and multicentric lesions are well demarcated from the surrounding liver in 65 percent of cases, with the remaining cases infiltrating the adjacent parenchyma by the vascular channels (90). Growth of the tumor appears to be by extension of the vascular channels along mesenchyme connecting portal triads. As the tumor extends, entrapped hepatocytes show pseudoglandular change, then degeneration or transformation to bile ducts (90). Areas of cavernous change are present in approximately 60 percent of cases, most frequently within the central portion of the tumor, but also near the periphery (fig. 4-20).

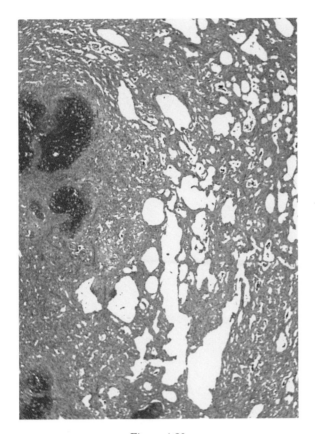

Figure 4-20
INFANTILE HEMANGIOENDOTHELIOMA
The vessels in the center of this tumor are cavernous.
Note the deeper areas of hemorrhage.

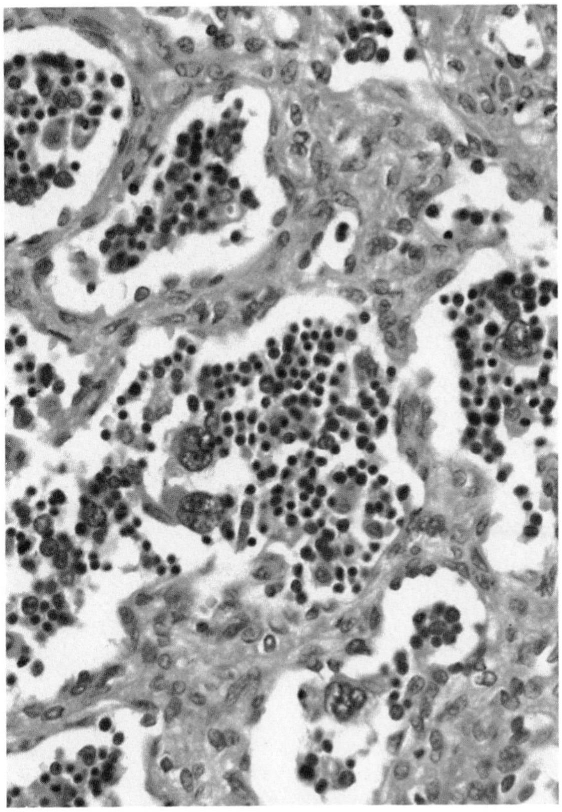

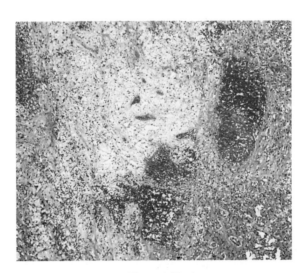

Figure 4-21
INFANTILE HEMANGIOENDOTHELIOMA
Marked extramedullary hematopoiesis.

These large channels are usually lined by an attenuated layer of endothelial cells.

Extramedullary hematopoiesis is seen in the majority of cases, with myeloid precursors and megakaryocytes within the vascular channels and/or the vascular stroma (fig. 4-21). Most lesions contain areas considered to be involutional, including thrombosis (fig. 4-22), fibrosis, calcification (fig. 4-23), and myxoid change. In cases treated with hepatic artery ligation or transarterial embolization, the entire lesion may be infarcted and necrotic with only a thin rim of viable tumor present at the margin, sometimes making a histologic diagnosis of infantile hemangioendothelioma difficult (94).

Immunohistochemical Findings. The endothelial cells of the tumor stain for factor VIII–related antigen, CD34, CD31, vimentin, and *Ulex europaeus* 1 (UEA-1) lectin (57). The cells underlying the endothelial cells are enveloped in basement membrane, and are positive for alpha-smooth

Figure 4-22
INFANTILE HEMANGIOENDOTHELIOMA
Thrombosis and hemorrhage deep in the tumor.

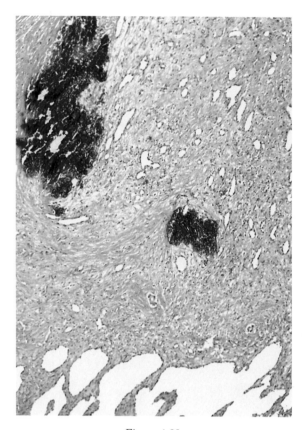

Figure 4-23
INFANTILE HEMANGIOENDOTHELIOMA
Dense fibrosis and plaque-like calcification in the depths of the tumor.

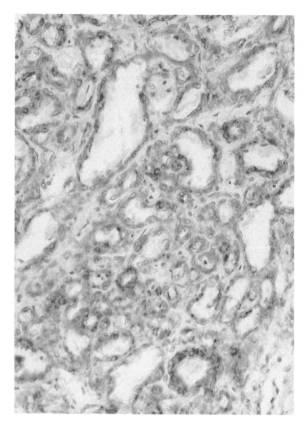

Figure 4-24
INFANTILE HEMANGIOENDOTHELIOMA
Cells surrounding the vascular spaces express smooth muscle actin (immunostain).

muscle actin (fig. 4-24) and negative for desmin, all characteristics of pericytes (57). Bile ducts within the lesion stain with cytokeratin (90).

Ultrastructural Findings. Electron microscopic examination of infantile hemangioendothelioma displays endothelial cells lining tumor vessels filled with red blood cells. The nuclei of the endothelial cells are irregular and the nucleoli prominent. An incomplete basal lamina separates the endothelial cells from the underlying stroma. Pericytes are not seen in the stroma, although bile ducts with normal-appearing epithelial cells may be present (62,90,101).

Flow Cytometry. Selby and colleagues (90) studied 21 cases and showed that 16 were DNA diploid and 3 aneuploid. Skin lesions were noted in 2 of the 3 aneuploid cases but only 1 of the diploid cases. On follow-up, all 3 patients with aneuploid tumors were dead while only 3 of the 16 patients with diploid tumors had died (90).

Treatment and Prognosis. The severity of the presenting symptoms and whether the lesion is single or multifocal determine the type of treatment employed. With single lesions in asymptomatic patients, surgical resection is often curative, although some authors suggest that initial treatment should be conservative, with surgery reserved for patients with intractable cardiac failure or refractory coagulopathy (89). For patients with large lesions or multifocal lesions spread throughout the liver, transplantation may be employed (56). Achilleos and colleagues (51), however, noted the recurrence of the lesion in a liver 41 months after transplantation.

For patients with larger single lesions or with multifocal tumors, hepatic artery ligation or transarterial embolization may be used (67,88). Hepatic artery embolization may also be used for the treatment of congestive heart failure and portal hypertension associated with the lesion (63).

Radiation therapy had been used in the past (59), but because of potential long-term side effects, is infrequently employed today. Favorable nonsurgical responses have also been reported with corticosteroids (54,102) and vincristine (83).

Infantile hemangiomas have been noted to regress spontaneously in 5 to 10 percent of cases (81,89,98,101). Hase and colleagues (65) reported the spontaneous regression of a lesion in the porta hepatis of a 4-month-old male who had his coagulopathy and obstructive jaundice treated by percutaneous transhepatic drainage only.

Overall survival is approximately 70 percent, with the majority of deaths (90 percent) occurring within 1 month following diagnosis, often associated with intraoperative or postoperative complications. The prognosis in patients with infantile hemangioendothelioma is adversely influenced by the presence of congestive heart failure, jaundice, and multiple tumor nodules, and by the absence of cavernous differentiation (90).

Relationship to Angiosarcoma of the Liver. The association of infantile hemangioendothelioma with angiosarcoma of the liver has been noted. Kirchner and colleagues (69) described the malignant degeneration of a liver lesion in a 4-year-old child who 3 1/2 years previously had received steroid therapy for multiple hepatic hemangioendotheliomas. An angiosarcoma of the left lobe was resected. Awan and colleagues (52) also noted the "malignant transformation" to an angiosarcoma of a lesion in a child whose infantile hemangioendothelioma had been resected from the right lobe of the liver and later from the left lobe. Other cases are discussed in chapter 12.

CAVERNOUS HEMANGIOMA

Definition. This is a single, less often multiple, benign lesion composed of communicating vascular spaces of varied size that are lined by a single layer of flat endothelial cells. The vascular spaces may contain thrombi, and the lesion can undergo sclerosis and calcification.

Clinical Features. Cavernous hemangioma is the most common benign hepatic tumor (134). Furthermore, the liver is the most common visceral site of hemangiomas; in one series of 570 hemangiomas from all sites, 19 percent occurred in the liver (126). The autopsy incidence in two series was 1 percent (117) and 7 percent (122).

Cavernous hemangioma is more frequent in women. In a series of 114 patients whose tumors were surgically excised, 87 were women (134). The mean age in that series was 46 years (range, 21 to 77 years).

The majority of patients with hemangiomas are asymptomatic. In one series of 89 cases reported from Memorial Hospital for Cancer and Allied Diseases, New York (142), only 12 patients (13.5 percent) had symptoms; the hemangiomas were an incidental finding at laparotomy or autopsy in 77 (86.5 percent) patients. About half of the symptomatic patients present with swelling of the abdomen or an upper abdominal mass; the other half have pain or symptoms referable to the gastrointestinal tract, probably related to pressure or displacement of adjacent viscera and organs. The symptoms may be of a few months' to many years' duration. Episodes of sudden pain may be due to intratumoral thrombosis or rupture with hemoperitoneum. Rupture may be spontaneous (116,125,134,159) or related to trauma (131). Portal hypertension, probably due to extrahepatic compression of the portal vein, was reported by Takahashi et al. (154). An unusual presentation, fever of unknown origin, has been reported in one instance (129). In another patient with a giant hepatic hemangioma, impaired humoral and cellular immunity was attributed to elevated plasma levels of TGF-β1 derived from the tumor tissue (133). Other complications include microangiopathic hemolytic anemia and consumption coagulopathy (*Kasabach-Merritt syndrome*) (151,157), and erythrocytosis due to secretion of erythropoietin by the tumor (153).

Other than during pregnancy and in patients taking estrogens, sudden, spontaneous enlargement of hepatic hemangioma has been observed in one patient (120). Doubling and tripling in size over time (34 months to 10.5 years) was demonstrated by follow-up imaging studies of four patients with cavernous hemangiomas (139). An 11-fold increase in volume in a decade was documented in another case (160).

Hepatic hemangioma has been reported in association with cysts of the liver and pancreas (122), von Meyenburg complex (114), tuberous sclerosis (124), and focal nodular hyperplasia (137,156).

The diagnosis of hemangioma of the liver is based largely on imaging studies, as noted later. Fine-needle aspiration biopsy has been used in

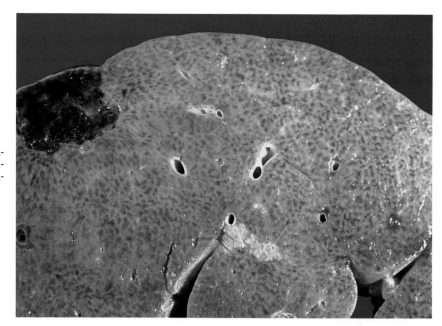

Figure 4-25
CAVERNOUS HEMANGIOMA
A small, dark brown, subcapsular lesion was an incidental finding in this liver affected by secondary amyloidosis.

diagnosis and is considered safe by some clinicians (113,118), but it can be complicated by bleeding (134). Liver tests are not helpful in diagnosis; they may be abnormal in some patients with giant hemangiomas, the most common finding being increased alkaline phosphatase activity.

Radiologic Findings. The various imaging modalities are compared in several publications (111,112). Ultrasound is of little value other than providing anatomic localization. Angiography is diagnostic but is an invasive technique whose use should be reserved for cases that cannot be confidently diagnosed by other means. MRI should be reserved for lesions smaller than 2.0 cm, and for those 2.5 cm and smaller that are adjacent to the heart and major hepatic vessels (110). The method of choice for diagnosing hepatic hemangioma is by Tc-99m blood pool single emission computed tomography (SPECT) (110,112,135).

Gross Findings. Hemangiomas of the liver may be single or multiple (135a,136). Single lesions are more frequently located in the right lobe. Pedunculation is an infrequent finding (2.3 percent) in autopsy cases (121), but was present in 15.2 percent of a surgically-treated series of cases (150), suggesting that pedunculation is more likely to occur with larger tumors.

Hemangiomas can be less than a centimeter to over 30 cm in diameter. They may partly project from the surface or can be deeply located (figs. 4-25, 4-26). They are usually well circumscribed, and the giant ones are partially separated from the liver substance by a distinct fibrous interface (161). Multiple lesions (*diffuse hemangiomatosis*) involve the entire liver (135a). Hemangiomas are fluctuant and compressible unless they have undergone regressive changes such as thrombosis, fibrosis, or calcification. When sectioned, they partially collapse due to the escape of blood, and have a spongy or honeycombed surface. Recent or organized thrombi, fibrosis, and calcification may be noted grossly (fig. 4-27). Fibrosis usually begins centrally but the entire lesion may appear as a firm, gray-white nodule (*sclerosed hemangioma*) (fig. 4-28). Rarely, the hemangioma may be necrotic, and appear firm and white or contain amorphous debris in the center (*solitary necrotic nodule*) (109,152).

Microscopic Findings. Cavernous hemangiomas contain no recognizable acinar landmarks, such as portal areas. They are composed of blood-filled spaces lined by a single layer of flat endothelial cells supported by a basement membrane (figs. 4-29, 4-30). The spaces may contain recent or organized thrombi (fig. 4-30). The basement membrane is supported by some collagen fibers and smooth muscle cells. Extensive fibrosis is seen in some areas (fig. 4-31), or may involve the entire lesion (sclerosed hemangioma) (fig. 4-32)

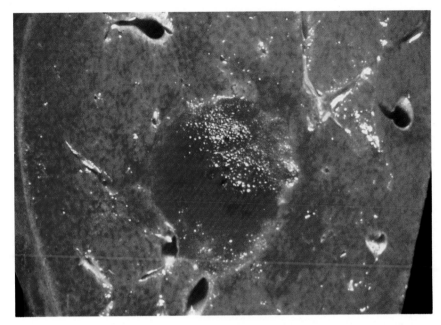

Figure 4-26
CAVERNOUS HEMANGIOMA
Section of the liver shows a small, deeply located, dark red hemangioma.

Figure 4-27
CAVERNOUS HEMANGIOMA
This sectioned tumor showed dark brown areas as well as white areas of fibrosis.

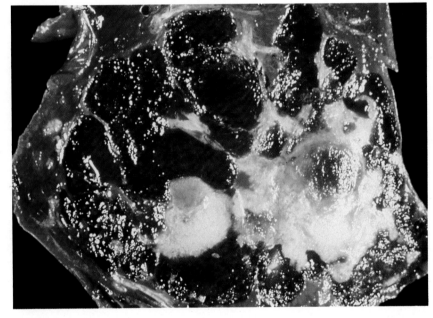

(128). Elastic fibers are scanty but are increased in areas of fibrosis, and in sclerosed hemangiomas (fig. 4-33). Calcification in areas of fibrosis may be spotty and granular or dense and plaque-like (fig. 4-34) (146). Phleboliths may be found in the lumen of some of the vascular channels.

Variants of hemangioma of the liver include *capillary "angioma"* reported by Edmondson (121), or *mixed capillary and cavernous hemangioma*

(117) which the authors have not encountered. Solitary necrotic nodules appear to arise in sclerosing hemangiomas and consist of acellular hyaline material; they may be single or multiple (109,152). Their chief importance is their possible confusion with metastatic liver lesions.

Immunohistochemical Findings. Immunohistochemical staining is of little value in diagnosis. As expected, the endothelial cells show

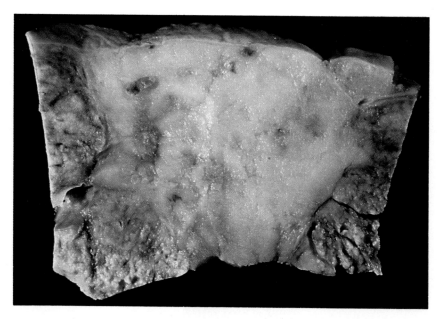

Figure 4-28
SCLEROSED HEMANGIOMA
Section of a subcapsular, gray-white nodule.

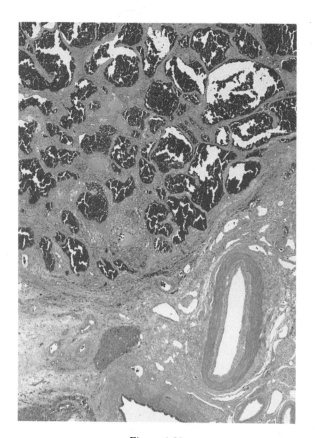

Figure 4-29
CAVERNOUS HEMANGIOMA
This well-circumscribed tumor is composed of multiple vascular spaces filled with liquid blood.

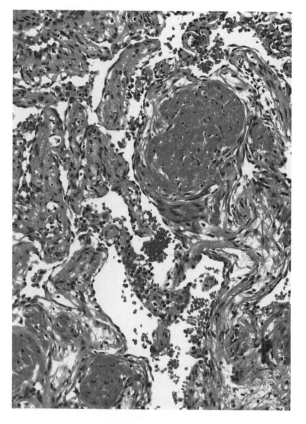

Figure 4-30
CAVERNOUS HEMANGIOMA
The cavernous spaces are lined by a single layer of benign, flat endothelial cells. Note the thrombus in one of the cavities.

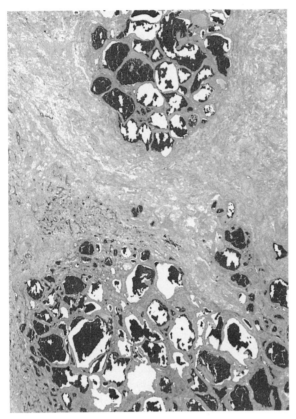

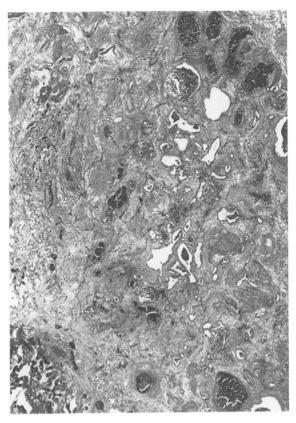

Figure 4-31
CAVERNOUS HEMANGIOMA
Left: This tumor is partially sclerosed.
Right: Connective tissue stain shows fibrosis of the hemangioma (Masson trichrome stain).

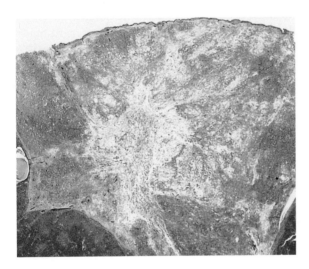

Figure 4-32
SCLEROSED HEMANGIOMA
The lesion consists of mature collagenous tissue. A few small vessels are present in the lower part (Masson trichrome stain).

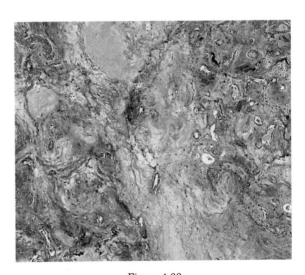

Figure 4-33
SCLEROSED HEMANGIOMA
Elastic fibers are present in the fibrous stroma.

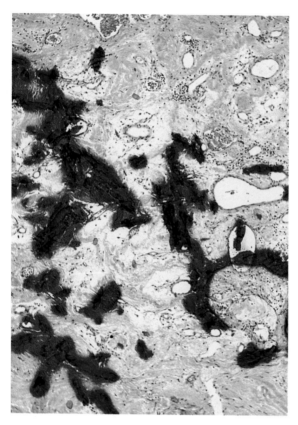

Figure 4-34
SCLEROSED HEMANGIOMA
There is dense, plaque-like calcification.

lectin binding (*Ulex europeaus antigen* [UEA-1]) and are strongly positive for factor VIII–related antigen, CD34, and CD31. The vessel wall exhibits slight staining for actin, myosin, and filamin (130).

Differential Diagnosis. This is very limited. Tumors that may be confused with cavernous hemangioma include lymphangioma, peliosis hepatis, and hereditary hemorrhagic telangiectasia.

Lymphangioma, a very rare tumor, is discussed in the next section. Histologically, the vascular spaces contain lymph, in contrast to cavernous hemangioma in which the spaces are filled with blood or recent or organized thrombi. Immunohistochemical staining for factor VIII–related antigen and UEA-1 does not differentiate blood from lymphatic vessels. However, the presence of a fragmented basal lamina and anchoring filaments appears to distinguish lymphatic vessels from blood vessels ultrastructurally (143). Peliosis hepatis is characterized grossly by multiple spaces of varied size that are filled with blood; the cavi-

ties are not lined by endothelium. The condition is most frequently a complication of anabolic steroid therapy, but it may be associated with other conditions. It is of unknown pathogenesis. Hereditary hemorrhagic telangiectasia is discussed in the next section.

Sclerosed hemangiomas may be mistaken for focal scars (e.g., healed granulomatous lesions) or small solitary fibrous tumors. Sclerosed hemangiomas contain numerous sclerosed vessels and often an elasticized stroma, which are not seen in focal scars. Solitary fibrous tumors, but not sclerosed hemangiomas, express CD34.

Etiology and Pathogenesis. Although cavernous hemangiomas occur in childhood (119) most are diagnosed in adults. They occur more frequently in women. Many years ago Ninard (140) drew attention to the number of hemangiomas that had been reported in multiparous women. Edmondson (121) raised the possibility of a role of female sex hormones in their development, especially since it is known that angiomatous lesions of the skin and gingiva do develop during pregnancy. Barter et al. (107) reported a series of cutaneous and mucosal hemangiomas which developed or caused symptoms during pregnancy. Cavernous hemangiomas of the liver can rapidly increase in size (132,149) or rupture (127) during pregnancy. Additionally, they have been known to enlarge (138) or recur (115) in patients on estrogen therapy. A case of extensive hemangiomatosis of the liver was reported during treatment with metoclopramide; the lesions regressed after the medication was stopped (123). It would thus appear that cavernous hemangiomas of the liver are acquired lesions, though a hamartomatous process cannot be dismissed entirely.

Treatment. There is general agreement that cavernous hemangioma of the liver should be treated conservatively. Only symptomatic lesions larger than 10 cm (giant hemangioma) should be treated by enucleation or resection (104,106,108, 145,147,155,158). Other treatment modalities have included hepatic artery ligation (144) or hepatic artery embolization (103,147,155), but the latter may be complicated by abscess formation (141,147). Orthotopic liver transplantation is an alternative procedure for unresectable hemangiomas (148). Radiotherapy now has no place in the management of this tumor.

HEREDITARY HEMORRHAGIC TELANGIECTASIA

Definition. This autosomal, dominantly inherited disease is characterized by telangiectases of the skin, mucosal surfaces, and multiple internal organs such as the lungs, brain, and liver. Synonyms include *Osler-Weber-Rendu disease* and *hepatic angiodysplasia*.

Clinical Features. The inheritance of the disease is autosomal dominant and the estimated frequency is 1 to 2 per 1,000,000 (174). Recent studies have shown mutations in endoglin, a receptor for transforming growth factor-β on chromosome 9 in some families (171,172), and linkage to chromosome 12q in others (182). The clinical and radiologic spectrums of hepatic manifestations have been reviewed by several authors (163,169,170,174–176,178,181). It is characterized by telangiectases (skin, mucous membranes); arteriovenous fistulas in the liver (in 30 percent of cases), lungs, and central nervous system; and aneurysms. Hepatic involvement is indicated by pain in the right upper quadrant of the abdomen and enlargement of the organ, which is sometimes pulsatile. High output cardiac failure may result from arteriovenous shunting in the liver (162). Portal hypertension and encephalopathy may develop (166,167). Liver failure is rare (173). Hereditary hemorrhagic telangiectasia may rarely co-exist with fibropolycystic disease of the liver (177).

Gross Findings. The liver shows spider-like arrangements of vessels on the surface (179). Sections reveal variable fibrosis and multiple, cavernous hemangioma–like foci. Nodular regenerative hyperplasia may be present (183,184).

Microscopic Findings. These have been reported by a number of investigators (164,167,180, 183) and are illustrated in figures 4-35 and 4-36. Three fibrovascular patterns were described by Daly and Schiller (164). One pattern was comprised of a honeycomb meshwork of dilated sinusoidal channels lined by endothelial cells set either directly upon hepatocyte plates or amid a loose fibrous stroma; the distribution of these foci was haphazard. A second pattern consisted of tortuous thick-walled veins flanked by numerous wide-caliber arteries that coursed randomly through the parenchyma amid variable amounts of fibrous tissue. A third pattern was evident in the enlarged

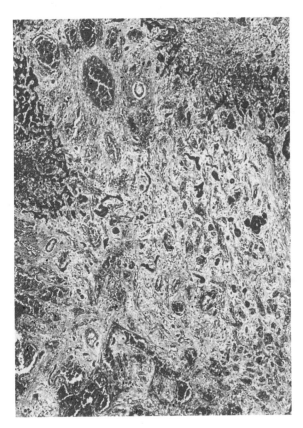

Figure 4-35
HEREDITARY HEMORRHAGIC TELANGIECTASIA
Multiple, small, thin-walled vascular channels are present in portal areas and within the acini (Masson trichrome stain).

portal areas in which numerous dilated vessels (veins, arteries, and lymphatics) showed prominently against a background of fibrous tissue. Regenerative nodules (partial nodular transformation) were described in the cases reported by Zelman (184) and Wanless and Gryfe (183).

Treatment and Prognosis. Arterial embolization has been used successfully to treat patients with dominant hepatic involvement (162, 165,168); it may prevent cardiac failure by lowering cardiac output. Hepatic transplantation was curative in three patients reported recently (161a). Death from hereditary hemorrhagic telangiectasia is rare, although a mortality rate of 10 percent is quoted by McDonald et al. (172). An unusual complication occurred in a 69-year-old woman treated with ethinylestradiol, multiple blood transfusions, and iron-dextran who developed hepatocellular carcinoma and acquired hepatocerebral degeneration (180).

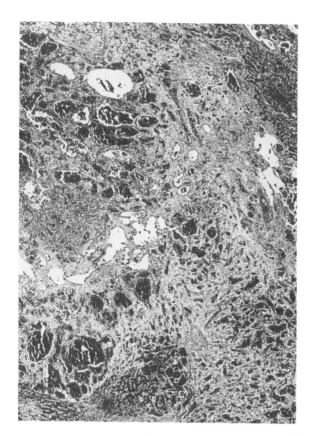 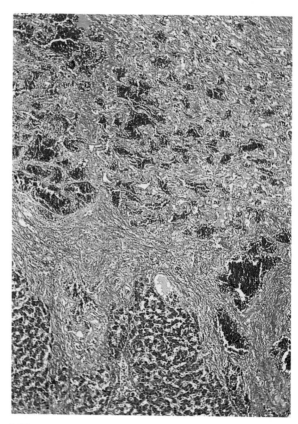

Figure 4-36
HEREDITARY HEMORRHAGIC TELANGIECTASIA
Left: There is extensive replacement of the acini by the vascular channels.
Right: Connective tissue stain demonstrates the supporting fibrous stroma of the vessels (Masson trichrome stain).

PELIOSIS HEPATIS AND BACILLARY PELIOSIS HEPATIS

Definition. Peliosis hepatis is characterized by cavities of varied size that contain liquid or clotted blood and are not lined by endothelium.

Clinical Features. Peliosis hepatis can occur at any age and in either sex. The liver is usually enlarged and may be tender. Severe abdominal pain may result from rupture and intraperitoneal hemorrhage (185). Hepatic failure is another recognized complication (187,196). Associated *extrahepatic peliosis,* e.g., involving the spleen (202) or multiple organs (190), has been reported. Imaging studies (ultrasound, CT, and MRI) are described by Jamadar et al. (191) and Maves et al. (195).

Gross Findings. The liver affected by peliosis hepatis shows multiple, varying-sized projections on the surface that are fluctuant and blue-

black. The lesions typically involve the entire liver, but "focal" peliosis hepatis has been described (200). The cut surface is riddled with cavities filled with liquid or clotted blood (fig. 4-37). The intervening parenchyma is usually not fibrotic or cirrhotic.

Microscopic Findings. The blood-filled cavities have ragged walls composed of liver cells; there is no endothelial lining (figs. 4-38, 4-39). The blood is often liquid but may be clotted; in a few instances the contents may be partially organized (fig. 4-39). The cavities may communicate with the surrounding sinusoids or terminal hepatic venules.

The lesions of bacillary peliosis hepatis have a histiocytoid appearance due to the presence of rounded cells with a purplish granular cytoplasm; these cells contain the microorganisms that are demonstrable with the Warthin-Starry

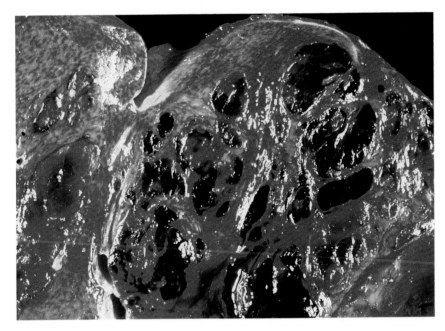

Figure 4-37
PELIOSIS HEPATIS
The liver section shows multiple cavities of varied size that are filled with clotted blood.

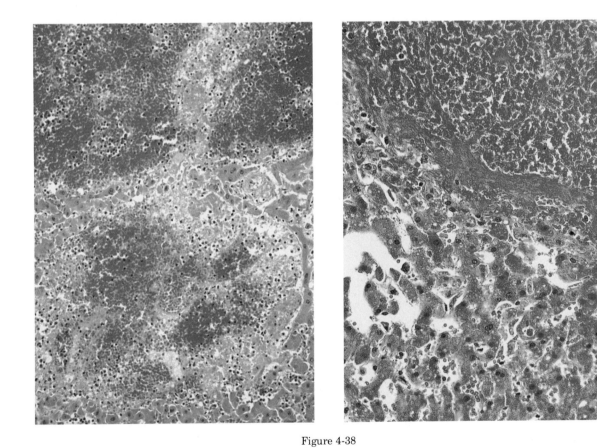

Figure 4-38
PELIOSIS HEPATIS
Left: Three almost confluent cavities are filled with blood.
Right: Higher magnification of a segment of one of the cavities shows no endothelial lining.

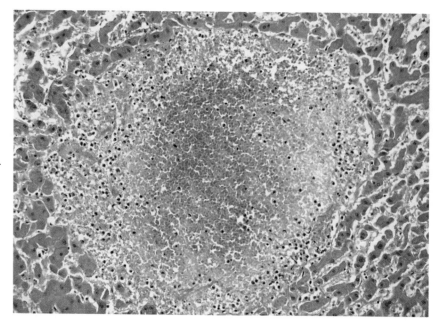

Figure 4-39
PELIOSIS HEPATIS
This cavity is partially organized at the periphery.

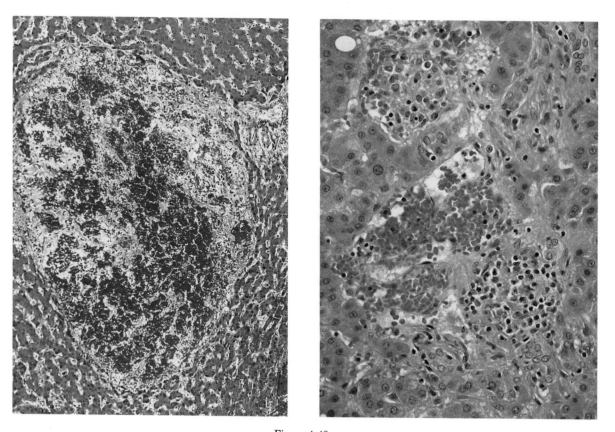

Figure 4-40
BACILLARY PELIOSIS
Left: The cavities are periportal and show a scanty fibrous stroma (Masson trichrome stain).
Right: There is focal inflammation.

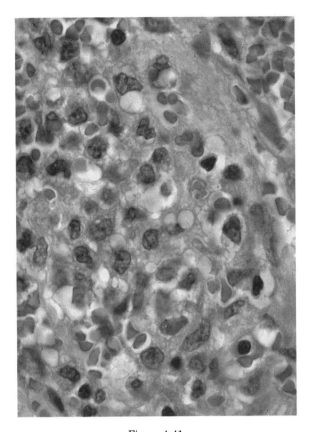

Figure 4-41
BACILLARY PELIOSIS
The inflammatory cells include large macrophages that
harbor the microorganisms (not shown).

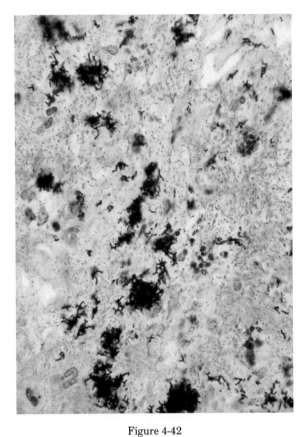

Figure 4-42
BACILLARY PELIOSIS
Hundreds of silvered bacilli are present in one of the
cavities (Warthin-Starry stain).

stain (figs. 4-40–4-42). The bacilli may also be
seen extracellularly. The cells are set in a loose
edematous stroma and are associated with inflammatory cells.

Etiology and Pathogenesis. Most cases of
peliosis hepatis are complications of anabolic steroid therapy (187,196). The steroids implicated in
this condition have included testosterone, methyltestosterone, oxymetholone, fluoxymesterone,
norethandrolone, and methandrostenolone.
Other drugs implicated in the etiology of peliosis
hepatis have included azathioprine (188), 6-thio-
guanine (193), tamoxifen (194), danazol (194a),
and oral contraceptives (203). Exposure to vinyl
chloride (198) and Thorotrast (197) has also led to
this condition. In the older literature, other recognized underlying conditions have included tuberculosis and malignant cachexia (185). Focal peliosis hepatis in five children, reported by Selby and
Stocker (200), has been attributed to asphyxial
death. Cases of bacillary peliosis hepatis in patients with the acquired immunodeficiency syndrome (AIDS) are due to infection with *Bartonella
(Rochalimaea) henselae* (184a,189,201).

Ultrastructural studies suggest that the initial injury in peliosis hepatis is to the endothelial
lining of the sinusoids, with escape of blood into
the spaces of Disse (199,204). There is also supporting in vitro evidence of cytotoxicity to endothelial cells by oxymetholone (192).

Treatment and Prognosis. Most cases of
peliosis hepatis are fatal. Rarely, recovery has
been reported after cessation of therapy with
anabolic steroids (196), following lobectomy after
rupture of a peliotic cavity (186), or after hepatic
transplantation (193). Erythromycin and doxy-
cycline have been used with excellent results in
the treatment of bacillary peliosis (184a).

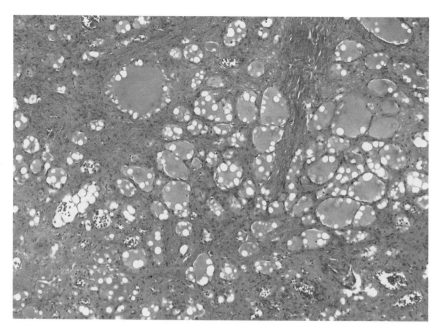

Figure 4-43
LYMPHANGIOMA
The vascular spaces contain lymph.

LYMPHANGIOMA
AND LYMPHANGIOMATOSIS

Definition. These are multiple, or less often single, benign lesions composed of spaces of varied size that contain lymph and are lined by endothelium. Hepatic involvement may be isolated or accompanied by lymphangiomatosis of the spleen, skeleton, or other organs and tissues. Synonyms include *hepatic lymphangiomatosis, hepatic cavernous lymphangioma, lymphangioendothelioma, generalized lymphangioma,* and *multiple lymphangiectasis.*

Clinical Features. Examples of lymphangiomas that only involved the liver are rare (206, 208–211,215); other reported cases have diffusely involved the liver and spleen (207,213), while in still other cases there was involvement of the liver, spleen, skeleton, and various other tissues and organs (205,206,212). The age at presentation has varied from the neonatal period (211) to old age, but most of the cases with diffuse visceral and skeletal involvement occur in children and young adults. The female to male ratio is 2 to 1 (206). Symptoms and signs depend on the organs and tissues involved. They include single or multiple fractures, abdominal swelling, hepatosplenomegaly, pleural effusions, ascites, or organ failure (e.g., liver or respiratory failure); a few patients are asymptomatic.

Imaging studies show lytic lesions of bones with or without fractures, hepatosplenomegaly, sonolucent areas on ultrasound, and multiple, varying-sized, hypodense lesions on CT scans.

Gross Findings. The liver is usually markedly enlarged and diffusely involved by multiple, whitish lesions of varied size that are cystic and contain a clear or chylous milky fluid (211,215).

Microscopic Findings. The lymphatic spaces are of varied size, with some cystically dilated, and are lined by a single layer of endothelium (fig. 4-43), but papillary projections or "tufting" may be seen (fig. 4-44). The endothelium rests on a basement membrane and the cystic spaces are surrounded by fibrous tissue (fig. 4-45). The endothelial lining cells express factor VIII–related antigen, CD31, and CD34.

Differential Diagnosis. Mesenchymal hamartoma may contain lymphatic channels, but is distinguishable from lymphangioma by the presence of bile ducts, a loose mesenchyme with cystic degeneration, hepatic parenchymal elements, and blood vessels. Hepatic lymphangiomatosis has been mistakenly diagnosed as polycystic liver disease (210). Lymphangiomas are distinguishable from cavernous hemangiomas by their content of lymph. Pseudoneoplastic and cystic dilatation of hepatic lymphatics, in one case secondary to post-traumatic infection of bile ducts, has been reported (213).

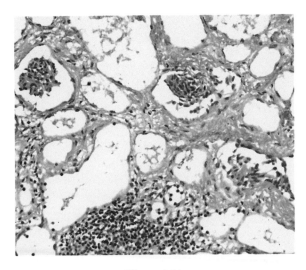

Figure 4-44
LYMPHANGIOMA
The spaces are empty and are lined by a single layer of flat endothelial cells. Three of the spaces reveal papillary proliferation of the endothelial lining.

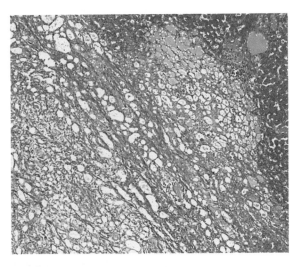

Figure 4-45
LYMPHANGIOMA
There is a variable fibrous stroma around the vascular spaces.

Pathogenesis. The cases with systemic involvement may represent a malformation of the lymphatic system, but supporting evidence is lacking.

Treatment and Prognosis. The prognosis of patients with visceral and skeletal involvement is poor, in particular those with pleural and lung involvement (212). For patients with massive splenomegaly, splenectomy can provide symptomatic relief (214). Hepatic resection is only feasible when the tumor is localized (208); successful hepatic transplantation for liver failure was reported in one instance (209). Three patients with hepatic involvement, whose tumors were only biopsied, had survived 2, 3, and 9 years at last follow-up (206,215).

ANGIOMYOLIPOMA

Definition. Angiomyolipoma is a benign tumor composed of variable admixtures of adipose tissue, smooth muscle (spindled or epithelioid), and thick-walled blood vessels. Most tumors display extramedullary hematopoiesis.

Clinical Features. Hepatic angiomyolipoma occurs equally in males and females. The age range is from 10 to 72 years (mean, 50 years); pediatric cases are rare (216). About two thirds of the patients are symptomatic: abdominal pain or discomfort, an upper abdominal mass, malaise, anorexia, and fever. Tuberous sclerosis is an associated finding in 6 percent of cases (228, 234). Many of the tumors are initially diagnosed by imaging studies.

Angiomyolipoma is hyperechoic on ultrasound examination. It presents as a low density mass on CT, and is hypervascular in angiographic studies. MRI has also been used in diagnosis (215a).

Gross Findings. In reference to location in the liver, 60 percent are in the right lobe, 30 percent in the left lobe, 20 percent in both lobes, and 8 percent in the caudate lobe (228). Angiomyolipomas can vary considerably in size, from less than a centimeter to 36 cm. The term *giant angiomyolipoma* has been used to designate unusually large tumors (226,231). Most of the tumors are solitary, but there is one report of multiple lesions (225). The tumors are smooth externally, usually globular, and well circumscribed. The color and consistency depend on the proportions of fat and smooth muscle: tumors that contain a large quantity of fat tend to be yellow (fig. 4-46) or mottled yellow and tan (fig. 4-47) and softer in consistency than tumors that contain much smooth muscle, which are firm and tan-white (fig. 4-48). Scattered foci of hemorrhage and necrosis may be evident.

Microscopic Findings. Angiomyolipomas are composed of admixtures of mature adipose tissue; tortuous, thick-walled and often hyalinized

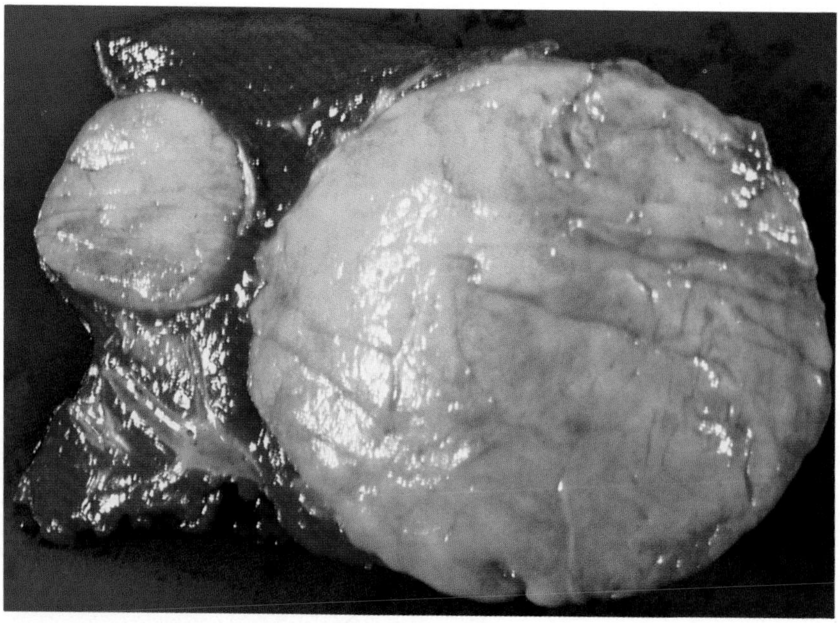

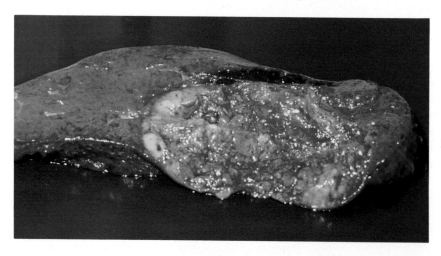

Figure 4-46
ANGIOMYOLIPOMA
The section of two tumors shows them to be well-circumscribed and bright yellow.

Figure 4-47
ANGIOMYOLIPOMA
This tumor has a variegated, yellow and tan cut surface.

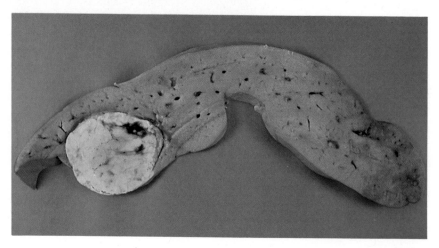

Figure 4-48
ANGIOMYOLIPOMA
This sharply defined tumor has a light tan cut surface, with two foci of hemorrhage.

vessels; and smooth muscle (figs. 4-49, 4-50). The tumors have a rich network of capillaries throughout. A trabecular arrangement of cells may be evident (fig. 4-51) (235a). The smooth muscle cells are either spindle shaped or epithelioid (figs. 4-52, 4-53). The latter may have an empty cytoplasm with perinuclear condensation of cytoplasmic material (fig. 4-54). The empty cytoplasm is rich in glycogen, as can be demonstrated by a periodic acid–Schiff (PAS) stain (fig. 4-55).

Ultrastructurally, the epithelioid cells are characterized by unusual cytoplasmic organelles such as myofilaments having focal densities and dense attachments, numerous large electron dense bodies, and a large number of glycogen particles and lipid droplets (232). Melanin pigment may be present in the epithelioid cells and can be demonstrated by a Fontana stain or a Warthin-Starry stain at pH 3.2 that is specific for melanin (fig. 4-56). Melanosomes have been

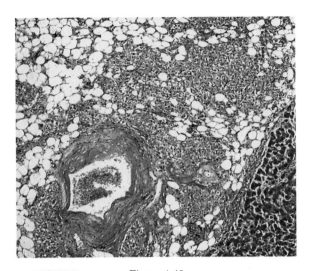

Figure 4-49
ANGIOMYOLIPOMA
The tumor is sharply circumscribed but nonencapsulated. It is composed of adipose tissue as well as areas of solid smooth muscle. Note the thick-walled vessels (Masson trichrome stain).

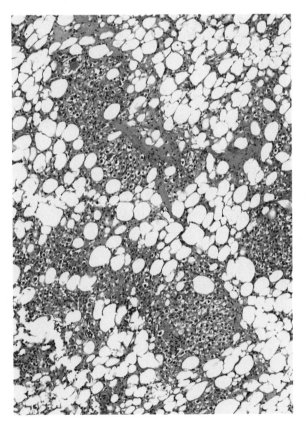 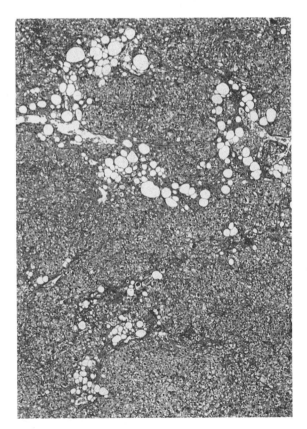

Figure 4-50
ANGIOMYOLIPOMA
Left: This tumor consists of approximately equal proportions of fat and aggregates of epithelioid smooth muscle cells.
Right: This tumor consists predominantly of smooth muscle.

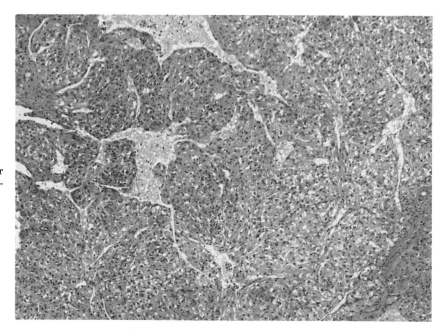

Figure 4-51
ANGIOMYOLIPOMA
The tumor has a trabecular pattern resembling that of hepatocellular carcinoma.

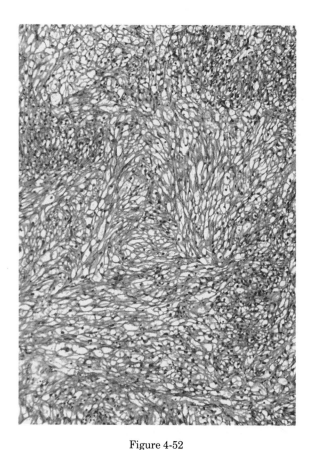

Figure 4-52
ANGIOMYOLIPOMA
Angiomyolipoma showing intersecting bundles of spindled smooth muscle cells. Most of the cells have an empty cytoplasm.

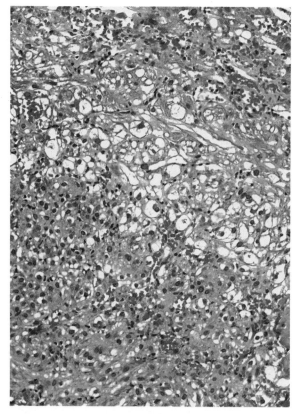

Figure 4-53
ANGIOMYOLIPOMA
The tumor cells are more rounded and epithelioid. The cells in the upper field have an empty cytoplasm.

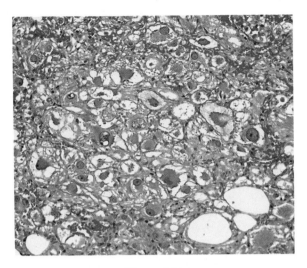

Figure 4-54
ANGIOMYOLIPOMA
The tumor cells are large. The cytoplasmic contents are condensed around the nuclei and there is a clear periphery. Note the often large nuclei with prominent nucleoli.

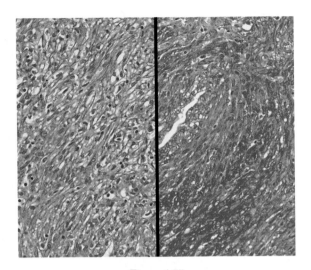

Figure 4-55
ANGIOMYOLIPOMA
The smooth muscle cells contain abundant glycogen (right) that is digested with diastase (left) (PAS stain).

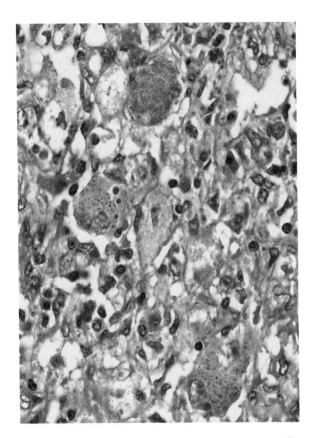

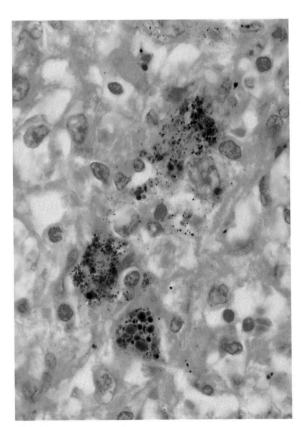

Figure 4-56
ANGIOMYOLIPOMA
Left: The smooth muscle cells contain brown melanin granules.
Right: The melanin granules are stained black with the Fontana stain.

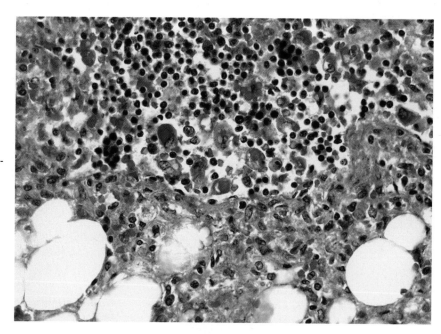

Figure 4-57
ANGIOMYOLIPOMA
Marked extramedullary hematopoiesis is seen.

identified ultrastructurally in one hepatic and two renal angiomyolipomas (224,237). The proportion of adipose tissue and smooth muscle is quite variable, and occasional tumors are composed largely of one or the other component (221, 223,230). Hematopoietic foci are frequently found in angiomyolipoma and may be prominent in some cases (fig. 4-57).

Some angiomyolipomas have clusters of smooth muscle cells with hibernoma-like (223) or oncocyte-like (234a) features. Other tumors contain aggregates of foam cells that represent lipidized smooth muscle cells (figs. 4-58, 4-59). Occasional tumors have large, irregular and hyperchromatic nuclei with prominent eosinophilic nucleoli (fig. 4-60) (221,228). The vessels in angiomyolipoma, particularly the arteries, are often thick-walled, with marked narrowing or obliteration of the lumen. The wall may contain an increased number of smooth muscle cells or a proliferation of elastic fibers, or it may be replaced by hyalinized fibrous tissue (figs. 4-61, 4-62). Calcification of the vessels or stroma may be present occasionally (fig. 4-63).

Immunohistochemical Findings. Most of the spindle cells and the cells with an empty cytoplasm are immunoreactive to antismooth muscle actin antibodies (muscle-specific and alpha-smooth muscle actin) (fig. 4-64). There is

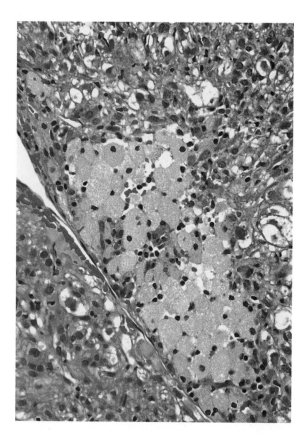

Figure 4-58
ANGIOMYOLIPOMA
There is a cluster of lipidized smooth muscle cells.

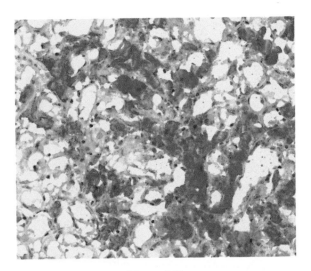

Figure 4-59
ANGIOMYOLIPOMA
The lipidized cells stain with oil red-O in this frozen section specimen.

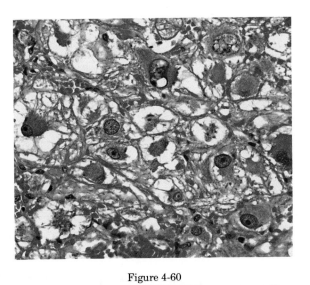

Figure 4-60
ANGIOMYOLIPOMA
A higher magnification of figure 4-54 demonstrates often large, hyperchromatic nuclei with prominent nucleoli.

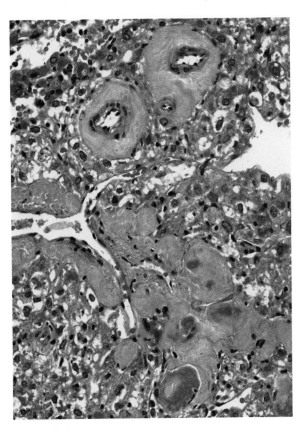
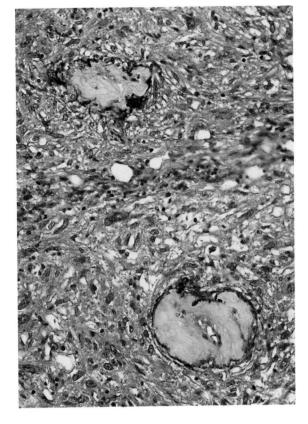

Figure 4-61
ANGIOMYOLIPOMA
Left: Markedly thick-walled and sometimes hyalinized vessels have a very narrow lumen.
Right: The Musto pentachrome stain shows the collagen (yellow) and the peripherally located elastica.

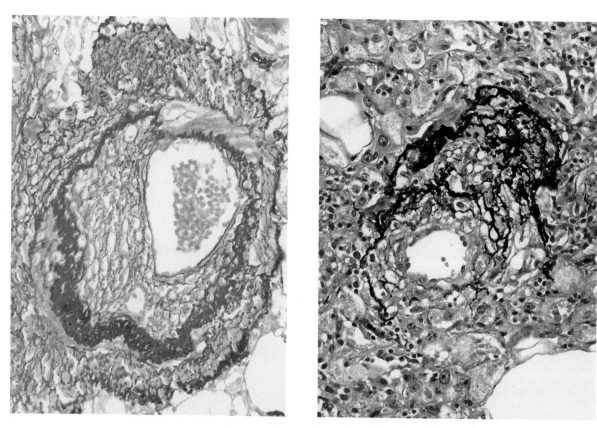

Figure 4-62
ANGIOMYOLIPOMA
The thick-walled vessels in this tumor contain abnormally proliferated and sometimes thick elastic fibers. (Victoria blue stain is on the left and Musto pentachrome stain is on the right.)

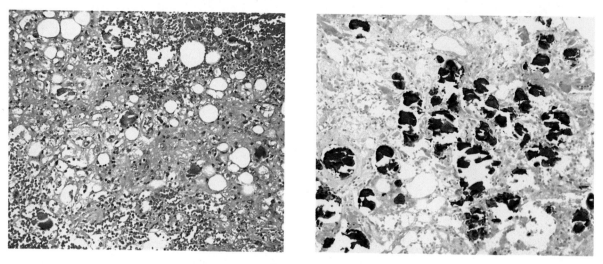

Figure 4-63
ANGIOMYOLIPOMA
Left: Focal calcification.
Right: Calcification is stained black with the von Kossa stain.

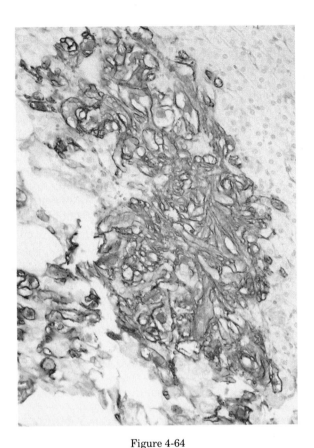

Figure 4-64
ANGIOMYOLIPOMA
The smooth muscle cells express smooth muscle actin (immunostain).

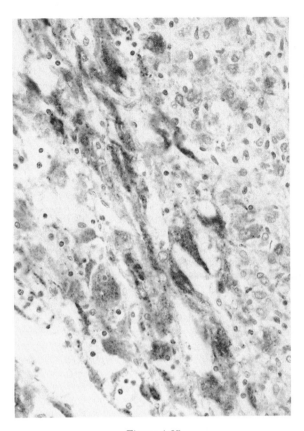

Figure 4-65
ANGIOMYOLIPOMA
The smooth muscle cells express the melanoma marker HMB-45 (immunostain).

also scattered, moderate to marked immunoreactivity to HMB-45 antibody (fig. 4-65), and, to a lesser degree, to S-100 protein antibody. Recently, expression of melan-A (MART-1), a melanoma marker, has been reported in angiomyolipoma (fig. 4-66) (220). The smooth muscle of the thick-walled vessels is immunoreactive to alpha-smooth muscle actin antibody but not to HMB-45 antibodies (fig. 4-67). In a recent study, 31 percent of renal angiomyolipomas were found to contain clusters of progesterone receptor-immunoreactive smooth muscle cells (222).

Differential Diagnosis. In large series, most cases, particularly needle biopsy specimens, are initially misdiagnosed (221,235). The problematic cases are tumors composed predominantly of smooth muscle cells (227,230), tumors with pleomorphic cells (229), and tumors that have a trabecular pattern (235a). Tumors composed predominantly of smooth muscle cells may be

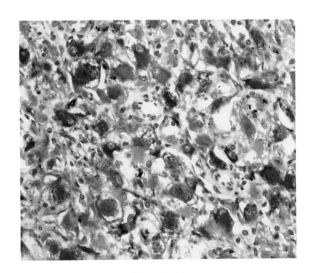

Figure 4-66
ANGIOMYOLIPOMA
The smooth muscle cells express melan-A (MART-1), a melanoma marker (immunostain).

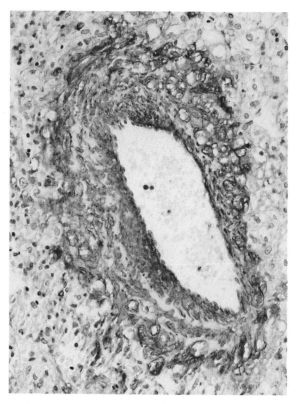

Figure 4-67
ANGIOMYOLIPOMA
This thick-walled vessel is composed of smooth muscle cells expressing smooth muscle actin (immunostain).

mistaken for leiomyomas, but those tumors are negative for the melanoma markers (HMB-45 and melan-A). Tumors with pleomorphic cells may be misdiagnosed as hepatocellular carcinoma, as may those with a trabecular pattern. Hepatocellular carcinomas usually have canaliculi (stainable with polyclonal carcinoembryonic antigen [CEA] antibody), produce bile, and do not express smooth muscle or melanoma antigens. Tumors with a large quantity of fat may be misdiagnosed as lipomas. All tumors that look like lipomas should be immunostained for smooth muscle markers and HMB-45; these immunostains will typically show perivascular clusters of positive cells. Angiomyolipomas with abundant extramedullary hematopoiesis may be mistaken for myelolipoma, a very rare hepatic tumor discussed in the following section. Other than the histopathologic differences, myelolipomas do not express smooth muscle or melanoma antigens. Focal fatty change, also discussed subsequently,

affects multiple contiguous hepatic acini that retain their underlying architecture.

Pathogenesis. Melanoma antigens are expressed by renal and hepatic angiomyolipomas, clear cell "sugar" tumor of the lung, clear cell tumor of the pancreas, and lymphangiomyomatosis, as well as tuberous sclerosis–associated brain lesions (217–220,223,224,230,236,238). It has been proposed that, morphologically and phenotypically, angiomyolipomas belong to a family of lesions characterized by proliferation of perivascular epithelioid cells (218,233,238).

Treatment and Prognosis. Surgical excision is curative. One patient whose tumor was not excised was followed for 4 years with CT examinations; the diameter of his tumor increased by 10 percent (231). We are aware of one published case of hepatic angiomyolipoma that underwent malignant change (219a).

MYELOLIPOMA

Definition. Myelolipoma is a benign tumor composed of fat and hematopoietic cells.

Clinical Features. Only a handful of hepatic myelolipomas have been reported (240–244). In fact, extra-adrenal myelolipomas are rare: in a literature survey up to 1994, Brietta and Watkins (239) found 25 cases. More than 50 percent of these tumors are found in the presacral region, followed in decreasing frequency by mediastinal, perirenal, hepatic, and gastric lesions. The reported hepatic myelolipomas have been associated with hepatomegaly or a palpable mass (241,244), right upper quadrant pain (245), or minimal abnormalities of liver tests (243), or they may be an incidental finding at autopsy (241). On CT examination the lesions have low or inhomogeneous attenuation (243,246). Most have occurred in middle-aged or elderly females.

Gross Findings. The size of hepatic myelolipomas varies from 2 to 12 cm in largest dimension. They are well circumscribed but nonencapsulated, and are composed of yellow, generally soft tissue.

Microscopic Findings. Myelolipomas consist of variable quantities of adipose tissue intermingled with nucleated erythrocytes, erythroblasts, megakaryocytes, and myeloid elements (figs. 4-68, 4-69). Rubin et al. (245) also described sheets and clusters of lipid-containing foamy histiocytes in their case.

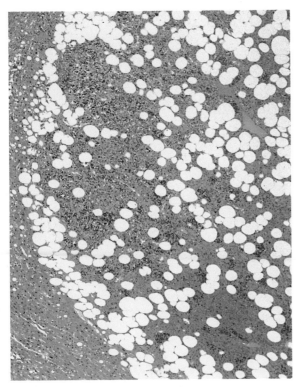

Figure 4-68
MYELOLIPOMA
This sharply circumscribed lesion is composed of fat and hematopoietic tissue.

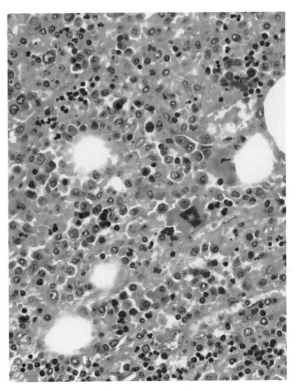

Figure 4-69
MYELOLIPOMA
The cells are of myeloid and erythroid lineage, and there is one megakaryocyte.

Differential Diagnosis. Hepatic myelolipomas can be differentiated from angiomyolipomas, which can show abundant hematopoiesis, by the absence of a smooth muscle component and the lack of expression of smooth muscle actin or HMB-45. Extramedullary hematopoietic tumors in the liver are exceptionally rare (239,246); they are composed entirely of hematopoietic elements.

Treatment. The treatment is surgical excision (245) or lobectomy (241).

FOCAL FATTY CHANGE

Definition. These are multiacinar foci of macrovesicular steatosis that occur in an architecturally normal liver. They are also termed *focal fat infiltration*.

Clinical Features. This condition was first described by Simon (260) as focal fat infiltration of the liver; he clearly distinguished it from lipoma of the liver. The largest series of 10 cases, with clinical and pathological findings, was reported by Brawer et al. (251). Most of the affected patients are adults from 21 to 79 years, but rare cases have been reported in children (251,255). More cases have occurred in females, with a 4 to 1 ratio in the series of Brawer et al. The condition has been associated with a bewildering variety of diseases, including alcoholic liver disease (254,257,261), diabetes mellitus (255), congestive heart failure (255), porphyria cutanea tarda (253), and metastases from malignant tumors of diverse organs and tissues (251,256) as well as being associated with continuous ambulatory peritoneal dialysis (255). In a review of 39 histologically documented cases of focal fatty change published up to 1991, Grove et al. (255) found that 17 (45 percent) occurred in patients with insulin dependent diabetes mellitus. These authors and Wanless et al. (262) also described three patients with diabetes mellitus and focal fatty change who had been on continuous ambulatory peritoneal dialysis and had received intraperitoneal insulin therapy.

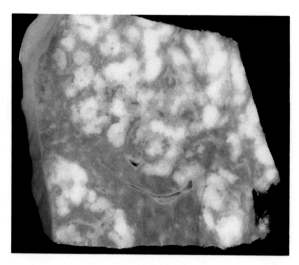

Figure 4-70
FOCAL FATTY CHANGE
The lesion has a mottled white and gray appearance; the white areas represent fat with zonal, multiacinar involvement. (Note: The white rather than yellow color of the fatty change is due to formalin fixation of the specimen.)

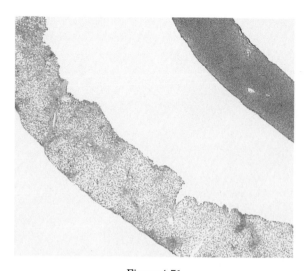

Figure 4-71
FOCAL FATTY CHANGE
Two sections of the same needle biopsy specimen show the marked focal fatty change (lower section) and the normal liver (top).

In view of the large number of underlying conditions, symptoms and signs specifically attributable to focal fatty change have not been forthcoming. The importance of the condition is its possible confusion in imaging studies with primary or metastatic tumors of the liver. The lesions are hyperechoic on ultrasound examination (252,254,258,263). Focal fatty change may display different appearances over time or disappear completely (252,258). The lesions appear as low attenuation areas on CT imaging (248, 249,263). The CT appearances of focal fatty change in patients with alcoholic liver disease have been classified into five types by Tang-Barton et al. (261): 1) lobar or segmental uniform lesions; 2) lobar or segmental nodular lesions; 3) perihilar lesions; 4) diffuse patchy lesions; and 5) diffuse nodular lesions. Resolution or changes in the appearance of the lesions has also been documented in CT studies (249,261). Enhanced dynamic CT scans are useful for differentiating focal fatty change from neoplasms (247).

The diagnosis of focal fatty infiltration of the liver is usually established by biopsy, which should include a sample of the unaffected liver parenchyma.

Gross Findings. The lesions may involve one or both lobes, and may be single or multiple. As

demonstrated in imaging studies, the lesions in alcoholics may be diffuse, segmental, or even lobar in distribution (261). They are well demarcated but nonencapsulated, and yellow or yellow-white (fig. 4-70). The size varies from less than 1 to 11 cm (255). They may be deeply located or subcapsular. In diabetics on continuous ambulatory peritoneal dialysis the lesions were restricted to a very thin subcapsular zone (255, 262). Some were located near the falciform ligament (251,263).

Microscopic Findings. Focal fatty change affects multiple contiguous acini that have recognizable portal areas and terminal hepatic veins (fig. 4-71). The steatosis is typically macrovesicular and usually involves the acini diffusely (fig. 4-72) but, as pointed out by Brawer et al. (251), there may be sparing of zone 3 or zone 1. The adjacent parenchyma may be congested but fibrosis or cirrhosis are exceptionally rare (251). In the cases reported by Wanless et al. (262), Mallory bodies were present in the subcapsular lesions, in addition to steatosis.

Differential Diagnosis. Focal fatty change can be distinguished from primary benign or malignant liver tumors that may contain variable quantities of fat, such as angiomyolipoma, hepatocellular adenoma, or hepatocellular carcinoma, by

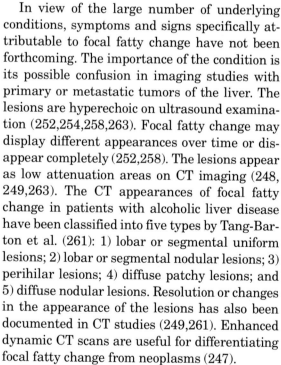

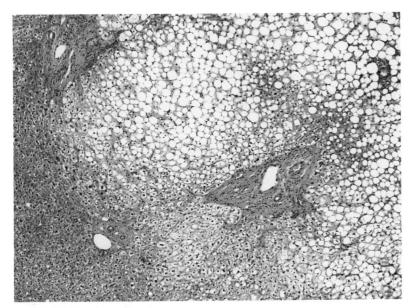

Figure 4-72
FOCAL FATTY CHANGE
The fatty change involves multiple contiguous acini.

the presence of an underlying acinar architecture. Additionally, true tumors have characteristic patterns and cytologic features.

Etiology and Pathogenesis. These remain unknown. Focal ischemia superimposed on conditions producing fatty change of the liver was proposed as the pathogenetic mechanism by Brawer et al. (251). In the cases associated with continuous ambulatory peritoneal dialysis with intraperitoneal insulin therapy, Wanless et al. (262) have suggested that the high insulin concentration in subcapsular liver cells leads to localized steatosis. An aberrant portal blood supply bringing more insulin to a sequestered segment of liver (that showed focal fatty change) was invoked in the pathogenesis of one reported case (250).

PSEUDOLIPOMA

Definition. This is an encapsulated mass of fat, often necrotic and sometimes calcified, which usually lies in a concavity on the surface of the liver.

Clinical Features. In 1985, Karhunen (266) collected 13 published cases of this pseudotumor and added 3 of his own. Another case, that of Inoue (264), was published in 1989. The prevalence of pseudolipomas was 0.2 percent in a series of 1,300 consecutive necropsies performed in Karhunen's department in Helsinki, Finland (266). Six cases of this lesion, including the three

previously reported (265), are on file at AFIP. Five cases were reported recently by Watanabe et al. (268a); four were incidental findings at surgery and one was an autopsy case. Imaging studies of the four surgically detected lesions were described by these authors; they were misdiagnosed as hepatic cysts. All pseudolipomas have been incidental findings at necropsy or laparotomy. They occur in males past the fourth decade of life; in the literature survey of Karhunen (266) the mean age was 60 years. Only one pseudolipoma was found in a pathologically altered liver, viz. cirrhosis (264).

Gross Findings. The majority of pseudolipomas have been located in the right lobe. They are usually solitary but in one of the AFIP cases there were two lesions, both in the right lobe. They are small, from a few millimeters up to 2 cm in diameter, and often appear to be embedded on the surface of the liver. They are yellow to yellow-white, and may have a gritty sensation when sectioned.

Microscopic Findings. Pseudolipomas are encapsulated, oval or spherical masses of mature adipose tissue, often showing necrosis (figs. 4-73, 4-74). Diffuse or focal calcification is often present and there may be osseous metaplasia.

Etiology and Pathogenesis. Rolleston and McNee (268) postulated that hepatic pseudolipoma represents an imprisoned or encapsulated appendix epiploica that had lost its moorings to the

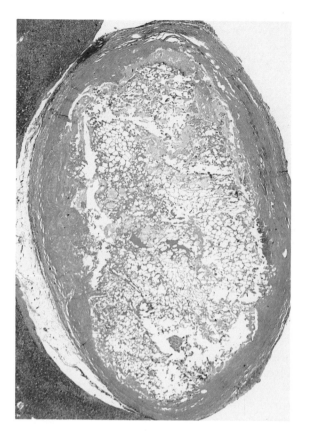
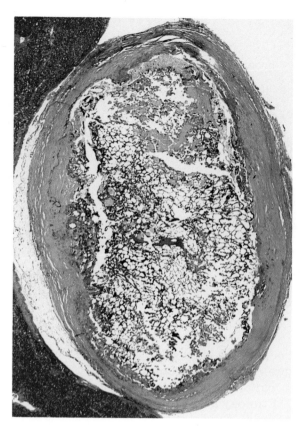

Figure 4-73
PSEUDOLIPOMA
Left: A dislodged lesion lies in a concavity on the surface of the liver.
Right: The thick fibrous capsule is yellow green in the Musto pentachrome-stained section.

Figure 4-74
PSEUDOLIPOMA
The lesion is composed of degenerated fat.

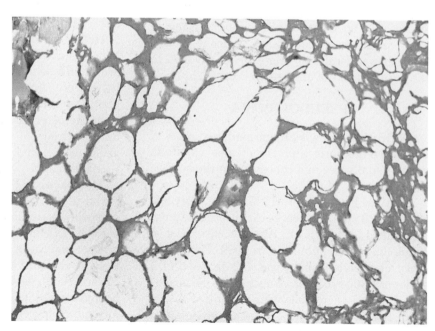

large bowel and migrated and became attached to Glisson's capsule. The occurrence of a similar nodule on the serosa of the stomach in one of the AFIP cases (265), and the finding of peritoneal "loose bodies" (266) support that hypothesis. Recently, membranous fat necrosis, thought to be ischemic in etiology, has been found to occur in appendices epiploicae (267). Such a mechanism could account for the detachment and subsequent migration of these structures. There was a history of previous abdominal surgery in half the AFIP cases; this may be of pathogenetic significance in some cases.

LEIOMYOMA

Definition. Leiomyoma is a benign tumor composed of interlacing bundles of smooth muscle fibers.

Clinical Features. This tumor is very rare in the liver; only 10 cases have been reported to date. Seven occurred in adults with an age range from 30 to 87 years (269–277a). Two tumors developed in children 3 and 4 years after liver transplantation (271) and heart transplantation (269), respectively. Most of the patients have presented with a mass in the upper abdomen, sometimes accompanied by pain. Imaging studies are described in the cases reported by Herzberg (272) and Reinertson (276).

Gross Findings. The tumors can be located in either lobe. The epithelioid leiomyoma reported by Ishak (273) was pedunculated. The leiomyomas can be large (up to 15 cm in maximum dimension), and two weighed more than a kilogram (1,070 g and 3,750 g) (271,277). They are well circumscribed and firm to rubbery in consistency. Sections disclose pink-white tissue with a whorled appearance. The tumors typically lack areas of necrosis or hemorrhage.

Microscopic Findings. Leiomyoma of the liver is composed of interlacing bundles of uniform spindle cells with plump, oval nuclei that have blunt ends (figs. 4-75, 4-76). Mitoses are absent or rare. The tumor cells have a brick-red color in Masson trichrome–stained sections, and longitudinal myofibrils may be discerned. There is a scanty fibrous stroma. A variant with a myxoid stroma has been described (277a). Ultrastructural studies have demonstrated filaments, some dense bodies, subplasmalemmal linear

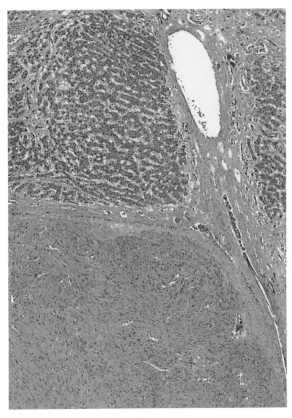

Figure 4-75
LEIOMYOMA
The tumor (bottom) is separated from the adjacent parenchyma by a thin capsule.

densities, and pinocytotic vesicles (271,277a). The one published example of an *epithelioid leiomyoma* consisted of nests of round or polygonal cells bounded by reticulin fibers, in addition to the spindle cells more typical of the usual leiomyoma (273). Immunohistochemical studies show expression of muscle-specific actin and smooth muscle actin by the tumor cells.

Differential Diagnosis. Leiomyoma must be differentiated from leiomyosarcoma, either primary or metastatic. Leiomyosarcomas are more cellular, and exhibit nuclear pleomorphism and hyperchromasia, areas of necrosis, and an increased mitotic rate (more than 1 per 10 high-power fields). However, in a small biopsy specimen differentiation of a benign from a malignant smooth muscle tumor may be difficult. Given the rarity of primary leiomyomas of the liver, the possibility of a metastasis from a primary in the gastrointestinal tract, retroperitoneum, or

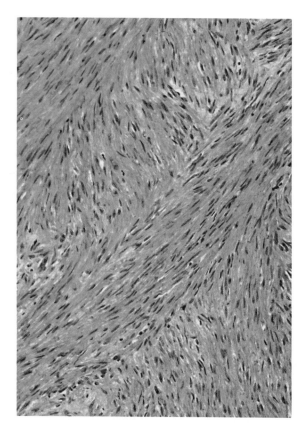 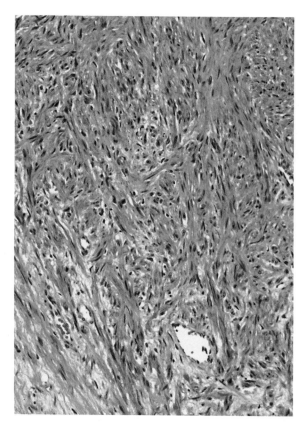

Figure 4-76
LEIOMYOMA
Left: Medium power view of the tumor shows intersecting bundles of benign smooth muscle cells.
Right: Higher magnification shows the typical fibrillar appearance of benign smooth muscle cells.

uterus should always be kept in mind. Differentiation of leiomyoma from solitary fibrous tumor is based on the cytologic features, expression of actin, and lack of expression of CD34.

SOLITARY FIBROUS TUMOR

Definition. Solitary fibrous tumor is a single, sometimes pedunculated tumor that resembles similar tumors arising in the pleura, mediastinum, or other sites. It is usually benign but can undergo malignant transformation. Synonyms include *localized fibrous tumor, localized* or *solitary fibrous mesothelioma, fibroma,* and *fibromatosis.*

Clinical Features. Solitary fibrous tumor is a rare tumor that occurs in adults, with an age range between 32 and 83 years (mean, 57 years) (290). More cases have been reported in females, in a ratio of 2 to 1 (290). The tumors can lead to

upper abdominal discomfort or pain, and a mass may be palpated. Symptoms may be related to pressure on adjacent viscera and organs. Some patients may be asymptomatic. Hypoglycemia has been reported rarely (290,291). Radiologic findings include a cold area in scintiscans, a low density mass on CT, and a hypervascular mass in celiac angiograms (285–287).

Gross Findings. In a series of nine cases from the AFIP, which is the largest reported to date, the tumors varied considerably in size, from 2 to 20 cm (290). Three of the largest reported tumors weighed over 3,000 g (281,284,286). They can arise in either lobe of the liver and are occasionally pedunculated. The external surface is typically smooth and the consistency firm. Sections reveal a light tan to gray-white cut surface with a whorled texture (fig. 4-77). Foci of cystic degeneration necrosis or hemorrhage may be present.

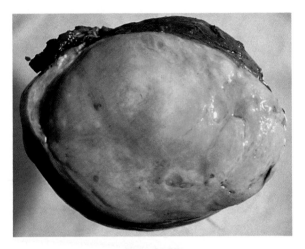

Figure 4-77
SOLITARY FIBROUS TUMOR
The section shows a bulging, well-circumscribed tumor with a vaguely nodular tan surface.

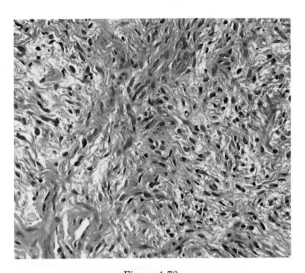

Figure 4-78
SOLITARY FIBROUS TUMOR
The tumor is composed of wavy, elongated spindle cells.

Microscopic Findings. The tumors often show alternating cellular and relatively acellular areas (figs. 4-78, 4-79). The former consist of bundles of spindle cells arranged haphazardly or in a storiform pattern. The cells have a lightly eosinophilic cytoplasm and fusiform nuclei lacking pleomorphism. In some cases the tumor cells are arranged around ectatic vessels in a hemangiopericytoma-like pattern. In the relatively acellular areas there are thick, intersecting bundles of collagen (fig. 4-79) that stain intensely blue with the Masson trichrome stain (fig. 4-80). There is a well-developed reticulin network in the tumor (fig. 4-81).

In our experience (290) and that of others (283), the tumors judged to have undergone malignant change show foci of necrosis, prominent cellular atypia, and mitotic activity in the range of 2 to 4 mitoses per 10 high-power fields (figs. 4-82, 4-83).

In a series of 10 extrahepatic solitary fibrous tumors, Yokoi et al. (294) found that malignant transformation may be associated with loss of expression of CD34 and with p53 mutation. Comparative genomic hybridization studies have recently been found useful for the evaluation of malignant transformation of solitary fibrous tumors (287): DNA copy number changes (mostly chromosomal gains) were found in tumors larger than 10 cm, including all tumors with more than 4 mitoses per 10 high-power fields.

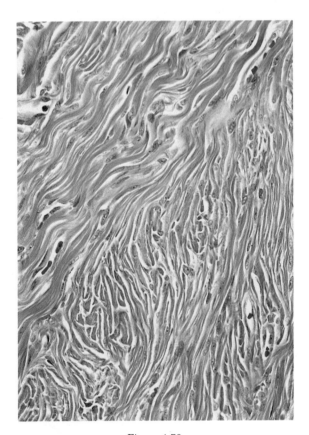

Figure 4-79
SOLITARY FIBROUS TUMOR
This tumor is relatively acellular with thick intersecting collagen bundles.

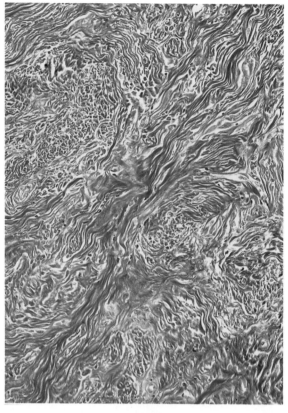

Figure 4-80
SOLITARY FIBROUS TUMOR
The intersecting bundles of collagen are shown to advantage by the Masson trichrome stain.

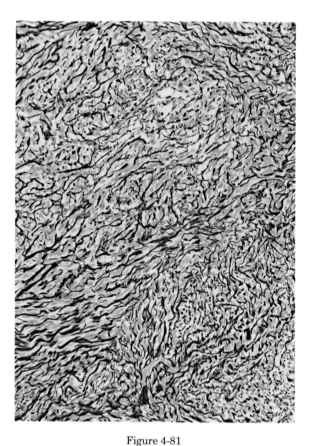

Figure 4-81
SOLITARY FIBROUS TUMOR
A network of reticulin fibers is demonstrated by the Manuel reticulin stain.

Figure 4-82
SOLITARY FIBROUS TUMOR
A benign part of a tumor (right) is compared with a much more cellular malignant area (left).

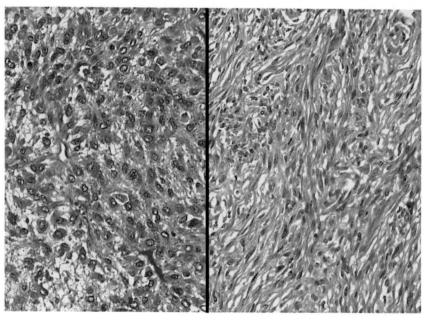

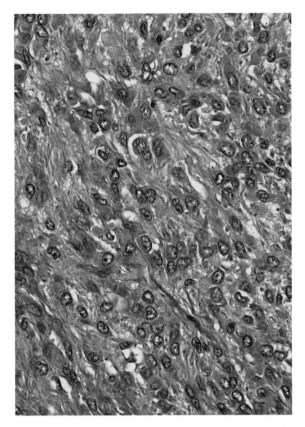 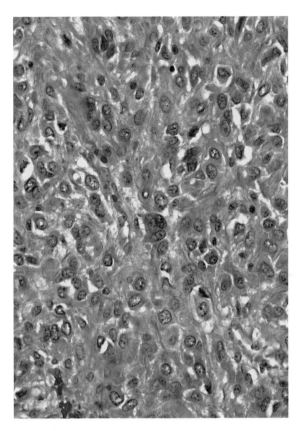

Figure 4-83
SOLITARY FIBROUS TUMOR, MALIGNANT
Left: The tumor is very cellular.
Right: Nuclear pleomorphism indicates malignancy.

Ultrastructurally, the majority of tumor cells are mesenchymal, with features of fibroblastic cells (278,287,288). Myofibroblastic differentiation of some cells has been observed in solitary fibrous tumors of soft tissue (292). A flow cytometric study of 16 tumors from serosal surfaces by El-Naggar et al. (282) showed a diploid pattern.

Immunohistochemical Findings. The staining reactions of solitary fibrous tumor of the liver are similar to those of such tumors arising in multiple other sites, such as the pleura, peritoneum, mediastinum, and soft tissues, to name but a few. The cells are immunoreactive for vimentin and CD34 (fig. 4-84), but are negative for keratin, smooth muscle actin, desmin, or S-100 protein (290). Other immunohistochemical reactions observed in some tumors are reviewed by Chan (279).

Histogenesis. This has been debated for decades, with current evidence (ultrastructural,

immunohistochemical) strongly supporting a mesenchymal (submesothelial) rather than mesothelial origin (280,282,287).

Differential Diagnosis. Benign tumors of the liver that may be mistaken for solitary fibrous tumor include sclerosed hemangioma, leiomyoma, inflammatory (myofibroblastic) pseudotumor, and hemangiopericytoma. Sclerosed hemangioma consists of dense collagen and elastic fibers with scattered, often hyalinized vessels; cavernous hemangiomatous foci may be present. Only the endothelial cells lining the vessels express CD34, CD31, and factor VIII–related antigen. Cells of leiomyoma of the liver express muscle-specific antigen and smooth muscle actin but not CD34. Inflammatory (myofibroblastic) pseudotumor of the liver is characterized by numerous plasma cells infiltrating fibrous tissue consisting of fibroblasts, myofibroblasts, and collagen fibers.

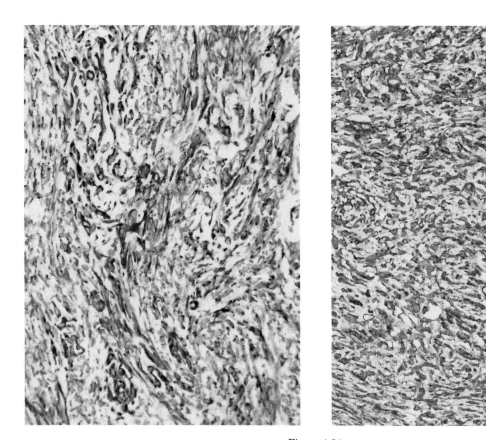

Figure 4-84
SOLITARY FIBROUS TUMOR
The tumor cells express vimentin (left) and CD34 (right).

Primary hemangiopericytoma of the liver is exceedingly rare; we are aware of only four such tumors (293). Two cases are on file at AFIP. A gross photograph of one case is shown in figure 4-85. Characteristically, hemangiopericytomas have ramifying or staghorn blood vessels, and a solid pattern: alveolar, trabecular, or myxoid (288). The neoplastic cells are uniform, polygonal to spindled, and have vesicular nuclei (fig. 4-86). Immunohistochemical stains are not helpful in the differential diagnosis since both solitary fibrous tumor and hemangiopericytoma show reactivity for CD34 and vimentin (fig. 4-87).

Treatment and Prognosis. The treatment of choice is surgical excision. Follow-up of several patients for 2 to 4 or more years has shown no evidence of recurrence (281,285,287). Although some tumors have shown cytologic evidence suggesting malignant change, there are no reports of metastases from hepatic solitary fibrous tumors.

LANGERHANS' CELL HISTIOCYTOSIS

Definition. This rare disorder is characterized by infiltration of various tissues and organs by Langerhans' cell histiocytes. Synonyms include *histiocytosis X* and *Langerhans' cell granulomatosis*.

Clinical Features. Langerhans' cell histiocytosis primarily affects bone but lung, skin, and lymph node involvement is not uncommon. Hepatic involvement is rare. Lieberman et al. (300), who collected 238 cases over a span of 50 years, did not mention any patients with liver disease. In a more recent series of 314 patients from the Mayo Clinic no hepatic involvement was noted although 5 of the patients had hepatosplenomegaly (297a).

Kaplan et al. (298) reported nine cases from the AFIP and found another 85 acceptable cases of hepatobiliary Langerhans' cell histiocytosis in the literature. The patients in the AFIP series ranged from 7 days to 62 years of age, with a

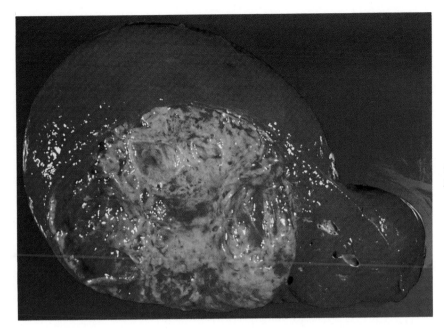

Figure 4-85
HEMANGIOPERICYTOMA
The section reveals an ill-defined tumor margin and a mottled yellow-tan and brown surface.

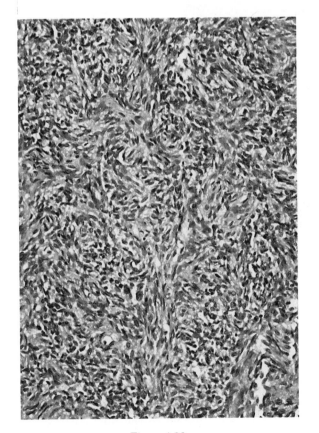

Figure 4-86
HEMANGIOPERICYTOMA
The tumor cells are spindled and form intersecting bundles.

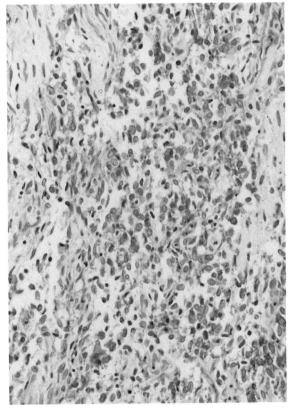

Figure 4-87
HEMANGIOPERICYTOMA
The tumor cells express CD34.

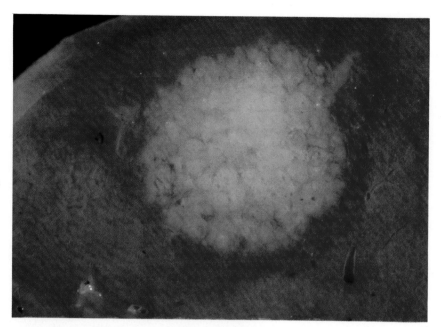

Figure 4-88
LANGERHANS'
CELL HISTIOCYTOSIS
The section shows a nodular,
light tan lesion.

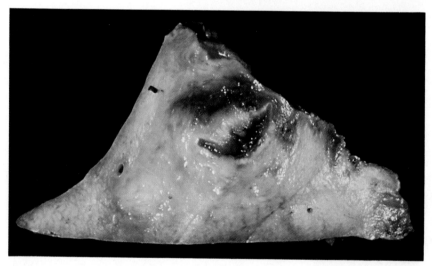

Figure 4-89
LANGERHANS'
CELL HISTIOCYTOSIS
The large portal area contains
a dilated necrotic bile duct with
surrounding fibrosis.

median of 18 months. Six were female and three were male. Hepatosplenomegaly, jaundice, liver dysfunction, and ascites were the most common clinical presentations. Two patients had previously been diagnosed with Langerhans' cell histiocytosis involving other organ systems. For six of the other seven patients, the diagnosis was first made by liver biopsy. One patient had a discrete hepatic mass, while another presented with multiple unilocular hepatic cysts.

Gross Findings. These vary with the stage of disease and type of hepatic involvement. Two patients in the AFIP series (298) had large ag-

gregates of Langerhans' cells, eosinophils, and other inflammatory cells that formed tumor-like masses (fig. 4-88). In two other cases infiltration of large ducts led to grossly visible cystic dilatation and rupture (fig. 4-89). Still other patients with biliary sclerosis showed irregular fibrosis; biliary cirrhosis was found in two patients.

Microscopic Findings. Three major patterns of hepatic involvement were observed, singly or in combination in the nine AFIP cases. These included: 1) small bile duct infiltration and destruction, producing clinicopathologic features of chronic cholestasis reminiscent of primary

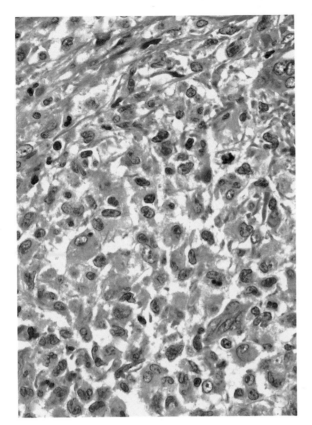 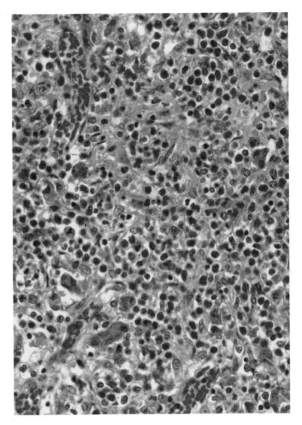

Figure 4-90
LANGERHANS' CELL HISTIOCYTOSIS
Left: The Langerhans' cells have ill-defined outlines, an eosinophilic cytoplasm, and vesicular nuclei.
Right: Numerous eosinophils are noted in the infiltrate.

sclerosing cholangitis. Two patients with this pattern had no Langerhans' cells in the liver, and the diagnosis was established in extrahepatic sites; 2) destructive cholangitis of large bile ducts, producing cystic dilatation, rupture, and bile extravasation; and 3) masses of Langerhans' cells, ranging from small granulomatoid foci to large tumor-like masses.

The diagnostic feature of all cases was the presence of Langerhans' cells. These cells typically have an abundant pink cytoplasm; lobulated, coffee-bean shaped or contorted nuclei with a fine chromatin pattern; and no discernible nucleoli (fig. 4-90). In all but one of the nine AFIP cases the Langerhans' cells were accompanied by varying numbers of eosinophils, lymphocytes, neutrophils, plasma cells, non-Langerhans' histiocytes, and occasional multinucleated giant cells. Immunostains were extremely useful in confirming the nature of the Langerhans' cells which were always deco-

rated by antibodies to S-100 protein (fig. 4-91) and CD1a (figs. 4-92, 4-93), as reported previously by others (296,299). Typical Birbeck granules were found ultrastructurally in one case.

Two patients, both with disseminated disease, had masses of Langerhans' cells that ranged from granulomatoid foci to large tumor-like lesions (figs. 4-94, 4-95). Eosinophils were present in abundance in these lesions. A similar case was reported recently by Cavazza et al. (295a).

All but two cases demonstrated some degree of active bile duct infiltration, injury, and destruction by Langerhans' cells (figs. 4-96, 4-97). In our experience, this is the most characteristic feature of hepatic involvement by this disease. Small and medium-sized bile ducts were often infiltrated by the Langerhans' cells with displacement of the epithelial cells. Some ducts were entirely replaced by masses of Langerhans' cells within the preexisting basement membrane. Two cases

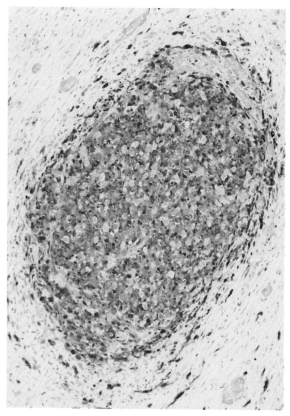

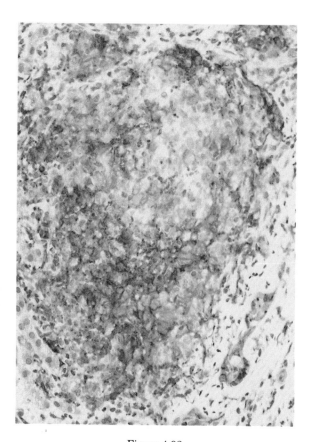

Figure 4-91
LANGERHANS' CELL HISTIOCYTOSIS
The Langerhans' cells express S-100 protein (immunostain).

Figure 4-92
LANGERHANS' CELL HISTIOCYTOSIS
The Langerhans' cells in the tumor-like aggregates express CD1a (immunostain).

Figure 4-93
LANGERHANS'
CELL HISTIOCYTOSIS
The Langerhans' cells that have infiltrated the bile duct express CD1a (immunostain).

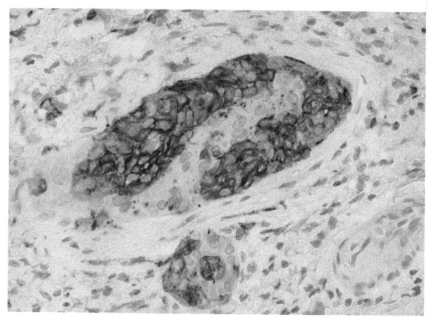

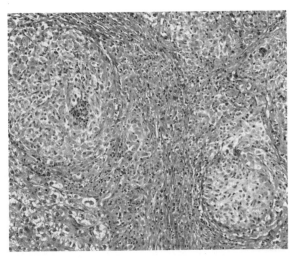

Figure 4-94
LANGERHANS' CELL HISTIOCYTOSIS
Two focal, granulomatoid aggregates of Langerhans' cells.

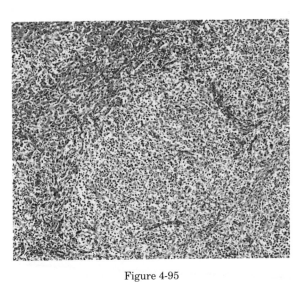

Figure 4-95
LANGERHANS' CELL HISTIOCYTOSIS
Extensive, pan-acinar involvement of the liver mimicking a neoplasm. This is the same case depicted in figure 4-88.

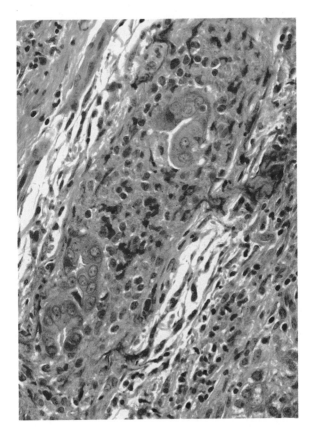

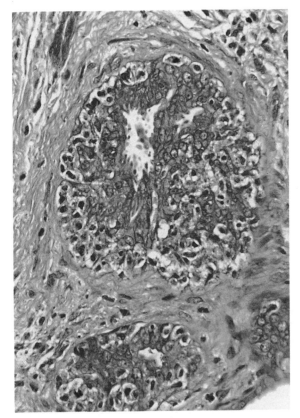

Figure 4-96
LANGERHANS' CELL HISTIOCYTOSIS
The bile ducts are surrounded and infiltrated by Langerhans' cells.

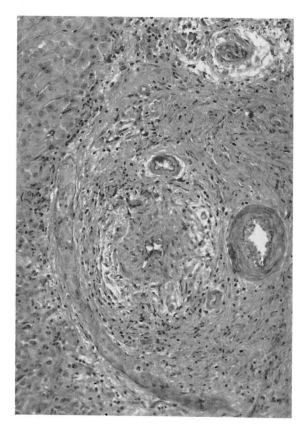

Figure 4-97
LANGERHANS' CELL HISTIOCYTOSIS
A destroyed bile duct is located adjacent to an artery in a portal area.

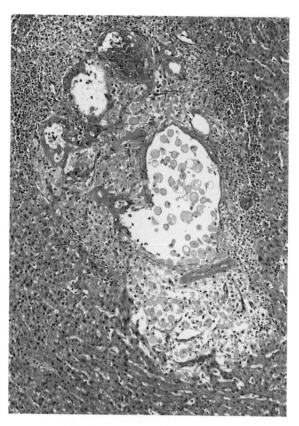

Figure 4-98
LANGERHANS' CELL HISTIOCYTOSIS
A ruptured bile duct contains and is surrounded by pseudoxanthomatous cells. The portal area also is infiltrated by inflammatory cells, and some Langerhans' cells were demonstrated by the CD1a immunostain (not shown). This is the same case depicted in figure 4-89.

showed injury to large ducts by the Langerhans' cells, producing cystic dilatation and rupture of the ducts, resulting in a xanthogranulomatous inflammatory response (fig. 4-98).

Concentric periductal fibrosis was a prominent feature in a majority of the cases (fig. 4-99). This was similar to the fibrosis that accompanies chronic obstructive biliary tract disease or primary sclerosing cholangitis. In cases where the ductal infiltration by Langerhans' cells was pronounced, there was often marked surrounding fibrosis with demonstrable Langerhans' cells in the fibrous tissue. Ducts at a distance from the Langerhans' cell lesions also sometimes showed epithelial injury and periductal fibrosis, indicating a secondary sclerosing cholangitis.

Changes secondary to the destructive and sclerotic lesions in the bile duct were nearly always present. In all cases there was periportal ductular proliferation, ranging from mild to se-

vere. Eight of the nine cases demonstrated chronic cholestatic features with periportal cholate stasis (pseudoxanthomatous change) and sometimes staining for copper or copper binding protein, as demonstrated by the rhodanine and Victoria blue stains, respectively. Some degree of periportal or bridging fibrosis was seen in seven of the nine cases. Two of these had progressed to an established "biliary" cirrhosis (fig. 4-100).

Differential Diagnosis. Primary sclerosing cholangitis, with or without chronic inflammatory bowel disease, can occur in childhood. In view of the morphologic overlap with Langerhans' cell histiocytosis we would recommend immunostains for S-100 protein and CD1a in all cases clinically or morphologically diagnosed as primary sclerosing cholangitis in children. *Rosai-Dorfman disease* rarely involves the liver

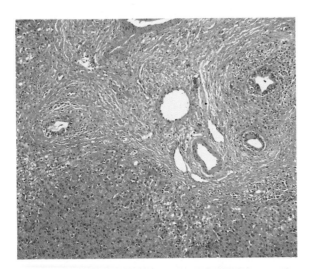 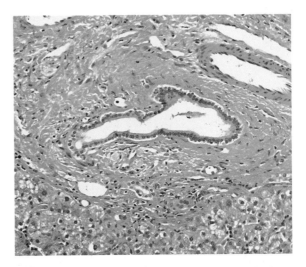

Figure 4-99
LANGERHANS' CELL HISTIOCYTOSIS
Left: The bile ducts are inflamed.
Right: There is periductal sclerosis.

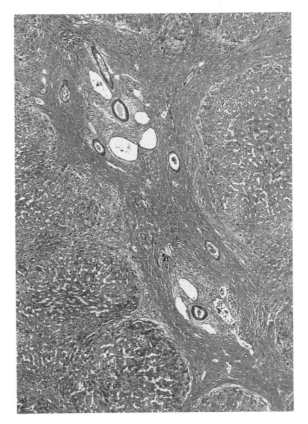

Figure 4-100
LANGERHANS' CELL HISTIOCYTOSIS
Left: Micronodular biliary cirrhosis (Masson trichrome stain).
Right: Marked ductopenia (Masson trichrome stain).

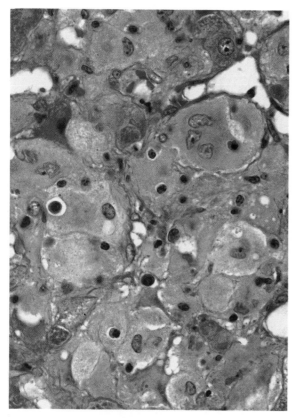

Figure 4-101
ROSAI-DORFMAN DISEASE

The sinusoids contain large cells with pale, eosinophilic cytoplasm and vesicular nuclei. Several have ingested mononuclear cells (arrows).

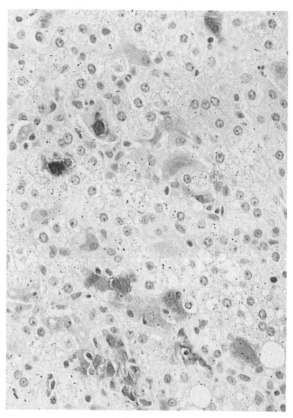

Figure 4-102
ROSAI-DORFMAN DISEASE

Several of the cells express S-100 protein. The CD1a immunostain (not shown) was negative in this case.

(297). Tumor-like lesions do not occur in this disease. Typically, there is sinusoidal and portal area infiltration by large histiocytes that show avid phagocytosis, including phagocytosis of lymphocytes, and sometimes plasma cells or red blood cells (fig. 4-101). The cells express S-100 protein but not CD1a (fig. 4-102) (295).

Etiology and Pathogenesis. These remain undetermined. Lieberman et al. (300) believe that the disease is a reactive rather than a neoplastic process, but William et al. (301) has presented evidence supporting a clonal proliferative disorder. Recently, human cytomegalovirus (HCMV) was detected immunohistochemically in 9 of 27 cases of Langerhans' cell histiocytosis by Kawakubo et al. (298a); HCMV-DNA was detected in 7 of 20 of those cases. This study requires confirmation by other investigators. Our concept of the pathogenesis of hepatobiliary

involvement in Langerhans' cell histiocytosis is schematically depicted in figure 4-103.

Treatment and Prognosis. According to Leiberman (300), patients with Langerhans' cell histiocytosis have a good overall prognosis. Based on the long-term follow-up of 238 patients for a median period of 10.5 years, no deaths were attributed to the disease itself. Virtually all patients recovered except for occasional residual orthopedic problems or diabetes insipidus. Howarth et al. (297a), however, found that 20 percent of patients with multisystem involvement have a progressive disease course despite treatment. Patients with hepatic involvement have considerable morbidity and mortality related to the disease. Follow-up information was available for eight of the nine AFIP patients: three patients underwent orthotopic liver transplantation; two were alive and well after 5 years while the third died a year

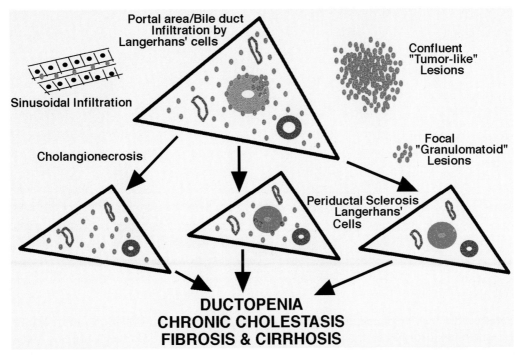

Figure 4-103
LANGERHANS' CELL HISTIOCYTOSIS
Pathogenesis of hepatic involvement (bile duct, green; portal vein, blue; hepatic artery, red; Langerhans' cells, orange). (Fig. 13 from Kaplan KJ, Goodman ZD, Ishak KG. Liver involvement in Langerhans cell histiocytosis. A study of nine cases. Mod Pathol 1999;12:370–8.)

later of disease. One patient with cystic lesions had these resected, followed by adjuvant chemotherapy; he was alive and well after 2 years with no evidence of recurrence. The remaining three patients died within weeks of diagnosis.

INFLAMMATORY PSEUDOTUMOR

Definition. This single, or less often multiple, tumor is composed of myofibroblasts, fibroblasts, and collagenized areas that are infiltrated with chronic inflammatory cells, predominantly polyclonal plasma cells, histiocytes, and macrophages. Synonyms include *inflammatory myofibroblastic tumor, inflammatory myofibrohistiocytic proliferation, plasma cell granuloma,* and *inflammatory fibrosarcoma.*

Clinical Features. Inflammatory pseudotumor is a relatively uncommon hepatic lesion; the lung is the most frequently affected organ. In a large series of 84 extrapulmonary pseudotumors reported by Coffin et al. (308) only 7 (8 percent) were located in the liver; the most fre-

quent sites were the mesentery and omentum (43 percent). Shek et al. (333) reviewed 47 reported cases of hepatic pseudotumors in 1993 and added 4 of their own. In 1990 we evaluated 31 cases on file at AFIP (311); data from these cases are noted in the succeeding sections.

In the AFIP series, 70 percent of the patients were male, with a mean age of 56 years (range, 3 to 77 years). The most frequent presenting symptoms were fever, right upper quadrant pain, and weight loss. Jaundice is usually a complication of inflammatory pseudotumor involving the extrahepatic bile ducts or pancreas. In 22 (73 percent) of the AFIP cases the hepatic mass was not the primary disease but was discovered during evaluation or treatment for another condition.

Laboratory findings in both the hepatic and extrahepatic tumors include leukocytosis, a raised erythrocyte sedimentation rate, an elevated C reactive protein level, and hypergammaglobulinemia (302,308). There may also be mild elevation of serum aminotransferases and alkaline phosphatase activity.

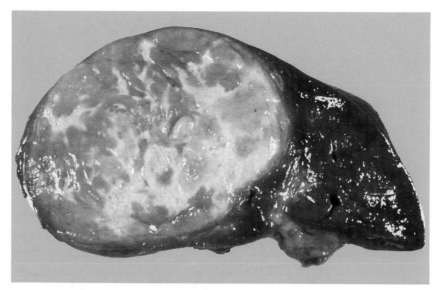

Figure 4-104
INFLAMMATORY
PSEUDOTUMOR
This tumor is well circumscribed and has a mottled yellow and tan cut surface.

Associated conditions were found in 22 of the 31 AFIP cases; hepatic abscesses or their remnants were present in 7. Cultures from four of these lesions yielded various bacteria (*Escherichia coli, Klebsiella, Bacteroides, Proteus,* and unidentified anaerobes). *Klebsiella pneumoniae* was isolated from one reported case (324) and *Bacteroides corrodens* from another (302). Other extrahepatic diseases in the AFIP series included pancreatitis (2 cases), diverticulitis/pericolonic abscess (2 cases), gastric ulcers (2 cases), choledocholithiasis with ascending cholangitis (1 case), and pneumonia (1 case). Four patients had mass lesions of the head of the pancreas (biopsy-proven to be nonmalignant in two instances), and one patient had chronic granulomatous disease of childhood. Antecedent diseases reported in the literature appear to be less common than in the AFIP series. Lyons et al. (323) found only 7 in the 45 cases that they culled from the literature. Other associated conditions not seen in the AFIP series but reported in the literature have included chronic cholangitis (325), primary sclerosing cholangitis (313,326), Caroli's disease (323), and acute myelomonocytic leukemia (321).

Imaging studies have been reported in some cases (318,322). Ultrasonography reveals a "mosaic" pattern with gas-like features suggesting an abscess (318). CT shows a low density lesion that does not enhance after the introduction of intravenous contrast material. The pseudotumors are hypovascular or less often avascular in hepatic angiograms. Radiologic examination of one pseudotumor in a 9-month-old boy revealed calcification and a heterogeneous tumor, amputation of the left portal vein, and dilatation of bile ducts, strongly suggesting malignancy (321a).

Gross Findings. The lesions may be solitary or multiple, and can vary in size from 1 cm to large masses involving an entire lobe (311). Of the 47 cases reviewed by Shek et al. (331), 81 percent were solitary while 19 percent were multiple. These authors noted that 53 percent of the tumors were located in the right lobe, 24 percent in the left lobe, and 13 percent involved both lobes. Hepatic hilar involvement occurs in 10 percent of cases; examples of such cases were reported by a number of investigators (308,314,317,319,325,329). The tumors, single or multiple, are usually well circumscribed, firm, and tan or yellow-white (figs. 4-104, 4-105). Sections disclose a solid or whorled pattern, but areas of necrosis or myxoid change may be evident.

Microscopic Findings. Inflammatory pseudotumors contain an admixture of inflammatory cells with a predominance of polyclonal plasma cells (figs. 4-106–4-108). Lymphocytes are also present, as are occasional lymphoid aggregates or follicles (302,303). Neutrophils, eosinophils, and macrophages (fig. 4-108) may also be seen. The inflammatory cells infiltrate a stroma composed of interlacing bundles of myofibroblasts, fibroblasts, and collagen bundles (figs. 4-109, 4-110). Dense areas of fibrosis may be seen. The tumors

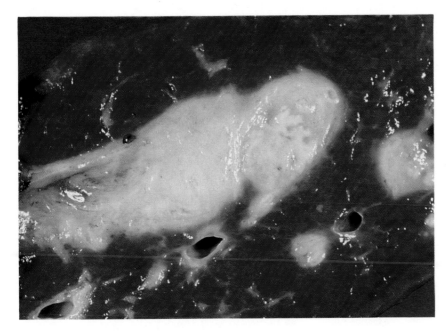

Figure 4-105
INFLAMMATORY
PSEUDOTUMOR
This tumor is glistening white
but has an irregular yellow focus
suggesting necrosis. Two other
smaller lesions are also noted.

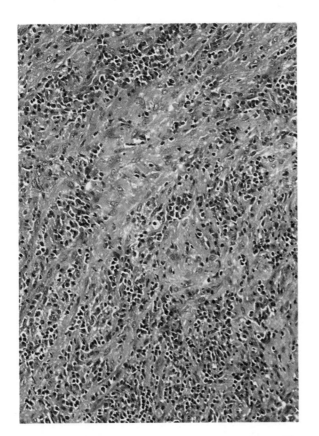
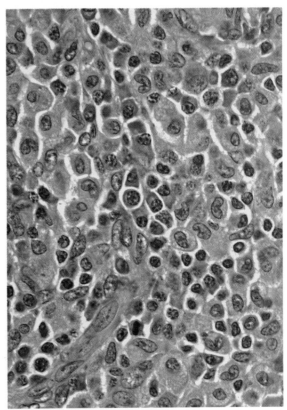

Figure 4-106
INFLAMMATORY PSEUDOTUMOR
Left: The clusters of plasma cells are intermingled with fibrous tissue.
Right: High-power view of an admixture of plasma cells and macrophages.

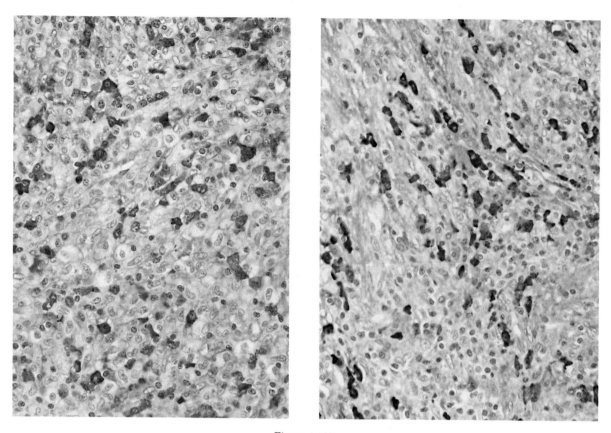

Figure 4-107
INFLAMMATORY PSEUDOTUMOR
Left: Plasma cells express IgG (immunostain).
Right: Other plasma cells express IgA (immunostain).

Figure 4-108
INFLAMMATORY
PSEUDOTUMOR
Macrophage cells in the tumor
express lysozyme (immunostain).

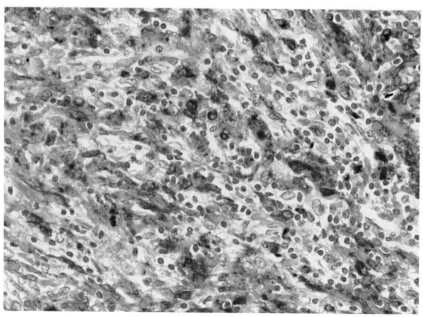

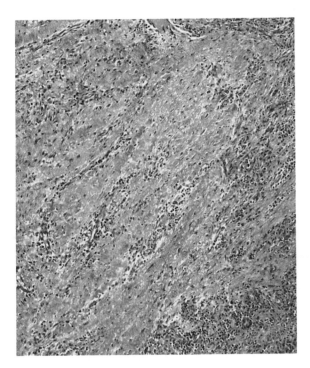

Figure 4-109
INFLAMMATORY PSEUDOTUMOR
The stroma in this tumor is densely collagenous (Masson trichrome stain).

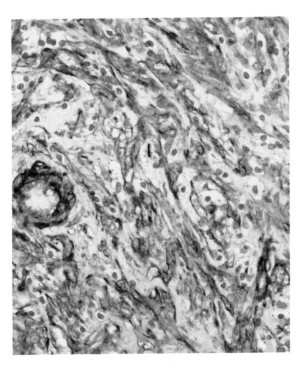

Figure 4-110
INFLAMMATORY PSEUDOTUMOR
The myofibroblasts in the tumor express smooth muscle actin (immunostain).

are usually richly supplied with vessels (fig. 4-111). A xanthogranulomatous inflammatory response may be present, as well as occasional areas of suppuration. An occlusive portal phlebitis was described in a number of reports (303,307, 318,332,334) and was also present in some of the AFIP cases (fig. 4-112). Bile ducts with an acute cholangitis may be trapped in the lesion. A unique case with invasion of the inferior vena cava was reported by Broughan et al. (306).

Differential Diagnosis. Confluent granulomas in hepatic sarcoidosis may produce a tumor-like lesion that can be confused with inflammatory pseudotumor in imaging studies and grossly (309, 320). Histopathologically, the granulomatous nature of these lesions should pose no problems in diagnosis. The paucity of inflammatory cells and the strong expression of CD34 antigen should readily distinguish solitary fibrous tumor from inflammatory pseudotumor. The benign appearance of the stromal cells and the abundance of plasma cells should allow differentiation of inflammatory pseudotumor from malignant fibrous histiocytoma and other sarcomas. Two liver tumors, initially thought to be inflammatory pseudotumor, later

proved to be Epstein-Barr virus–related *follicular dendritic cell tumors* (330,331). These very rare tumors can be distinguished ultrastructurally and immunohistochemically from inflammatory pseudotumor by the positive staining with CD21, CD35, R4/23, and Ki-M4. This entity was reviewed recently by Perez-Ordonez and Rosai (327). The differential diagnosis of inflammatory pseudotumor in general is extensively discussed in a recent review by Ritter et al. (329).

Pathogenesis. As noted earlier, some inflammatory pseudotumors of the liver are clearly related to a variety of bacterial infections. Epstein-Barr virus RNA has been detected by Arber et al. (304) in 7 of 18 inflammatory pseudotumors (41.2 percent), including two hepatic tumors. However, Epstein-Barr virus could not be incriminated in the etiology of three pseudotumors of the pancreaticobiliary region (336). The relationship between Epstein-Barr virus and inflammatory pseudotumor is critically reviewed by Arber et al. (305). Recently, human herpesvirus-8 genes were found to be expressed in five pulmonary inflammatory pseudotumors (312a). Whether the virus is a passive bystander or has an active role in the

131

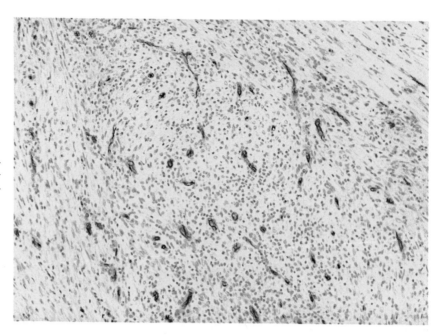

Figure 4-111
INFLAMMATORY
PSEUDOTUMOR
This tumor contains a rich network of capillaries that is demonstrated by the CD34 immunostain.

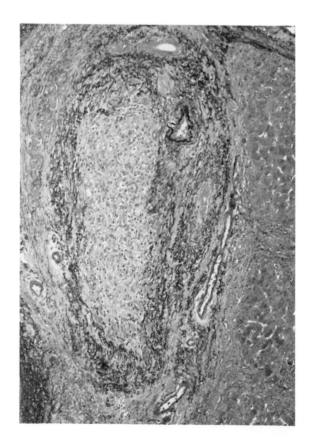 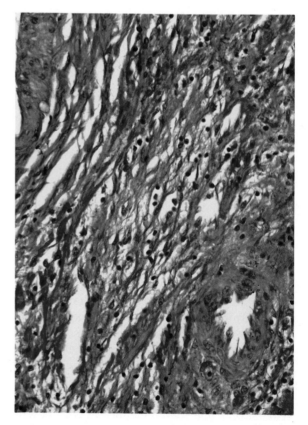

Figure 4-112
INFLAMMATORY PSEUDOTUMOR
Left: Portal vein branches show pylephlebitis (Victoria blue stain).
Right: Portal vein branch with an old organized thrombus (Masson trichrome stain).

pathogenesis of the tumor remains to be determined. Coffin et al. (308) believe that inflammatory pseudotumor is a benign nonmetastasizing proliferation of myofibroblasts with a potential for recurrence and persistent local growth, similar in some respects to the fibromatoses. However, recent cytogenetic studies of three nonhepatic cases have shown clonal aberrations, indicating a neoplastic process (335). It would appear that the majority of inflammatory pseudotumors are reactive (some to an infectious process) but some may be neoplastic.

Treatment and Prognosis. Excision has been performed in a number of cases and has generally been curative. Rare tumors have recurred (308,318a). Transplantation was successful in one case (313). Cases located in the hilum may not be amenable to resection, and surgery may lead to persistent problems with biliary drainage (302). Biliary stenting, resulting in survival for 5 years, was performed in a patient reported by Pokorny et al. (328). A few patients have shown improvement following steroid (317) or nonsteroidal anti-inflammatory drug therapy (315). Spontaneous regression occurred in the case reported by Gollapudi et al. (312). Transformation to sarcoma has been reported for soft tissue pseudotumors (310) and for hepatic inflammatory pseudotumors (326a,336). The combination of atypia, ganglion-like cells, and p53 expression, as well as DNA ploidy analysis may help identify tumors that might undergo malignant change or pursue a more aggressive clinical course with recurrences (318a).

MISCELLANEOUS BENIGN MESENCHYMAL TUMORS

Xanthomatous Neuropathy. A macroscopically identifiable xanthomatous neuropathy involving the unmyelinated nerves in the hilum of the liver and all portal tracts was reported by Ludwig et al. (343). Microscopically, accumulations of xanthomatous cells were found beneath the perineurium of the affected nerves. The etiology could not be ascertained.

Nerve Sheath Tumors. *Plexiform neurofibromatosis* has been reported in several patients with neurofibromatosis (337,340,342,345). There may be simultaneous involvement of the extrahepatic bile ducts (338) or the mesentery (345). A patient reported by Lederman (342) also had a

malignant schwannoma and an angiosarcoma of the liver, while in the case reported by Andreu et al. (337) the plexiform neurofibromatosis was associated with an angiosarcoma. A solitary *benign schwannoma* occurring in a patient without neurofibromatosis was described by Hytiroglou et al. (341). These authors also found five other published examples of nerve sheath tumors of the liver in patients without neurofibromatosis. Another case was recently described by Flemming et al. (338a). On rare occasions, *neurofibromas* may involve the duodenum or ampulla of Vater in patients with neurofibromatosis (344) and can cause obstructive jaundice. A case of plexiform neurofibromatosis of the liver is illustrated in figures 4-113 to 4-115 (345).

Chondroma. A single large tumor was described in the liver of a 44-year-old woman by Fried et al. (339). It was followed-up by CT imaging for 6 years and then excised because of a recent increase in size. The tumor occupied the entire right lobe, measured 16 cm in maximum diameter, and was multilobulated. Histologically, it consisted of a chondroid matrix in which were scattered chondrocyte-like cells. This patient had a history of parotid mixed tumor, raising the possibility that the "chondroma" was a late hepatic metastasis.

Myxoma. Three examples of this exceedingly rare tumor have been reported; they are discussed by Craig et al. (338) in the previous AFIP Fascicle on tumors of the liver. However, there are no examples in the files of the AFIP.

Benign Multicystic Mesothelioma. Three mesotheliomas of the liver have been reported (273, 338). One was a firm fibrous tumor attached to Glisson's capsule by a broad base (338). Microscopically, it was composed of moderately cellular tissue indented by deep clefts lined with mesothelial cells. Two other examples on file at the AFIP were incidental autopsy findings in a 34-year-old female. Her liver showed two well-circumscribed, yellowish tan nodules (0.5 cm and 2 cm in diameter) protruding from the surface of the right lobe. Both tumors had a similar microscopic appearance, with multiple cystically dilated spaces lined by cuboidal or flat endothelial cells and occasional papillary projections (figs. 4-116, 4-117). These projections were supported by fibrous tissue in which cords of liver cells and an occasional portal area were trapped. The tumors were classified as benign multicystic mesotheliomas.

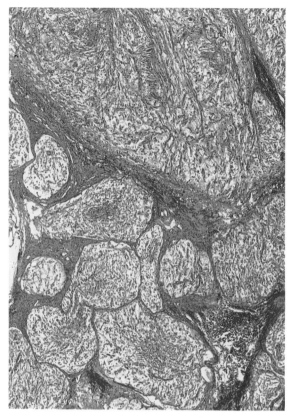

Figure 4-113
PLEXIFORM NEUROFIBROMATOSIS
There is a tumor-like aggregate of hypertrophied neural elements.

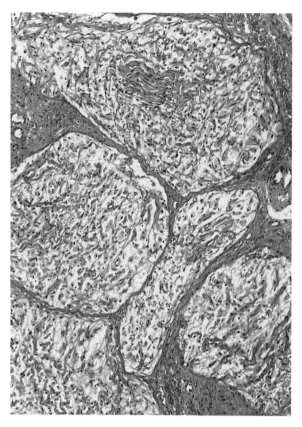

Figure 4-114
PLEXIFORM NEUROFIBROMATOSIS
Higher magnification of the neural elements.

Figure 4-115
PLEXIFORM
NEUROFIBROMATOSIS
Expression of S-100 protein by the neural elements (immunostain).

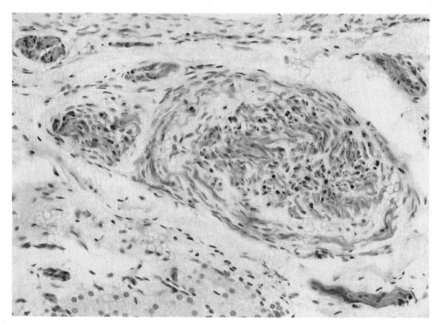

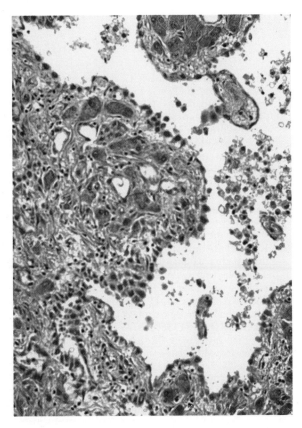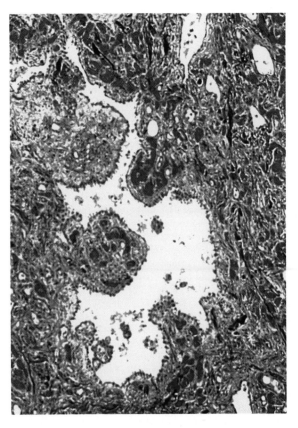

Figure 4-116
BENIGN MULTICYSTIC MESOTHELIOMA

Left: The irregular cystic space is lined by a single layer of mesothelial cells. The supporting connective tissue contains some isolated liver cells and a few inflammatory cells.

Right: The supporting collagenous stroma and groups of liver cells are noted to surround the mesothelial-lined cystic space (Masson trichrome stain).

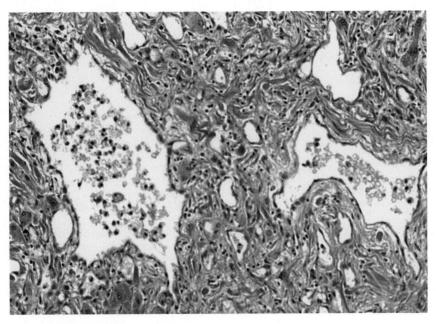

Figure 4-117
BENIGN MULTICYSTIC
MESOTHELIOMA

Higher magnification of several cystic spaces lined by mesothelial cells with interspersed, randomly oriented collagen bundles and some mononuclear inflammatory cells.

REFERENCES

Mesenchymal Hamartoma

1. Alanen A, Katevuo K, Toikkanen S. A non-cystic mesenchymal hamartoma of the liver—an unusual case of an unusual entity. Case report and review of the literature. Bildgebung 1987;56:181–4.
2. Alkalay AL, Puri AR, Pomerance JJ, et al. Mesenchymal hamartoma of the liver responsive to cyclophosphamide therapy: therapeutic approach. J Pediatr Surg 1985;20:125–8.
3. Balmer B, Le Coultre C, Feldges A, Hanimann B. Mesenchymal liver hamartoma in a newborn; case report. Eur J Pediatr Surg 1996;6:303–5.
4. Bartho S, Schulz HJ, Bollmann R, Specht U. Prenatally diagnosed mesenchymal hamartoma of the liver. Zentralbl Pathol 1992;138:141–4.
5. Bejvan SM, Winter TC, Shields LE, et al. Prenatal evaluation of mesenchymal hamartoma of the liver: gray scale and power Doppler sonographic imaging. J Ultrasound Med 1997;16:227–9.
6. Chau KY, Ho JW, Wu PC, Yuen WK. Mesenchymal hamartoma of liver in a man: comparison with cases in infants. J Clin Pathol 1994;47:864–6.
7. Cooper K, Hadley G, Moodley P. Mesenchymal hamartoma of the liver. A report of 5 cases. S Afr M J 1989;75:295–8.
8. de Chadarevian JP, Pawel BR, Faerber EN, Weintraub WH. Undifferentiated (embryonal) sarcoma arising in conjunction with mesenchymal hamartoma of the liver. Mod Pathol 1994;7:490–3.
9. De Maioribus CA, Lally KP, Sim K, Isaacs H, Mahour GH. Mesenchymal hamartoma of the liver. A 35-year review. Arch Surg 1990;125:598–600.
10. Dehner LP, Ewing SL, Sumner HW. Infantile mesenchymal hamartoma of the liver. Histologic and ultrastructural observations. Arch Pathol 1975;99:379–82.
11. Donovan AT, Wolverson MK, de Mello D, Craddock T, Silverstein M. Multicystic hepatic mesenchymal hamartoma of childhood. Computerized tomography and ultrasound characteristics. Pediatr Radiol 1981;11:163–5.
12. Dooley JS, Li AK, Scheuer PJ, et al. A giant cystic mesenchymal hamartoma of the liver: diagnosis, management, and study of cyst fluid. Gastroenterology 1983;85:958–61.
13. Drachenberg CB, Papadimitriou JC, Rivero MA, Wood C. Distinctive case. Adult mesenchymal hamartoma of the liver: report of a case with light microscopic, FNA cytology, immunohistochemistry, and ultrastructural studies and review of the literature. Mod Pathol 1991;4:392–5.
14. Edmondson HA. Differential diagnosis of tumors and tumor-like lesions of liver in infancy and childhood. Am J Dis Child 1956;91:168–86.
15. Edmondson HA. Tumors of the liver and intrahepatic bile ducts. Atlas of Tumor Pathology, Vol. 25. Armed Forces Institute of Pathology, Washington, D.C., 1958.
16. Ehren H, Mahour GH, Isaacs H Jr. Benign liver tumors in infancy and childhood. Am J Surg 1983;145:325–9.
17. Federici S, Galli G, Sciutti R, Cuoghi D. Cystic mesenchymal hamartoma of the liver. Pediatr Radiol 1992;22:307–8.
18. Giyanani VL, Meyers PC, Wolfson JJ. Mesenchymal hamartoma of the liver: computed tomography and ultrasonography. J Comput Assist Tomogr 1986;10:51–4.
19. Gramlich TL, Killough BW, Garvin AJ. Mesenchymal hamartoma of the liver: report of a case in a 28-year-old. Hum Pathol 1988;19:991–2.
20. Grases PJ, Matos-Villalobos M, Arcia-Romero F, Lecuna-Torres V. Mesenchymal hamartoma of the liver. Gastroenterology 1979;76:1466–9.
21. Gutierrez OH, Burgener FA. Mesenchymal hamartoma of the liver in an adult: radiologic diagnosis. Gastrointest Radiol 1988;13:341–4.
22. Hirata GI, Matsunaga ML, Medearis AL, Dixon P, Platt LD. Ultrasonographic diagnosis of a fetal abdominal mass: a case of a mesenchymal liver hamartoma and a review of the literature. Prenat Diagn 1990;10:507–12.
23. Kaufman RA. Is cystic mesenchymal hamartoma of the liver similar to infantile hemangioendothelioma and cavernous hemangioma on dynamic computed tomography? Pediatr Radiol 1992;22:582–3.
24. Lack EE. Mesenchymal hamartoma of the liver. A clinical and pathologic study of nine cases. Am J Pediatr Hematol Oncol 1986;8:91–8.
25. Lai FM, Jayakumar CR, Saw L, Kumar G. Hepatic mesenchymal hamartoma: a case report and radiological findings. Singapore Med J 1996;37:226–8.
25a. Lauwers GY, Grant LD, Donnelly WH, et al. Hepatic undifferentiated (embryonal) sarcoma arising in a mesenchymal hamartoma. Am J Surg Pathol 1997;21:1248–54.
26. Lennington WJ, Gray GF Jr, Page DL. Mesenchymal hamartoma of liver. A regional ischemic lesion of a sequestered lobe. Am J Dis Child 1993;147:193–6.
27. Maresch R. Ueber ein lymphangiom der liber. Ztschr Heilk Wiern Hepid 1903;24:30–40.
28. Mascarello JT, Krous HF. Second report of a translocation involving 19q13.4 in a mesenchymal hamartoma of the liver. Cancer Genet Cytogenet 1992;58:141–2.
29. Megremis S, Sfakianaki E, Voludaki A, Chroniaris N. The ultrasonographic appearance of a cystic mesenchymal hamartoma of the liver observed in a middle-aged woman. J Clin Ultrasound 1994;22:338–41.
30. Okeda R. Mesenchymal hamartoma of the liver—an autopsy case with serial sections and some comments on its pathogenesis. Acta Pathol Jpn 1976;26:229–36.
31. Otal TM, Hendricks JB, Pharis P, Donnelly WH. Mesenchymal hamartoma of the liver. DNA flow cytometric analysis of eight cases. Cancer 1994;74:1237–42.
32. Rao SP, Bhagavath S, Chen CK, Tolete-Velcek F. Mesenchymal hamartoma of the liver in an older child: association with disseminated intravascular coagulation. Med Pediatr Oncol 1984;12:112–5.
33. Rey MJ, Ordi J, Ribe A, Garcia-Valdecasas JC, Ayuso JR, Cardesa A. Hepatic mesenchymatous hamartoma presenting in an adult patient (see comments). Med Clin (Barc) 1995;104:180–2.
34. Roberts EA, Liu P, Stringer D, Superina RA, Mancer K. Mesenchymal hamartoma in a 10-month-old infant: appearance by magnetic resonance imaging. Can Assoc Radiol J 1989;40:219–21.
35. Ros PR, Goodman ZD, Ishak KG, et al. Mesenchymal hamartoma of the liver: radiologic-pathologic correlation. Radiology 1986;158:619–24.

36. Salisbury JR, Darby AJ, Portmann BC. Mesenchymal hamartoma of the liver—report of an unusual case. Postgrad Med J 1986;62:757–60.

37. Shuto T, Kinoshita H, Yamada C, et al. Bilateral lobectomy excluding the caudate lobe for giant mesenchymal hamartoma of the liver. Surgery 1993;113:215–22.

38. Smith WL, Ballantine TV, Gonzalez-Crussi F. Hepatic mesenchymal hamartoma causing heart failure in the neonate. J Pediatr Surg 1978;13:183–5.

39. Speleman F, De Telder V, De Potter KR, et al. Cytogenetic analysis of a mesenchymal hamartoma of the liver. Cancer Genet Cytogenet 1989;40:29–32.

40. Stanley P, Hall TR, Woolley MM, Diament MJ, Gilsanz V, Miller JH. Mesenchymal hamartomas of the liver in childhood: sonographic and CT findings. Am J Roentgenol 1986;147:1035–9.

41. Stocker J. Hepatic tumors in children. In: Stocker JT, ed. Liver disease in children. St. Louis: Mosby, 1994.

42. Stocker J, Conran R, Selby D. Tumor and pseudotumors of the liver. In: Stocker TJ, Askin F, eds. Pathology of solid tumors in children. London: Chapman & Hall, 1998:83–110.

43. Stocker JT, Ishak KG. Mesenchymal hamartoma of the liver: report of 30 cases and review of the literature. Pediatr Pathol 1983;1:245–67.

44. Tovbin J, Segal M, Tavori I, et al. Hepatic mesenchymal hamartoma: a pediatric tumor that may be diagnosed prenatally. Ultrasound Obstet Gynecol 1997;10:63–5.

45. Turlin B, Deugnier Y, Kerneis J, et al. Liver mesenchymal hamartoma in adulthood. Report of a new case. Ann Pathol 1996;16:192–5.

46. Vandendriessche L, Bonhomme A, Breysem L, et al. Mesenchymal hamartoma: radiological differentiation from other possible liver tumors in childhood. J Belge Radiol 1996;79:74–5.

47. Velasquez G, Katkov H, Formanek A. Primary liver tumors in the pediatric age group: an angiographic challenge. ROFO Fortschr Geb Roentgenstr Nuklearmed 1979;130:408–17.

48. Wada M, Ohashi E, Jin H, et al. Mesenchymal hamartoma of the liver: report of an adult case and review of the literature. Intern Med 1992;31:1370–5.

49. Wholey MH, Wojno KJ. Pediatric hepatic mesenchymal hamartoma demonstrated on plain film, ultrasound and MRI, and correlated with pathology. Pediatr Radiol 1994;24:143–4.

50. Yamamoto M, Hagihara H, Mogaki M, et al. Adult mesenchymal hamartoma of the liver mimicking bile duct cystadenoma. J Gastroenterol 1994;29:518–24.

Infantile Hemangioendothelioma

51. Achilleos OA, Buist LJ, Kelly DA, et al. Unresectable hepatic tumors in childhood and the role of liver transplantation. J Pediatr Surg 1996;31:1563–7.

52. Awan S, Davenport M, Portmann B, Howard ER. Angiosarcoma of the liver in children. J Pediatr Surg 1996;31:1729–32.

53. Battaglino F, Cappellari F, Criscino A, Salvo R, Comisi F, Termini C. Hemangioendothelioma of the liver in the newborn: description of 2 cases. Pediatr Med Chir 1993;15:605–8.

54. Berger TM, Berger MF, Hoffman AD, Zimmermann D, Tonz O. Imaging diagnosis and follow-up of infantile hepatic haemangioendothelioma: a case report. Eur J Pediatr 1994;153:100–2.

55. Burke DR, Verstandig A, Edwards O, Meranze SG, McLean GK, Stein EJ. Infantile hemangioendothelioma: angiographic features and factors determining efficacy of hepatic artery embolization. Cardiovasc Intervent Radiol 1986;9:154–7.

56. Calder CI, Raafat F, Buckels JA, Kelly DA. Orthotopic liver transplantation for type 2 hepatic infantile haemangioendothelioma. Histopathology 1996;28:271–3.

57. Cerar A, Dolenc-Strazar ZD, Bartenjev D. Infantile hemangioendothelioma of the liver in a neonate. Immunohistochemical observations. Am J Surg Pathol 1996;20:871–6.

58. Chan YF, Choi AC, Ma L, Leung MP. Infantile hemangioendothelioma of the liver: ultrastructural study of a type II case. Pathology 1986;18:463–8.

59. Corbella F, Arico M, Podesta AF, Villa A, Beluffi G, Bianchi E. Infantile hepatic hemangioendothelioma treated by radiotherapy. Pediatr Radiol 1983;13:297–300.

60. Coronado Perez, H Angulo Hernandez O. Liver neoplasms in children. Bol Med Hosp Infant Mex 1981;38:723–40.

61. Dehner LP, Ishak KG. Vascular tumors of the liver in infants and children. A study of 30 cases and review of the literature. Arch Pathol 1971;92:101–11.

62. Feldman PS, Shneidman D, Kaplan C. Ultrastructure of infantile hemangioendothelioma of the liver. Cancer 1978;42:521–7.

63. Fellows KE, Hoffer FA, Markowitz RI, Neill JA. Multiple collaterals to hepatic infantile hemangioendotheliomas and arteriovenous malformations: effect on embolization [see comments]. Radiology 1991;181:813–8.

64. Hanchard B, Persaud V, Kerr G, Baum P. Primary infantile haemangioendothelioma of the liver. West Indian Med J 1983;32:44–7.

65. Hase T, Kodama M, Kishida A, et al. Successful management of infantile hepatic hilar hemangioendothelioma with obstructive jaundice and consumption coagulopathy. J Pediatr Surg 1995;30:1485–7.

66. Ito H, Yamasaki T, Okamoto O, Tahara E. Infantile hemangioendothelioma of the liver in patient with interstitial deletion of chromosome 6q: report of an autopsy case. Am J Med Genet 1989;34:325–9.

67. Itoh K, Itoh S, Fukuoka H, et al. Therapeutic embolization of infantile hemangioendothelioma of the liver. Rinsho Hoshasen 1989;34:933–6.

68. Keslar PJ, Buck JL, Selby DM. From the archives of the AFIP. Infantile hemangioendothelioma of the liver revisited. Radiographics 1993;13:657–70.

69. Kirchner SG, Heller RM, Kasselberg AG, Greene HL. Infantile hepatic hemangioendothelioma with subsequent malignant degeneration. Pediatr Radiol 1981;11:42–5.

70. Konja J, Belicza M, Krstulovic B, Tiefenbach A. Infantile hemangioendothelioma of the liver in a 5-month-old infant (author's transl). Lijec Vjesn 1977;99:218–24.

71. Lin HJ, Lin CC, Chen SH, et al. Infantile hemangioendothelioma of the liver. Taiwan I Hsueh Hui Tsa Chih 1978;77:120–6.

72. Lucaya J, Enriquez G, Amat L, Gonzalez-Rivero MA. Computed tomography of infantile hepatic hemangioendothelioma. Am J Roentgenol 1985;144:821–6.

73. Mahboubi S, Sunaryo FP, Glassman MS, Patel K. Computed tomography, management, and follow-up in infantile hemangioendothelioma of the liver in infants and children. J Comput Tomogr 1987;11:370–5.

74. Marton T, Silhavy M, Csapo Z, et al. Multifocal hemangioendothelioma of the fetus and placenta. Hum Pathol 1997;28:866–9.

75. Maruiwa M, Nakamura Y, Motomura K, et al. Cornelia de Lange syndrome associated with Wilms' tumour and infantile haemangioendothelioma of the liver: report of two autopsy cases. Virchows Arch [A] 1988;413:463–8.

76. McHugh K, Burrows PE. Infantile hepatic hemangioendotheliomas: significance of portal venous and systemic collateral arterial supply. J Vasc Interv Radiol 1992;3:337–44.

77. Morita Y, Saito H, Hiromura T, et al. Image diagnosis of infantile hemangioendothelioma of the liver. Rinsho Hoshasen 1988;33:1677–83.

78. Noel AW, Heyman S. Scintigraphic findings in infantile hemangioendothelioma. Clin Nucl Med 1986;11:413–6.

79. Noronha R, Gonzalez-Crussi F. Hepatic angiosarcoma in childhood. A case report and review of the literature. Am J Surg Pathol 1984;8:863–71.

80. Novak D, Suchy F, Balistreri W. Disorders of the liver and biliary system relevant to clinical practice. In: Oski F, ed. Principles and practice of pediatrics. Philadelphia: JB Lippincott, 1990:1746–77.

81. Pardes JG, Bryan PJ, Gauderer MW. Spontaneous regression of infantile hemangioendotheliomatosis of the liver: demonstration by ultrasound. J Ultrasound Med 1982;1:349–53.

82. Park CH, Hwang HS, Hong J, Pak MS. Giant infantile hemangioendothelioma of the liver. Scintigraphic diagnosis. Clin Nucl Med 1996;21:293–5.

83. Perez Payarols J, Pardo Masferrer J, Gomez Bellvert C. Treatment of life-threatening infantile hemangiomas with vincristine [Letter]. N Engl J Med 1995;333:69.

84. Pethe VV, Kalgutkar AD, Mondkar J, Oak SN, Deodhar KP, Deshmukh SS. Hepatic hemangioendothelioma of infancy with congestive cardiac failure—report of a case. Indian J Cancer 1995;32:186–8.

85. Powers C, Ros PR, Stoupis C, et al. Primary liver neoplasms: MR imaging with pathologic correlation. Radiographics 1994;14:459–82.

86. Presedo A, Martinez-Ibanez V, Castellote A, et al. Infantile hepatic hemangioendothelioma of the liver: report of 11 cases. Chir Pediatr 1996;9:51–4.

87. Ramadwar RH, Deshmukh SS, Oak SN, Karmarkar SJ. Infantile hemangioendothelioma of the liver in a neonate. Indian Pediatr 1993;30:1441–4.

88. Robbins RC, Chin C, Yun KL, et al. Arterial switch and resection of hepatic hemangioendothelioma. Ann Thorac Surg 1995;59:1575–7.

89. Samuel M, Spitz L. Infantile hepatic hemangioendothelioma: the role of surgery. J Pediatr Surg 1995;30:1425–9.

90. Selby DM, Stocker JT, Waclawiw MA, Hitchcock CL, Ishak KG. Infantile hemangioendothelioma of the liver. Hepatology 1994;20:39–45.

91. Shah KD, Beck AR, Jhaveri MK, Keohane M, Weinberg B, Gerber MA. Infantile hemangioendothelioma of heterotopic intrathoracic liver associated with diaphragmatic hernia. Hum Pathol 1987;18:754–6.

92. Skopec LL, Lakatua D. Non-immune fetal hydrops with hepatic hemangioendothelioma and Kasabach-Merritt syndrome: a case report. Pediatr Pathol 1989;9:87–93.

93. Stocker J. Hepatic tumors in children. In: Suchy FS, ed. Liver disease in children. St. Louis: Mosby, 1994:901–29.

94. Stocker J, Conran R, Selby D. Tumor and pseudotumors of the liver. In: Stocker J, Askin F, eds. Pathology of solid tumors in children. London: Chapman & Hall, 1998:83–110.

95. Strate SM, Rutledge JC, Weinberg AG. Delayed development of angiosarcoma in multinodular infantile hepatic hemangioendothelioma [Letter]. Arch Pathol Lab Med 1984;108:943–4.

96. Suh YL, Cho KJ, Chi JG, Park KW. Infantile hemangioendothelioma of the liver—a case report. J Korean Med Sci 1987;2:195–200.

97. Szymanowicz J, Podraza W, Talerczyk M, Witkowska-Ozogowska J. Infantile hemangioendothelioma in a 10-week-old girl. Pediatr Pol 1989;64:189–92.

98. Wong DC, Masel JP. Infantile hepatic haemangioendothelioma. Australas Radiol 1995;39:140–4.

99. Wood BP, Putnam TC, Chacko AK. Infantile hepatic hemangioendotheliomas associated with hemihypertrophy. Pediatr Radiol 1977;5:242–5.

100. Yasunaga C, Sueishi K, Ohgami H, Suita S, Kawanami T. Heterogenous expression of endothelial cell markers in infantile hemangioendothelioma. Immunohistochemical study of two solitary cases and one multiple one. Am J Clin Pathol 1989;91:673–81.

101. Zerbini MC, Vianna MR, Ribeiro D, Ayoub AA, Porta G, Sesso A. Is there a role for pericytic cells in the vascular bed of infantile hemangioendothelioma of the liver? J Submicrosc Cytol Pathol 1991;23:141–5.

102. Zurcher B, Caflisch U, Hofer B, Scharli A, Laissue J. Hemangioendothelioma of the liver (case report) (author's transl). Z Kinderchir 1982;35:26–31.

Cavernous Hemangioma

103. Allison DJ, Jordan H, Hennessy O. Therapeutic embolisation of the hepatic artery: a review of 75 procedures. Lancet 1985;1:595–9.

104. Alper A, Ariogul O, Emre A, et al. Treatment of liver hemangiomas by enucleation. Arch Surg 1988;123:660–1.

105. Aspray M. Calcified hemangiomas of the liver. Am J Roentgenol Rad Ther 1945;53:446–53.

106. Baer HU, Dennison AR, Mouton W, Stain SC, Zimmermann A, Blumgart LH. Enucleation of giant hemangiomas of the liver. Technical and pathologic aspects of a neglected procedure. Ann Surg 1992;216:673–6.

107. Barter RH, Letterman GS, Schurter M. Hemangiomas in pregnancy. Am J Obstet Gynecol 1963;87:625–34.

108. Belli L, De Carlis L, Beati C, et al. Surgical treatment of symptomatic giant hemangiomas of the liver. Surg Gynecol Obstet 1992;174:474–8.

109. Berry CL. Solitary "necrotic nodule" of the liver: a probable pathogenesis. J Clin Pathol 1985;38:1278–80.

110. Birnbaum BA, Weinreb JC, Megibow AJ, et al. Definitive diagnosis of hepatic hemangiomas: MR imaging versus Tc–99m–labeled red blood cell SPECT. Radiology 1990;176:95–101.

111. Bradley M, Stewart I, Metraweli C. Diagnosis of peripheral cavernous haemangioma: comparison of ultrasound, CT, and RBC scintigraphy. Clin Radiol 1991;44:34–7.

112. Brant WE, Floyd JL, Jackson DE, Gilliland JD. The radiological evaluation of hepatic cavernous hemangioma. JAMA 1987;257:2471–4.

113. Caturelli E, Rapaccini GL, Sabelli C, et al. Ultrasound-guided fine-needle aspiration biopsy in the diagnosis of hepatic hemangioma. Liver 1986;6:326–30.

114. Chung EB. Multiple bile-duct hamartomas. Cancer 1970;26:287–96.

115. Conter RL, Longmire WP Jr. Recurrent hepatic hemangiomas. Possible association with estrogen therapy. Ann Surg 1988;207:115–9.

116. Cozzi PJ, Morris DL. Two cases of spontaneous liver rupture and literature review. HPB Surgery 1996;9:257–60.

117. Craig JR, Peters RL, Edmondson HA. Tumors of the liver and intrahepatic bile ducts. Atlas of Tumor Pathology, Second Series, Fascicle 26. Washington D.C., Armed Forces Institute of Pathology, 1989.

118. Cronan JJ, Esparza AR, Dorfiman GS, Ridlen MS, Paolella LP. Cavernous hemangioma of the liver. Role of percutaneous biopsy. Radiology 1988;166:133–8.

119. Dehner LP, Ishak KG. Vascular tumors of the liver in infants and children. A study of 30 cases and review of the literature. Arch Pathol 1971;92:101–11.

120. Dupre CT, Fincher RM. Case report: cavernous hemangioma of the liver. Am J Med Sci 1992;303:241–4.

121. Edmondson HA. Tumors of the liver and intrahepatic bile ducts. Atlas of Tumor Pathology, Section VII. Fascicle 25. Washington D.C., Armed Forces Institute of Pathology, 1958.

122. Feldman M. Hemangioma of the liver. Special reference to its association with cysts of the liver and pancreas. Am J Clin Pathol 1958;29:160–2.

123. Feurle GE. Arteriovenous shunting and cholestasis in hepatic hemangiomatosis associated with metoclopramide. Gastroenterology 1990;99:258–62.

124. Fleury P, Smits N, Van-Baal S. The incidence of hepatic hamartomas in tuberous sclerosis. Evaluation by ultrasonography. ROFO 1987;146:694–6.

125. Garcia Reinoso G, Saez-Royuela F, Gómez Rubio M, et al. Formas de presentación y procedimientos diagnósticos del hemangioma hepàtico gigante. Rev Esp Enf Ap Digest 1989;76:617–21.

126. Geschickter CF, Keasbey LE. Tumors of blood vessels. Am J Cancer 1935;23:568–91.

127. Graham E, Cohen AW, Soulen M, Fay R. Symptomatic liver hemangioma with intra-tumor hemorrhage treated by angiography and embolization during pregnancy. Obstet Gynecol 1993;81:813–6.

128. Haratake J, Horie A, Nagafuchi Y. Hyalinized hemangioma of the liver. Am J Gastroenterol 1992;87:234–6.

129. Hopkins K, Bailey RJ. Hepatic hemangioma: an unusual cause of fever of unknown origin. Can J Gastroenterol 1990;4:227–9.

130. Hosaka M, Murase N, Orito T, Mori M. Immunohistochemical evaluation of factor VIII related antigen, filament proteins and lectin binding in haemangiomas. Virchows Arch [A] 1986;407:237–47.

131. Hotokezaka M, Kojima M, Nakamura M, et al. Traumatic rupture of hepatic hemangioma. J Clin Gastroenterol 1996;23:69–71.

132. Issa P. Cavernous hemangioma of the liver. The role of radiotherapy Br J Radiol 1968;41:26–32.

133. Ito N, Kawata S, Tsushima H, et al. Increased circulating transforming growth factor b1 in a patient with giant hepatic hemangioma: possible contribution to an impaired immune function. Hepatology 1997;25:93–6.

134. Iwatsuki S, Todo S, Starzl TE. Excisional therapy for benign hepatic lesions. Surg Gynecol Obstet 1990;171:240–6.

135. Langsteger W, Lind P, Eber B, Koltinger P, Behan A, Eber O. Diagnosis of hepatic hemangioma with 99m Tc-labeled red cells: single photon emission computed tomography (SPECT) versus planar imaging. Liver 1989;9:288–93.

135a. Lehmann FS, Beglinger C, Schnabel K, Terracciano L. Progressive development of diffuse liver hemangiomatosis. J Hepatol 1999;30:951–4.

136. Levitt LM, Coleman M, Yarvis J. Multiple large hemangiomas of the liver. N Engl J Med 1955;252:854–5.

137. Mathieu D, Zafrani ES, Anglada MC, Dhumeaux D. Association of focal nodular hyperplasia and hepatic hemangioma. Gastroenterology 1989;97:154–7.

138. Morley JE, Myers JB, Sack FS, Kalk F, Epstein EE, Lennon J. Enlargement of cavernous haemangioma associated with exogenous administration of oestrogens. S Afr Med J 1974;48:695–7.

139. Nghiem HV, Bogost GA, Ryan JA, Lund P, Freeny PC, Rice KM. Cavernous hemangiomas of the liver: enlargement over time. AJR Am J Roentgenol 1997;169:137–40.

140. Ninard B. Tumeurs du Foie. Paris, Librarie le Francois, 1950.

141. Panis Y, Fagniez PL Cherqui D, et al. Successful arterial embolization of giant liver haemangioma. Report of a case with five year computed tomography follow up. HPB Surgery 1993;7:141–6.

142. Park WC, Phillips R. The role of radiation therapy in the management of hemangiomas of the liver. JAMA 1970;212:1496–8.

143. Pearson JM, McWilliam LJ. A light microscopical, immunohistochemical, and ultrastructural comparison of hemangiomata and lymphangiomata. Ultrastr Pathol 1990;14:497–504.

144. Peveretos P, Panoussopoulos D. Giant hepatic hemangioma: treatment by ligation of the hepatic artery. J Surg Oncol 1986;31:48–51.

145. Pietrabissa A, Giulianotti R, Campatelli A, et al. Management and follow-up of 78 giant haemangiomas of the liver. Br J Surg 1996;83:915–8.

146. Plachta A. Calcified cavernous hemangioma of the liver. Radiology 1996;79:783–8.

147. Reading NG, Forbes A, Nunnerly HB, Williams R. Hepatic haemangioma: a critical review of diagnosis and management. Q J Med (New Series) 1988;67:431–5.

148. Russo MW, Johnson MW, Fair JH, Brown RS. Orthotopic liver transplantation for giant hepatic hemangioma. Am J Gastroenterol 1997;92:1940–1.

149. Saegusa T, Ito K, Oba N, et al. Enlargement of multiple cavernous hemangioma of the liver in association with pregnancy. Int Med 1995;34:207–11.

150. Schumacker HB. Hemangioma of the liver. Discussion of symptomatology and report of patients treated by operation. Surgery 1942:11:209–22.

151. Shimizu, M, Miura J, Itoh H, Soitoh Y. Hepatic giant cavernous hemangioma with microangiopathic hemolytic anemia and consumption coagulopathy. Am J Gastroenterol 1990;85:1411–3.

152. Sundaresan M, Lyons B, Akosa AB. "Solitary" necrotic nodules of the liver: an aetiology reaffirmed. Gut 1991;32:1378–80.

153. Taillan B, Sanderson F, Fuzibet JG, et al. Association polyglobulie angiome hépatique. Mise en évidence d'une activité "érythropoïétine-like" intratumorale. Presse Méd 1990;19:1319–20.

154. Takahashi T, Katoh H, Dohke M, Okushiba S. A giant hepatic hemangioma with secondary portal hypertension: a case report of successful surgical treatment. Hepatogastroenterology 1997;44:1212–4.

155. Vishnevsky VA, Mohan VS, Pomelov VS, Todua FI, Guseinov EK. Surgical treatment of giant cavernous hemangioma of the liver. HPB Surgery 1991;4:69–79.

156. Wanless IR, Mawdsley C, Adams R. On the pathogenesis of focal nodular hyperplasia of the liver. Hepatology 1985;5:1194–200.

157. Watzke HH, Linkesch W, Hay U. Giant hemangioma of the liver (Kasabach-Merritt syndrome): successful suppression of intravascular coagulation permitting surgical removal. J Clin Gastroenterol 1989;11:347–50.

158. Yamagata M, Kanematsu T, Matsumata T, Utsonomiya T, Ikeda Y, Sugimachi K. Management of haemangioma of the liver: comparison of results between surgery and observation. Br J Surg 1991;78:1223–5.

159. Yamamoto T, Kawarada Y, Yano T, Noguchi T, Mizumoto R. Spontaneous rupture of hemangioma of the liver: treatment with transcatheter hepatic arterial embolization. Am J Gastroenterol 1991;86:1645–9.

160. Yoshida J, Yamasaki S, Yamamoto J, et al. Growing cavernous hemangioma of the liver: 11-fold increase in volume in a decade. J Gastroenterol Hepatol 1991;6:414–6.

161. Zimmermann A, Baer HU. Fibrous tumor-liver interface in large hepatic neoplasms: its significance for tumor resection and enucleation. Liver Transpl Surg 1996;2:192–9.

Hereditary Hemorrhagic Telangiectasia

161a. Boillot O, Bianco F, Viale JP, et al. Liver transplantation resolves the hyperdynamic circulation in hereditary hemorrhagic telangiectasia with hepatic involvement. Gastroenterology 1999;116:187–92.

162. Caselitz M, Wagner S, Chavan A, et al. Clinical outcome of transfemoral embolisation in patients with arteriovenous malformations of the liver in hereditary haemorrhagic telangiectasia (Weber-Rendu-Osler disease). Gut 1998;42:123–6.

163. Cloogman HM, DiCapo RD. Hereditary hemorrhagic telangiectasia: sonographic findings in the liver. Radiology 1984;1505:521–2.

164. Daly JJ, Schiller AL. The liver in hemorrhagic telangiectasia (Osler-Weber-Rendu disease). Am J Med 1976;60:723–6.

165. Derauf BJ, Hunter DW, Sirr SA, Cardella JF, Castaneda-Zuniga W, Amplatz K. Peripheral embolization of diffuse hepatic arteriovenous malformations in a patient with hereditary hemorrhagic telangiectasia. Caridovasc Intervent Radiol 1987;10:80–3.

166. Fagel WJ, Perlberger R, Kauffmann RH. Portosystemic encephalopathy in hereditary hemorrhagic telangiectasia. Am J Med 1988;85:858–60.

167. Feizi O. Hereditary hemorrhagic telangiectasia presenting with portal hypertension and cirrhosis of the liver. A case report. Gastroenterology 1972;63:660–4.

168. Gothlin JH, Nordgard K, Jonsson K, Nyman U. Hepatic telangiectasia in Osler's disease treated with arterial embolization. Eur J Radiol 1982;2:27–30.

169. Haitjema T, Wastermann CJ, Overtoom TT, et al. Hereditary hemorrhagic telangiectasia (Osler-Weber-Rendu disease). New insights in pathogenesis, complications and treatment. Arch Intern Med 1996;156:714–9.

170. Martini GA. Cirrhosis of the liver in hereditary hemorrhagic telangiectasia. Proceedings of the first world congress of gastroenterology. Baltimore: Williams & Wilkins, 1959:857–8.

171. McAllister KA, Grogg KM, Johnson DW, et al. Endoglin, a TGF-binding protein of endothelial cells, is the gene for hereditary hemorrhagic telangiectasia type 1. Nat Gent 1994;8:345–51.

172. McDonald MT, Papenberg KA, Ghosh S, et al. A disease locus for hereditary hemorrhagic telangiectasia maps to chromosome 9q 33–34. Nat Genet 1994;6:197–204.

173. Mukasa C, Nakamura K, Chijiiwa Y, Sakai H, Nawata H. Liver failure caused by hepatic angiodysplasia in hereditary hemorrhagic telangiectasia. Am J Gastroenterol 1998;93:471–3.

174. Peery WH. Clinical spectrum of hereditary hemorrhagic telangiectasia (Osler–Weber–Rendu disease). Am J Med 1987;82:989–97.

175. Ralls PW, Johnson MB, Radin R, Lee KP, Boswell WD. Hereditary hemorrhagic telangiectasia: findings in the liver with color Doppler sonography. AJR Am J Roentgenol 1992;159:59–61.

176. Reilly PJ, Nostrant TT. Clinical manifestations of hereditary hemorrhagic telangiectasia. Am J Gastroenterol 1984;79:363–7.

177. Saxena R, Hytiroglou P, Atillasoy EO, Cakaloglu Y, Emre S, Thung SN. Coexistence of hereditary hemorrhagic telangiectasia and fibropolycystic liver disease. Am J Surg Pathol 1998;22:368–72.

178. Smith JL, Lineback ML. Hereditary hemorrhagic telangiectasia: 9 cases in one Negro family, with special reference to hepatic lesions. Am J Med 1954;17:41–9.

179. Solis-Herruzo JA, Garcia-Cabezudo J, Santalla-Pecina F, Duran-Aguado A, Olmedo-Camacho J. Laparoscopic findings in hereditary haemorrhagic telangiectasia (Osler-Weber-Rendu disease). Endoscopy 1984;16:137–9.

180. Sussman EB, Sternberg SS. Hereditary hemorrhagic telangiectasia, a case with hepatocellular carcinoma and acquired hepatocerebral degeneration. Arch Pathol 1975;99:95–100.

181. Thomas ML, Carty H. Hereditary hemorrhagic telangiectasia of the liver demonstrated angiographically. Acta Radiol 1974;15:433–8.

182. Vincent P, Plauchu H, Hazan J, Faure S, Weissenbach J, Godet J. A third locus for hereditary haemorrhagic telangiectasia maps to chromosome 12q. Hum Mol Genet 1996;4:945–9.

183. Wanless IR, Gryfe A. Nodular transformation of the liver in hereditary hemorrhagic telangiectasia. Arch Pathol Lab med 1986;110:331–5.

184. Zelman S. Liver fibrosis in hereditary hemorrhagic telangiectasia. Fibrosis of diffuse insular character. Arch Pathol 1962;74:66–72.

Peliosis Hepatis and Bacillary Peliosis

184a. Adal KA, Cockerell CJ, Petri WA Jr. Cat scratch disease, bacillary angiomatosis, and other infections due to Rochalimaea. N Engl J Med 1994;330:1509–15.

185. Bagheri SA, Boyer JL. Peliosis hepatitis associated with androgenic-anabolic steroid therapy. A severe form of hepatic injury. Ann Intern Med 1974;81:610–8.

186. Bird DR, Vowles KD. Liver damage from long-term methyltestosterone. Lancet 1977;2:400–1.

187. Boyer JL. Androgenic-anabolic steroid associated peliosis hepatis in man. A review of 38 reported cases. Adv Pharmacol Therap 1978;8:175–84.

188. Degott C, Rueff B, Kreis H, Duboust A, Potet F, Benhamou JP. Peliosis hepatis in recipients of renal transplants. Gut 1978;19:748–53.

189. Granter SR, Barnhill RL. Bacillary angiomatosis. Adv Pathol Lab Med 1993;6:491–504.

190. Ichijima K, Kobashi Y, Yamabe H, Fuiji Y, Inoue Y. Peliosis hepatis. An unusual case involving multiple organs. Acta Pathol Jpn 1980;30:109–20.

191. Jamadar DA, D'Souza SP, Thomas EA, Giles TE. Case report: radiological appearance in peliosis hepatis. Br J Radiol 1994;67:102–4.

192. Kosek JC, Smith DL. Cytotoxicity of oxymetholone to endothelial cells in vitro. Arch Pathol Lab Med 1980;104:405–8.

193. Larrey D, Freneaux E, Berson A. Peliosis hepatis induced by 6-thioguanine. Gut 1988;29:1265–9.

194. Loomus GN, Aneja P, Bota RA. A case of peliosis hepatis in association with tamoxifen therapy. Am J Clin Pathol 1983;80:881–3.

194a. Makdisi WJ, Cherian R, Vanveldhuizen PJ, Talley RL, Stark SP, Dixon AY. Fatal peliosis of the liver and spleen of a patient with agnogenic myeloid metaplasia treated with danazol. Am J Gastroenterol 1994;90:317–8.

195. Maves CK, Caron KH, Bisset GS III, Agarwal R. Splenic and hepatic peliosis: MR findings. AJR Am J Roentgenol 1992;158:75–6.

196. Nadell J, Kosek J. Peliosis hepatis. Twelve cases associated with oral androgen therapy. Arch Pathol Lab Med 1977;101:405–10.

197. Okuda K, Omata M, Itoh Y, Ikezaki H, Nakashima T. Peliosis hepatis is a late and fatal complication of thorotrast liver disease. Report of five cases. Liver 1981;1:110–22.

198. Paliard P, Valette PJ, Berger F, Contassot JC, Partensky C. Péliose hépatique tardive après traitement dun angiosarcome hépatique chez un sujet exposé au chlorure de vinyl monomére. Gastroenterol Clin Biol 1991;15:445–8.

199. Ross RC, Kovacs K, Horvath E. Ultrastructure of peliosis hepatis in a percutaneous biopsy. Pathol Europ 1972;7:273–82.

200. Selby DM, Stocker JT. Focal peliosis hepatis, a sequela of asphyxial death? Pediatr Pathol Lab Med 1995;15:589–96.

201. Slater LN, Welch DF, Min KW. Rochalimaea henselae causes bacillary angiomatosis and peliosis hepatis. Arch Intern Med 1992;152:602–6.

202. Taxy JB. Peliosis: a morphologic curiosity becomes an iatrogenic problem. Hum Pathol 1978;9:331–40.

203. van Erpecum KJ, Janssens AR, Kreuning J, Ruiter DJ, Kroon HM, Grond AJ. Generalized peliosis hepatis after long–term use of oral contraceptives. Am J Gastroenterol 1988;83:572–5.

204. Zafrani ES, Cazier A, Baudelot AM, Feldmann G. Ultrastructural lesions of the liver in human peliosis. A report of 12 cases. Am J Pathol 1984;114:349–59.

Lymphangioma and Lymphangiomatosis

205. Asch MJ, Cohen AH, Moore TC. Hepatic and splenic lymphangiomatosis with skeletal involvement: report of a case and review of the literature. Surgery 1974;76:334–9.

206. Delamarre J, Lamblin G, Sevestre H, et al. Lymphangiome caverneux du foie. Étude de 2 cas et revue de la littérature. Gastroenterol Clin Biol 1990;14:576–80.

207. Dupuy JP, Catanzano G, Bouchet JB, Le Goff JJ. Le lymphangiome kystique hépato-splénique. Sem Hop 1984;60:2327–30.

208. Haratake J, Koide O, Takeshita H. Hepatic lymphangiomatosis: report of two cases, with an immunohistochemical study. Am J Gastroenterol 1992;87:906–9.

209. Miller C, Mazzaferro V, Makowka L, et al. Orthotopic liver transplantation for massive hepatic lymphangiomatosis. Surgery 1988;103:490–5.

210. O'Sullivan D, Torres VE, De Groen PC, et al. Hepatic lymphangiomatosis mimicking polycystic liver disease. Mayo Clin Proc 1998;73:1188–92.

211. Peters ME, Gilbert-Barness EF, Rao B, Odell GB. Lymphangioendothelioma of the liver in a neonate. J Pediatr Gastroenterol Nutr 1989;9:115–8.

212. Ramani P, Shah A. Lymphangiomatosis. Histologic and immunohistochemical analysis of four cases. Am J Surg Pathol 1993;17:329–35.

213. Sathyavagiswaran L, Sherwin RP. Acute and chronic pericholangiolitis with multifocal hepatic lymphangiomatosis. Hum Pathol 1989;20:601–3.

214. Schmid C, Beham A, Uranus S, et al. Non-systemic diffuse lymphangiomatosis of spleen and liver. Histopathology 1991;18:478–80.

215. van Steenbergen W, Joosten E, Marchal G, et al. Hepatic lymphangiomatosis. Report of a case and review of the literature. Gastroenterology 1985;88:1968–72.

Angiomyolipoma

215a. Ahmadi T, Itai Y, Takahashi M, et al. Angiomyolipoma of the liver: significance of CT and MR dynamic study. Abdomin Imaging 1998;23:620–6.

216. Ben-Izhak O, Groissman G, Lichtig C, et al. Hepatic angiomyolipoma in childhood: association with tuberous sclerosis. Pediatr Pathol Lab Med 1995;15:213–7.

217. Bonetti F, Pea M, Martignoni G, et al. Clear cell ("sugar") tumor of the lung is a lesion strictly related to angiomyolipoma—the concept of a family of lesions characterized by the presence of the perivascular epithelioid cells (PEC). Pathology 1994;26:230–6.

218. Bonetti F, Pea M, Martignoni G, et al. The perivascular epithelioid cell and related lesions. Adv Anat Pathol 1997;4:343–58.

219. Chan JK, Tsang WY, Pari MY, Tang MC, Pang SW, Fletcher CD. Lymphangiomyomatosis and angiomyolipoma: closely related entities characterized by hamartomatous proliferation of HMB-45 positive smooth muscle. Histopathology 1993;22:445–55.

219a. Dalle I, Sciot R, de Vos R, et al. Malignant angiomyolipoma of the liver: a hitherto unreported variant. Histopathology 2000;36:443–50.

220. Fetsch PA, Fetsch JE, Marincola FM, Travis W, Batts KP, Abati A. Comparison of melanoma antigen recognized by T cells (MART-1) to HMB-45: additional evidence to support a common lineage for angiomyolipoma, lymphangiomyomatosis, and clear cell sugar tumor. Mod Pathol 1998;11:699–703.

221. Goodman ZD, Ishak KG. Angiomyolipoma of the liver. Am J Surg Pathol 1984;8:745–50.

222. Henske EP, Ao X, Short P, et al. Frequent progesterone receptor immunoreactivity in tuberous sclerosis-associated renal angiomyolipomas. Mod Pathol 1998;11:665–8.

223. Ishak KG. Mesenchymal tumors of the liver. In: Okuda K, Peters RL, eds. Hepatocellular carcinoma. New York: John Wiley & Sons, 1976:247–307.

224. Kaiserling E, Kröber S, Xiao JC, Schamburg-Lever G. Angiomyolipoma of the kidney. Immunoreactivity with HMB-45. Light- and electron-microscopic findings. Histopathology 1994;25:41–8.

225. Kyokane T, Akita Y, Katayama M, et al. Multiple angiomyolipomas of the liver (case report). Hepatogastroenterology 1995;42:510–5.

226. Miyahara M, Kobayashi M, Tada I, et al. Giant hepatic angiomyolipoma simulating focal nodular hyperplasia. Jap J Surg 1988;18:346–50.

227. Nonomura A, Minato H, Kurumaya H. Angiomyolipoma predominantly composed of smooth muscle cells: problems in histological diagnosis. Histopathology 1998;33:20–7.

228. Nonomura A, Mizukami Y, Kodaya N. Angiomyolipoma of the liver: a collective review. J Gastroenterol 1994;29:95–105.

229. Nonomura A, Mizukami Y, Muraoks K, Yajima M, Oda K. Angiomyolipoma of the liver with pleomorphic histological features. Histopathology 1994;24:279–81.

230. Nonomura A, Mizukami Y, Takayanagi N, et al. Immunohistochemical study of hepatic angiomyolipoma. Pathol Int 1996;46:24–32.

231. Ohmori T, Arita N, Uraga N, et al. Giant hepatic angiomyolipoma. Histopathology 1989;15:540–3.

232. Okada K, Yokoyama S, Nakayama I, Tada I, Kobayashi M. An electron microscopic study of hepatic angiomyolipoma. Acta Pathol Jpn 1989;39:743–9.

233. Pea M, Martignoni G, Zamboni G, et al. Perivascular epithelioid cell [Letter]. Am J Surg Pathol 1996;20:1149–53.

234. Robinson JD, Grant EG, Haller JO, Cohen HL. Hepatic angiomyolipoma in tuberous sclerosis. J Ultrasound Med 1989;8:575–8.

234a. Shintaku M. Hepatic angiomyolipoma with "oncocyte-like" features. Histopathology 1998;33:581–3.

235. Tsui WM, Colombari R, Portmann BC, et al. Hepatic angiomyolipoma: a clinicopathologic study of 30 cases and delineation of unusual morphologic variants. Am J Surg Pathol 1999;23:34–48.

235a. Tsui WM, Yuen AK, Ma KF, Tse H. Hepatic angiomyolipomas with a deceptive trabecular pattern and HMB-45 reactivity. Histopathology 1992;21:569–73.

236. Weeks DA, Chase DR, Malott RL, et al. HMB-45 staining in angiomyolipoma, cardiac rhabdomyoma, other mesenchymal processes, and tuberous sclerosis–associated brain lesions. Int J Surg Pathol 1994;1:191–8.

237. Weeks DA, Malott RL, Arneson M, Zuppan C, Aitken D, Mierau G. Hepatic angiomyolipomas with striated granules and positivity with melanoma-specific antibody (HMB-45): a report of two cases. Ultrastr Pathol 1991;15:563–71.

238. Zamboni G, Pea M, Martignoni G, et al. Clear cell sugar tumor of the pancreas. A novel member of a family of lesions characterized by the presence of perivascular epithelioid cells. Am J Surg Pathol 1996;20:722–30.

Myelolipoma

239. Brietta LK, Watkins D. Giant extra-adrenal myelolipoma. Arch Pathol Lab Med 1994;118:188–90.

240. Dewar G, Leung NW, Ng HK, et al. Massive solitary, intrahepatic, extramedullary hematopoietic tumor in thalassemia. Surgery 1990;107:704–7.

241. Grosdidier J, Boissel P, Macinot C. Myélipome hépatique. A propos dune observation. Nouv Presse Med 1973;2:1777–9.

242. Ishak KG. Mesenchymal tumors of the liver. In Okuda K, Peters RL, eds. Hepatocellular carcinoma. New York: John Wiley & Sons, 1976:247–307.

243. Kaurich JD, Combs RJ, Zeiss J. Myelolipoma of the liver: CT features. J Comput Assist Tomogr 1988;12:660–1.

244. Mali SP, Gratama S, Mulder H. Myelolipoma of the liver. Fortschr Geb Rontgenstr Nulkearmed Erganzungsband 1986;144:610–1.

245. Rubin E, Russinovich NA, Luna RF, Tishler JM, Wilkerson JA. Myelolipoma of the liver. Cancer 1984;54:2043–6.

246. Wiener D, Halvorsen RA, Vollmer RT, Foster WL, Roberts L Jr. Focal intrahepatic extramedullary hematopoiesis mimicking neoplasm. AJR Am J Roentgenol 1987;149:1171–2.

Focal Fatty Change

247. Alpern MB, Lawson TL, Foley WD, et al. Focal hepatic masses and fatty infiltration detected by enhanced dynamic CT. Radiology 1986;158:45–9.

248. Baker ME, Silverman PM. Nodular focal fatty infiltration of the liver: CT appearances. AJR Am J Roentgenol 1985;145:79–80.

249. Bashist B, Hecht HL, Harley WD. Computed tomographic demonstration of rapid changes in fatty infiltration of the liver. Radiology 1982;142:691–2.

250. Battaglia DM, Wanless IR, Brady AP, Mackenzie RL. Intrahepatic sequestered segment of liver presenting as focal fatty change. Am J Gastroenterol 1995;90:2238–9.

251. Brawer MK, Austin GE, Lewin KJ. Focal fatty change of the liver, a hitherto poorly recognized entity. Gastroenterology 1980;78:247–52.

252. Clain JE, Stephens DH, Charboneau JW. Ultrasonography and computed tomography in focal fatty liver. Report of two cases with special emphasis on changing appearances over time. Gastroenterology 1984;87:948–52.

253. Flueckiger F, Steiner H, Leitinger G, Hoedl S, Deu E. Nodular focal fatty infiltration of the liver in acquired porphyria cutanea tarda. Gastrointestest Radiol 1991;16:237–9.

254. Giorgio A, Francica G, Aloisio T, et al. Multifocal fatty infiltration of the liver mimicking metastatic disease. Gastroenterol Int 1991;4:169–72.

255. Grove A, Vyberg B, Vyberg M. Focal fatty change of the liver. A review and a case associated with continuous ambulatory peritoneal dialysis. Virchows Arch [A] 1991;419:69–75.

256. Ishioka T, Shiotsu H, Kuwabara N, et al. A case of focal fatty change of the liver associated with gastric carcinoma. Acta Hepatol Jpn 1986;27:373–6.

257. Kudo M, Ikekubo K, Yamamoto K, et al. Focal fatty infiltration of the liver in acute alcoholic liver injury: hot spots with radiocolloid SPECT scan. Am J Gastroenterol 1989;84:948–52.

258. Livraghi T, Mattoni C, Sangalli G, Vettori C. Focal fatty liver change by sonography. Diagn Imag Clin Med 1984;53:226–30.

259. Quinn SF, Gosink BB. Characteristic sonographic signs of hepatic fatty infiltration. AJR Am J Roentgenol 1985;145:753–5.

260. Simon MA. Focal fat infiltration in the liver. Am J Pathol 1934;10:799–804.

261. Tang-Barton P, Vas W, Weissman J, Salimi Z, Patel R, Morris L. Focal fatty liver lesions in alcoholic liver disease: a broadened spectrum of CT appearances. Gastrointest Radiol 1985;10:133–7.

262. Wanless IR, Bargman JM, Oreopoulos DG, Vas SI. Subcapsular steatonecrosis in response to peritoneal insulin delivery: a clue to the pathogenesis of steatonecrosis in obesity. Mod Pathol 1989;2:69–74.

263. Yoshikawa J, Matsui O, Takashima T, et al. Focal fatty change of the liver adjacent to the falciform ligament: CT and sonographic findings in five surgically confirmed case. AJR Am J Roentgenol 1987;149:491–4.

Pseudolipoma

264. Inoue T, Shiga J, Machinami R. Hepatic pseudolipoma. A hitherto undescribed hyperchoic hepatic nodule. Direct correlation between ultrasonography and histology. Acta Hepatol Jpn 1989;30:1533–6.

265. Ishak KG. Mesenchymal tumors of the liver. In: Okuda K, Peters RL, eds. Hepatocellular carcinoma. New York: John Wiley & Sons, 1976:247–305.

266. Karhunen PJ. Hepatic pseudolipoma. J Clin Pathol 1985;38:877–9.

267. Ramdial PK, Singh B. Membranous fat necrosis in appendices epiploicae. A clinicopathologic study. Virchows Arch 1998;432:223–7.

268. Rolleston H, McNee JW. Diseases of the liver, gall bladder and bile ducts. London: MacMillan, 1929:487.

268a. Watanabe J, Nakashima O, Noguchi K, Kojiro M. Imaging and pathology findings of pseudolipoma in the liver. Hepatol Res 1998;12:225–32.

Leiomyoma

269. Davidoff AM, Hebra A, Clark III BJ, et al. Epstein-Barr virus-associated hepatic smooth muscle neoplasm in a cardiac transplant recipient. Transplantation 1996;61:515–7.

270. Demel R. Ein Operierter Fall von Leber-Myom. Virchows Arch [A] 1926;261:881–4.

271. Hawkins EP, Jordan GL, McGavran MH. Primary leiomyoma of the liver. Successful treatment by lobectomy and presentation of criteria for diagnosis. Am J Surg Pathol 1980;4:301–4.

272. Herzberg AJ, MacDonald JA, Tucker JA, Humphrey PA, Myers WC. Primary leiomyoma of the liver. Am J Gastroenterol 1990;85:1642–5.

273. Ishak KG. Mesenchymal tumors of the liver. In: Okuda K, Peters RL, eds. Hepatocellular carcinoma. New York: John Wiley & Sons, 1976:247–307.

274. Lee ES, Locker J, Nalesnik M, et al. The association of Epstein-Barr virus with smooth-muscle tumors occurring after organ transplantation. N Engl J Med 1995;332:19–25.

275. McClain KL, Leach CT, Jenson HB, et al. Association of Epstein-Barr virus with leiomyosarcomas in young people with AIDS. N Engl J Med 1995;332:12–8.

276. Reinertson TE, Fortune JB, Peters JC, Pagnotta I, Balint JA. Primary leiomyoma of the liver. A case report and review of the literature. Dig Dis Sci 1992;37:622–7.

277. Rios-Dalenz JL. Leiomyoma of the liver. Arch Pathol 1965;79:54–6.

277a. Yoon GS, Kang GH, Kim OJ. Primary myxoid leiomyoma of the liver. Arch Pathol Lab Med 1998;122:1112–5.

Solitary Fibrous Tumor

278. Barnoud R, Arvieux C, Pasquier D, Pasquier B, Letoublon C. Solitary fibrous tumour of the liver with CD34 expression. Histopathology 1996;28:551–4.

279. Chan JK. Solitary fibrous—everywhere, and a diagnosis in vogue. Histopathology 1997;31:568–76.

280. Dervan PA, Tobin B, O'Connor M. Solitary (localized) fibrous mesothelioma: evidence against mesothelial cell origin. Histopathology 1986;10:867–75.

281. Edmondson HA. Tumors of the liver and intrahepatic bile ducts. Atlas of Tumor Pathology, Section VII, Fascicle 25. Washington, D.C., Armed Forces Institute of Pathology, 1958.

282. El-Naggar AK, Ro JY, Ayala AG, Ward R, Ordonez NG. Localized fibrous tumor of the serosal surfaces. Immunohistochemical, electron-microscopic, and flow-cytometric DNA study. Am J Clin Pathol 1989;92:561–5.

283. Flint A, Weiss SW. CD-34 and keratin expression distinguishes solitary fibrous tumor (fibrous mesothelioma) of pleura from desmoplastic mesothelioma. Hum Pathol 1995;26:428–31.

284. Ishak KG. Mesenchymal tumors of the liver. In: Okuda K, Peters RL, eds. Hepatocellular carcinoma. New York: John Wiley & Sons, 1976:247–307.

285. Kasano Y, Tanimura H, Tabuse K, Nagai Y, Mori K, Minami K. Giant fibrous mesothelioma of the liver. Am J Gastroenterol 1991;86:379–80.

286. Kim H, Damjanov I. Localized fibrous mesothelioma of the liver. Report of a giant tumor studied by light and electron microscopy. Cancer 1983;52:1662–5.

287. Kottke-Marchant K, Hart W, Broughan T. Localized fibrous tumor (localized fibrous mesothelioma) of the liver. Cancer 1989;64:1096–102.

288. Middleton LP, Duray PH, Merino MJ. The histological spectrum of hemangiopericytoma: application of immunohistochemical analysis including proliferation markers to facilitate diagnosis and predict prognosis. Hum Pathol 1998;29:636–40.

289. Miettinen MM, El-Refai W, Sarlomo-Rikala M, et al. Tumor-size-related DNA copy number changes occur in solitary fibrous tumors but not in hemangiopericytomas. Mod Pathol 1997;10:1194–200.

290. Moran CA, Ishak KG, Goodman ZG. Solitary fibrous tumor of the liver: a clinicopathologic and immunohistochemical study of nine cases. Ann Diagn Pathol 1998;2:19–24.

291. Nevius DB, Friedman NB. Mesotheliomas and extraovarian thecomas with hypoglycemia and nephrotic syndromes. Cancer 1956;12:1263–9.

292. Nielsen GP, O'Connell JX, Dickersin GR, Rosenberg AE. Solitary fibrous tumor of soft tissue: a report of 15 cases, including 5 malignant examples with light microscopic, immunohistochemical, and ultrastructural data. Mod Pathol 1997;10:1028–37.

293. Weitzner S. Primary hemangiopericytoma of the liver associated with hypoglycemia. Report of a case. Dig Dis 1970;15:673–8.

294. Yokoi T, Tsuzuki T, Yatabe Y, et al. Solitary fibrous tumour: significance of P53 and CD 34 immunoreactivity in its malignant transformation. Histopathology 1998;32:423–32.

Langerhans' Cell Histiocytosis

295. Bonetti F, Chilosi M, Menestrina F, et at. Immunohistochemical analysis of Rosai-Dorfman histiocytosis. A disease of S-100-CD1-histiocytes. Virchows Arch [A] 1987;411:129–35.

295a. Cavazza A, Pasquinelli G, Carlinfante G, Cenini E, Bonvicini U, Gardini G. Nodular Langerhans cell histiocytosis of the liver in an adult with colonic adenocarcinoma. Histopathology 1999;34:273–5.

296. Emile JG, Wechsler J, Brousse N, et al. Langerhans' cell histiocytosis: definitive diagnosis with the use of monoclonal antibody 010 on routinely paraffin-embedded samples. Am J Surg Pathol 1995;6:636–41.

297. Foucar E, Rosai J, Dorfman R. Sinus histiocytosis with massive lymphadenopathy (Rosai-Dorfman disease): review of an entity. Semin Diagn Pathol 1990;7:19–73.

297a. Howarth DM, Gilchrist GS, Mullan BP, Wiseman GA, Edmonson JH, Schumberg PJ. Langerhans cell histiocytosis. Diagnosis, natural history, management, and outcome. Cancer 1999;85:2278–90.

298. Kaplan KJ, Goodman ZD, Ishak KG. Liver involvement in Langerhans cell histiocytosis. A study of nine cases. Mod Pathol 1999;12:370–8.

298a. Kawakubo Y, Kishimoto H, Sato Y, et al. Human cytomegalovirus infection in foci of Langerhans cell histiocytosis. Virchows Arch 1999;434:109–15.

299. Krenacs L, Tiszaluicz L, Krenacs T, Boumsell L. Immunohistochemical detection of CD1a antigen in formalin-fixed and paraffin-embedded tissue sections with monoclonal antibody 010. J Pathol 1993;171:99–104.

300. Lieberman PH, Jones CR, Steinman RM, et al. Langerhans cell (eosinophilic) granulomatosis: a clinicopathologic study encompassing 50 years. Am J Surg Pathol 1996;20:519–22.

301. Willman CL, Busque L, Griffith BB. Langerhans' cell histiocytosis (histiocytosis X)—a clonal proliferative disease. N Engl J Med 1994;331:154–60.

Inflammatory Pseudotumor

302. Anthony PP. Inflammatory pseudotumour (plasma cell granuloma) of lung, liver and other organs. Histopathology 1993;23:501–3.

303. Anthony PP, Telesinghe PU. Inflammatory pseudotumour of the liver. J Clin Pathol 1986;39:761–8.

304. Arber DA, Kamel OW, van de Rijn M, et al. Frequent presence of Epstein-Barr virus in inflammatory pseudotumor. Hum Pathol 1995;26:1093–8.

305. Arber DA, Weiss LM, Chang KL. Detection of Epstein-Barr virus in inflammatory pseudotumor. Sem Diagn Pathol 1998;15:155–60.

306. Broughan TA, Fischer WL, Tuthill RJ. Vascular invasion by hepatic inflammatory pseudotumor. Cancer 1993;71:2934–40.

307. Chen KT. Inflammatory pseudotumor of the liver. Hum Pathol 1984;15:694–6.

308. Coffin CM, Watterson J, Priest JR, Dehner LP. Extrapulmonary myofibroblastic tumor (inflammatory pseudotumor). A clinicopathologic and immunohistochemical study of 84 cases. Am J Surg Pathol 1995;19:859–72.

309. Devaney K, Goodman ZD, Epstein MS, Zimmerman HJ, Ishak KG. Hepatic sarcoidosis. Clinicopathologic features in 100 patients. Am J Surg Pathol 1993;17:1272–80.

310. Donner LR, Trompler RA, White R. Progression of inflammatory myofibroblastic tumor (inflammatory pseudotumor) of soft tissue into sarcoma after several recurrences. Hum Pathol 1996;27:1095–8.

5

MISCELLANEOUS BENIGN TUMORS AND PSEUDOTUMORS

TERATOMA

Definition. Teratoma of the liver is a rare benign neoplasm composed of tissues of mesodermal, ectodermal, and endodermal origin.

Clinical Features. Fewer than 30 cases of teratoma of the liver have been reported, with the majority occurring in children, often at birth or in the first year of life (2,9,11,13). Winter and Freeny (12), however, described a slowly progressive lesion in a 44-year-old woman whom they followed for 17 years. There is a female predominance, and the lesion usually presents as an abdominal mass. Conditions associated with hepatic teratomas include anencephaly (8), trisomy 13 (2), and a previous history of ovarian dysgerminoma (11), ruptured mature cystic teratoma (3), or immature ovarian teratoma (1). The occurrence of hepatic teratoma in older patients following the resection of an ovarian dysgerminoma or immature teratoma, or rupture of a mature ovarian teratoma, suggests a possible "seeding" of the tumor (3) or "maturation" or "transformation" of tissue from the first malignancy, rather than a "true" teratoma as seen in infants (1,11).

Most patients present with an abdominal mass. Ultrasound shows a mixed echogenic pattern with areas of intense echogenicity reflecting the calcification and ossification present in the lesion (4). Alpha-fetoprotein may be elevated in some patients reflecting immature elements in the lesion (10). Care must be taken to consider the normal alpha-fetoprotein level of infants which at birth may be in the range of 25 to 50,000 ng/ml and not fall to "adult" levels of less than 25 ng/ml until 6 months of age (5). Resection may be curative although large size is associated with a high morbidity and mortality rate (2,6,7,12,13).

Gross Findings. Teratomas of the liver may be large (up to 20 cm and 500 g) (9) and involve either or both lobes (fig. 5-1). They may vary from soft to firm and solid to cystic depending on the component tissues. Areas of hemorrhage and necrosis may be present and the lesion may have a fibrous capsule (13).

Microscopic Findings. The component tissues reflect all three germ cell layers: ectoderm, mesoderm, and endoderm (fig. 5-2). Features seen with some consistency include areas of well-differentiated squamous cell epithelium, gastrointestinal mucosa and smooth muscle wall, respiratory epithelium and associated cartilage plates, renal glomeruli and tubules, skeletal muscle, fatty tissue, bone, nerve trunks, and primitive neural tissue (figs. 5-3–5-5). Less frequently seen are pancreatic acini, teeth, and hair (9). Watanabe and colleagues (11) noted the presence of normal hepatic tissue with extramedullary hematopoiesis within the teratoma. The presence of areas of hepatoblastoma within or adjacent to the other tissues is diagnostic of a teratoid hepatoblastoma rather than a teratoma (see chapter 6). Osteoid-like material, cartilage, primitive mesenchyme, and fibrous tissue are components frequently seen in mixed (epithelial and mesenchymal) hepatoblastoma.

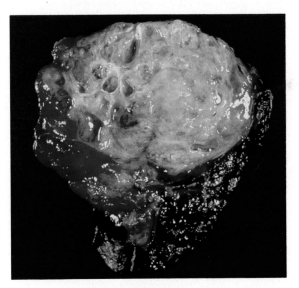

Figure 5-1
TERATOMA
Multiple cystic structures are intermixed with solid and gelatinous tissue in this section of teratoma from a 1-year-old male.

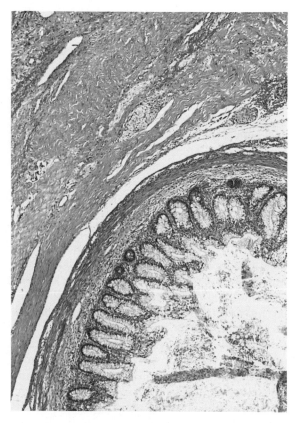

Figure 5-2
TERATOMA

One of the cystic structures from the lesion in figure 5-1 consists of a well-differentiated section of colon with an intact mucosa, submucosa, and muscular wall.

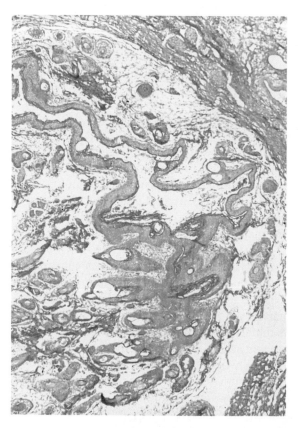

Figure 5-3
TERATOMA

Ribbons of cornified, stratified, squamous epithelium surround loose connective tissue containing adnexal structures.

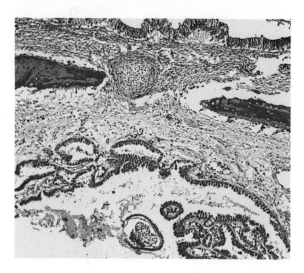

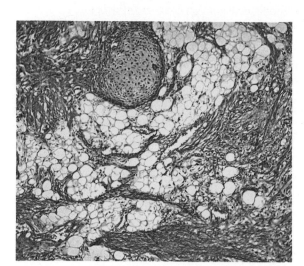

Figure 5-4
TERATOMA

Left: Mesenchymally derived components including mature cartilage plates lie adjacent to slit-like spaces lined by respiratory epithelium (ciliated pseudostratified columnar epithelium).

Right: Cartilage plates are adjacent to fat and smooth muscle.

PRIMARY HEPATIC PREGNANCY

Definition. Implantation of a fertilized ovum on the surface of the liver may lead to the formation of a placenta and growth of the embryo. While the pregnancy may rarely result in a liveborn fetus, more frequently, bleeding occurs leading to an acute hemoperitoneum.

Clinical Features. Approximately 1 percent of all pregnancies result in implantation of the conceptus outside the uterine cavity; the vast majority (95 to 97 percent) implant in the fallopian tube, with most of the remaining on the ovary, cervix, or peritoneal cavity (15). Only rarely do they occur in the vagina, liver, or spleen (14). Fewer than a dozen cases of hepatic pregnancy have been reported in the past 30 years (14,16–23).

Women with hepatic implantation usually present with acute abdominal pain as a result of bleeding from the implantation site (14). Diagnosis may be difficult since pregnancy may not be suspected. Most ectopic hepatic pregnancies are detected in the first trimester and resected because of abdominal bleeding, although birth by laparotomy of a 1,300 g liveborn infant has been reported (22).

Gross and Microscopic Findings. Most implantation sites are on the surface of the right lobe of the liver and vary in size according to the gestational age (fig. 5-6) (14,17,23). Hemorrhage

may be prominent at the implantation site (fig. 5-7) and simple oversewing of the hemorrhagic area after removal of the embryo/fetus may be sufficient treatment (18), although lobectomy may be required to control bleeding (16). In cases in which the placental tissue is not removed, treatment with methotrexate has been used to inactivate the trophoblastic tissue (19). Microscopically, when the implantation site is resected,

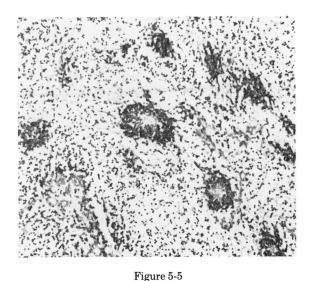

Figure 5-5
TERATOMA
Immature neural tissue contains clusters of neuroblast-like cells.

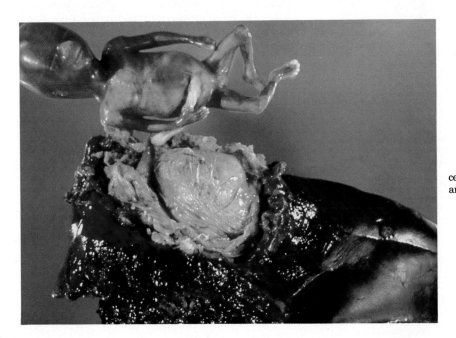

Figure 5-6
HEPATIC PREGNANCY
The fetus is attached to the placenta (embedded in the liver) by an umbilical cord.

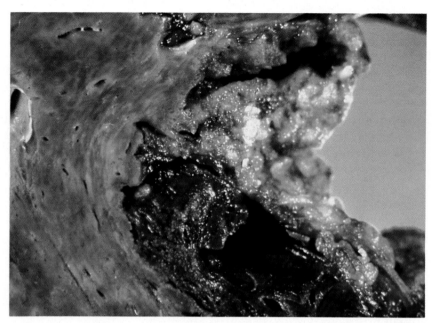

Figure 5-7
HEPATIC PREGNANCY
Area of hemorrhage at the implantation site.

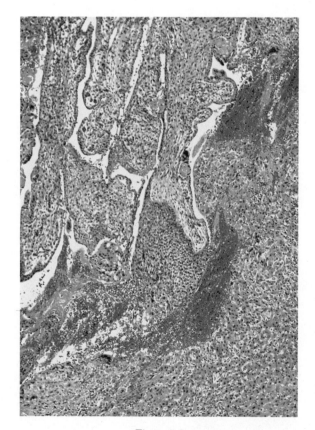

Figure 5-8
HEPATIC PREGNANCY PLACENTAL
VILLI AND ADJACENT LIVER

chorionic villi and trophoblastic cells infiltrate the hepatic parenchyma in the area immediately adjacent to the implantation site (fig. 5-8) (23).

HEPATIC ECTOPIA AND HETEROTOPIC TISSUES WITHIN OR FUSED TO THE LIVER

Definition. Hepatic ectopia consists of hepatic parenchyma not contiguous with the liver. Heterotopias are tissues of nonhepatic origin found partially "fused" to or entirely within the liver.

Clinical Features. With the exception of large masses or functioning tissue, heterotopic tissues within the liver are often incidental findings at surgery or autopsy.

Gross and Microscopic Findings. Fusion may occur between the liver and the adrenal gland, pancreas, or spleen (29,30,33). Tissues that may be found entirely within the liver include adrenal, pancreas, spleen, thyroid, and celomic fat (25,26, 34,37,39,40,47–49). Adreno-hepatic fusion has been described in nearly 10 percent of 636 autopsies reported by Honma (33). The incidence increases with age and is not associated with the pathologic conditions of either organ (30,33). A case on file at the Armed Forces Institute of Pathology (AFIP) is illustrated in figure 5-9. Fusion of the liver with the spleen or pancreas is extremely rare (29), although Lacerda and colleagues (34) found a

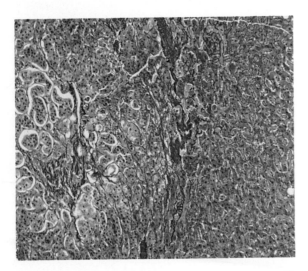

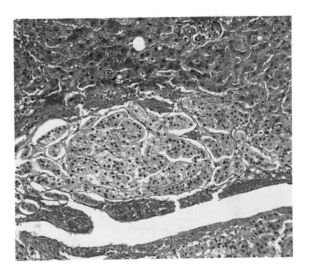

Figure 5-9
HEPATOADRENAL FUSION
Left: Adrenal cortex (left) is clearly demarcated from the liver (right).
Right: Higher magnification shows the lightly stained adrenal cortical cells and the smaller and darker liver cells.

6.2 cm mass of splenic tissue entirely within the liver. Intrahepatic pancreatic tissue has been reported rarely (figs. 5-10, 5-11) (37,39,42). The presence of microscopic foci of exocrine pancreatic tissue in the liver of 41-year-old patient with cirrhosis led Wolf et al. (50) to suggest pancreatic metaplasia rather than a true heterotopia.

Hepatic tissue may be found in the thorax as an extension of the liver through the diaphragm (38,41,43). Hepatic parenchyma not contiguous with the liver may also occur in other sites including the thorax, lung, splenic capsule, adrenal gland, pancreas, abdominal wall, gallbladder, esophago-gastric junction, omphalocele sac, placenta, and retroperitoneum (24,27,28,31,32, 35,36,44–46,48). This ectopic liver tissue may show the same pathologic changes (e.g., cirrhosis) that affect the liver and is prone to hepatocarcinogenesis (24,35).

Portions of liver may also be found in the thorax either as a separate structure or as a mass with a thin pedicle extending through the diaphragm (38,41,46). Mendoza and colleagues (36) noted an isolated nodule of liver within the lung of an infant with multiple cardiac anomalies. Shapiro and Metlay (44) reported another infant with cardiac anomalies and a supradiaphragmatic liver nodule. Shah and colleagues (43) described an infant with a diaphragmatic hernia who had an infantile hemangioendothelioma within an intrathoracic

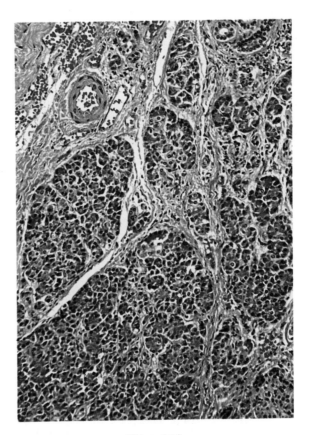

Figure 5-10
HETEROTOPIC PANCREAS IN LIVER
Pancreatic acinar tissue with no islets or ducts. Note the portal area in upper right corner.

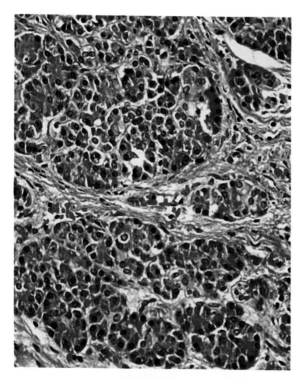

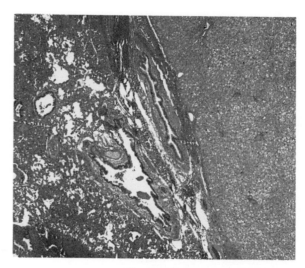

Figure 5-13
ECTOPIC LIVER IN AN
EXTRALOBAR PULMONARY SEQUESTRATION
Pulmonary parenchyma with a bronchus (center) abuts a nodule of hepatic parenchyma (right). (Courtesy of Dr. Liliane Boccon-Gibod, Paris, France.)

Figure 5-11
HETEROTOPIC PANCREAS IN LIVER
High magnification of pancreatic acinar tissue.

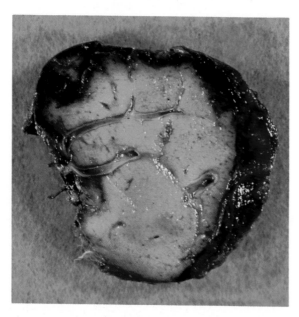

Figure 5-12
ECTOPIC LIVER IN AN
EXTRALOBAR PULMONARY SEQUESTRATION
Pale tan hepatic parenchyma is surrounded by deep red pulmonary parenchyma in a left-sided extralobar sequestration in an infant with a left-sided diaphragmatic hernia. (Courtesy of Dr. Liliane Boccon-Gibod, France.)

liver mass that was connected by a thin pedicle to the normal liver in the abdomen. Hepatic parenchyma has also been noted within an extralobar sequestration which lay between the liver and the left lower lobe of the lung in a newborn female with a diaphragmatic hernia (figs. 5-12, 5-13). Hepatic tissue may also be found within omphalocele sacs as separate structures or as extensions from the normal liver (31). Heterotopic hepatic tissue has been reported in the wall of the gallbladder (26,43). Buck and Koss (28) noted the presence of a 1.5 cm nodule of hepatic tissue within the right adrenal gland of an 8-year-old girl.

ADRENAL REST TUMORS

Definition. Adrenal rests are heterotopic adrenocortical cells within the capsule of the liver, excluding portions of the adrenal gland as a result of hepatoadrenal fusion or metastasis from a primary adrenal gland neoplasm (52). Diagnosis requires proof of steroid hormone production or excretion.

Clinical Features. Localized collections of adrenocortical tissue occasionally occur outside of the adrenal gland, most frequently in abdominal and pelvic sites. Rarely, these rests may be present in the liver and secrete adrenocorticosteroids,

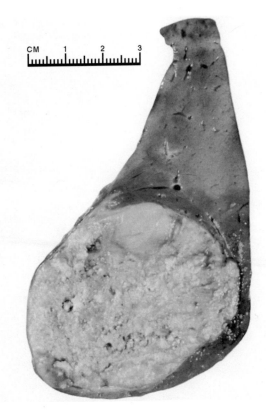

Figure 5-14
ADRENAL REST TUMOR
This cut surface of a large adrenocortical tumor arising in the liver shows abundant calcification within the encapsulated gray-yellow tumor. (Figure 130 from Fascicle 26, 2nd Series.)

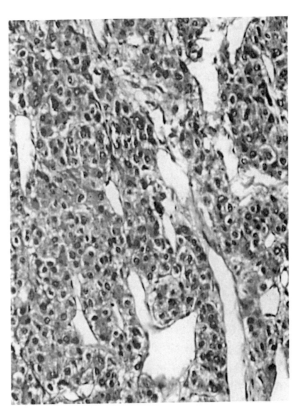

Figure 5-15
ADRENAL REST TUMOR
A trabecular pattern of growth is present with cords of cells separated by vascular channels lined by endothelial cells. (Figure 133 from Fascicle 26, 2nd Series).

resulting in features of Cushing's syndrome and, in women, virilization. Only five cases of functioning adrenal rest tumors have been reported up to 1998 (51,52,54).

Corticosteroid-producing adrenal rest tumors result in the features of Cushing's syndrome, including acne, amenorrhea, central obesity, diffuse scalp hair loss, fatigue, hirsutism, moon facies, muscle weakness, striae of the skin, and weight gain. Serum and urinary cortisol levels are elevated along with other steroid hormones associated with hypercortisolism (51,55). Patient ages range from 17 months to 23 years (53,55). Imaging studies including ultrasound, computed tomography (CT) and arteriography may reveal hepatomegaly or a mass within the liver, with or without calcification. Surgical resection of the tumor in a 21-year-old woman with no recurrence of hormonal activity (for a limited period of months) was reported by Contreras and colleagues (51).

Gross Findings. The tumors may be lobulated and encapsulated (fig. 5-14). Contreras and colleagues (51) described a 450 g tumor of the right lobe whose cut surface was "reminiscent of normal adrenal cortex." Wallace et al. (55) reported a 2,650 g, multilobulated, grayish white mass that extended from the right lobe into the left.

Microscopic Findings. The tumors are composed of cord-like arrangements of round to polygonal cells separated by vascular channels or bands of collagen (figs. 5-15, 5-16). The tumor cells vary in size and contain round to oval nuclei, occasionally multiple, with loose to dense chromatin, but no nucleoli (fig. 5-17). Marked pleomorphism may be noted, with the cytoplasm varying from finely granular to clear. While the tumor may appear encapsulated in some areas, infiltration of normal parenchyma at the margin of the tumor may be present along with areas of entrapped hepatocytes within the main mass.

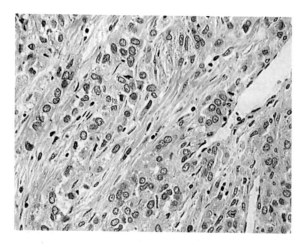

Figure 5-16
ADRENAL REST TUMOR
Fibrous strands separate columns of polygonal cells.
(Figure 134A from Fascicle 26, 2nd Series.)

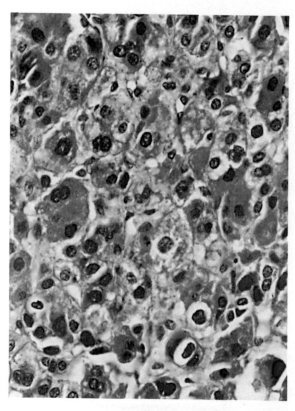

Figure 5-17
ADRENAL REST TUMOR
Tumor cells display anisocytosis and hyperchromasia.
The cytoplasm is finely granular and nucleoli are absent.
(Figure 132 from Fascicle 26, 2nd Series.)

Contreras and colleagues (51) noted "a piece of ectopic, otherwise normal adrenal cortex" adjacent to, but separated from, the tumor by a thin fibrous capsule.

RIEDEL'S LOBE
AND ACCESSORY LOBES

Riedel's lobe is a tongue-like caudal projection from the right lobe of the liver which may be palpated in the right upper quadrant. In the series of 31 cases reported by Reitemeier et al. (62) all the patients except 1 were women, their ages ranging from 31 to 77 years. Supernumerary lobes are relatively frequent findings, particularly on the inferior surface of the liver. They are connected to the liver by hepatic tissue or by a mesentery containing branches of the portal vein, hepatic vein and hepatic artery, and a bile duct (57). Intrathoracic accessory lobes, with their vascular supply perforating the diaphragm, have been reported (59,60). Accessory lobes may occasionally require surgical intervention because of their large size, torsion of a pedicle, or the presence of other associated defects (58,61). Radiographically, such cases may mimic intramural gastric or perigastric masses (56). A case of an accessory lobe on file at the AFIP is illustrated in figures 5-18 and 5-19.

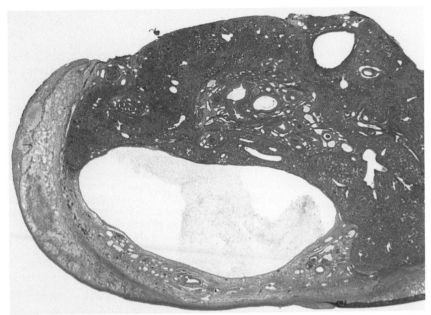

Figure 5-18
ACCESSORY LOBE
The lobe is surrounded by a layer of mesothelial cells and contains portal areas of varied size, a cyst, and hepatic parenchyma (Masson trichrome stain).

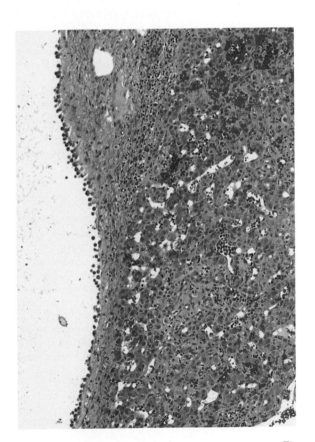

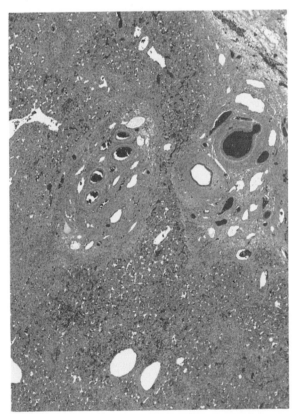

Figure 5-19
ACCESSORY LOBE
Left: Part of the large cyst is lined by mesothelial cells. The adjacent hepatic parenchyma shows a small portal area and dilated sinusoids containing hematopoietic cells.
Right: Two portal areas are surrounded by hepatic parenchyma.

REFERENCES

Teratoma

1. Caldas C, Sitzmann J, Trimble CL, McGuire WP. Synchronous mature teratomas of the ovary and liver: a case presenting 11 years following chemotherapy for immature teratoma. Gynecol Oncol 1992;47:385–90.
2. Dische MR, Gardner HA. Mixed teratoid tumors of the liver and neck and trisomy 13. Am J Clin Pathol 1978;69:631–7.
3. Kommoss F, Emond J, Hast J, Talerman A. Ruptured mature cystic teratoma of the ovary with recurrence in the liver and colon 17 years later. A case report. J Reprod Med 1990;35:827–31.
4. Kraudel K, Williams CH. Ultrasound case report of hepatic teratoma in newborn. J Clin Ultrasound 1984;12:89–101.
5. Novak D, Suchy F, Balistreri W. Disorders of the liver and biliary system relevant to clinical practice. In: Oski F, ed. Principles and practice of pediatrics. Philadelphia: JB Lippincott 1990:1746–77.
6. Pear BL, Boline JE. Teratoma of the liver. Cancer Sem 1972;4:229–33.
7. Rao PL, Venkatesh A, Murthy VS. Cystic teratoma in the bare area of liver. Indian J Pediatr 1987;54:275–8.
8. Robinson RA, Nelson L. Hepatic teratoma in an anencephalic fetus. Arch Pathol Lab Med 1986;110:655–7.
9. Stocker JT. Hepatic tumors. In: Balistreri WF, Stocker JT, eds. Pediatric hepatology. New York: Hemisphere Publishing, 1990;399–488.
10. Todani T, Tabuchi K, Watanabe Y, Tsutsumi A. True hepatic teratoma with high alpha fetoprotein in serum. J Pediatr Surg 1977:12:591–2.
11. Watanabe I, Kasai M, Suzuki S. True teratoma of the liver– report of a case and review of the literature. Acta Hepatogastroenterol 1978;25:40–4.
12. Winter TC III, Freeny P. Hepatic teratoma in an adult. Case report with a review of the literature. J Clin Gastroenterol 1993;17:308–10.
13. Witte DP, Kissane JM, Askin FB. Hepatic teratomas in children. Pediatr Pathol 1983;1:81–92.

Primary Hepatic Pregnancy

14. Borlum KG, Blom R. Primary hepatic pregnancy. Int J Gynaecol Obstet 1988;27:427–9.
15. Fox H, Buckley CH. The female genital tract and ovaries. In: McGee JO, Isaacson PG, Wright NA, eds. Oxford textbook of pathology, vol 2a. Oxford: Oxford University Press, 1992:1635–6.
16. Harris GJ, Al-Jurf AS, Yuh WT, Abu-Yousef MM. Intrahepatic pregnancy. A unique opportunity for evaluation with sonography, computed tomography, and magnetic resonance imaging. JAMA 1989;261:902–4.
17. Hietala SO, Andersson M, Emdin SO. Ectopic pregnancy in the liver. Report of a case and angiographic findings. Acta Chir Scand 1983;149:633–5.
18. Mitchell RW, Teare AJ. Primary hepatic pregnancy. A case report and review. S Afr Med J 1984;65:220.
19. Nichols C, Koong D, Faulkner K, Thompson G. A hepatic ectopic pregnancy treated with direct methotrexate injection. Aust N Z J Obstet Gynaecol 1995;35:221–3.
20. Paulino-Netto A, Roselli A. Hepatic ectopic pregnancy: successful surgical treatment of a patient with hepatic pregnancy and acute hemorrhage. Mt Sinai J Med 1986;53:514–7.
21. Pollice L, Pagliarulo G. Primary hepatic infantile hemangioendothelioma (author's transl). Tumori 1975;61:565–74.
22. Shukla VK, Pandey S, Pandey LK, et al. Primary hepatic pregnancy. Postgrad Med J 1985;61:831–2.
23. Veress B, Wallmander T. Primary hepatic pregnancy. Acta Obstet Gynecol Scand 1987;66:563–4.

Hepatic Ectopia and Heterotopic Tissues Within or Fused to the Liver

24. Arakawa M, Kimura Y, Sakata K, Kubo Y, Fukushima T, Okuda K. Propensity of ectopic liver to hepatocarcinogenesis: case reports and a review of the literature. Hepatology 1999;29:57–61.
25. Ballinger J. Hypoglycemia from metastasizing insular carcinoma of aberrant pancreatic tissue in the liver. Arch Pathol 1941;32:277–85.
26. Barbosa JJ, Dockerty MB, Waugh JM. Pancreatic heterotopia. Surg Gynecol Obstet 1946;82:527–41.
27. Boyle L, Gallivan MV, Chun B, Lack EE. Heterotopia of gastric mucosa and liver involving the gallbladder. Report of two cases with literature review. Arch Pathol Lab Med 1992;116:138–42.
28. Buck FS, Koss MN. Heterotopic liver in an adrenal gland. Pediatr Pathol 1988;8:535–40.
29. Cotelingam JD, Saito R. Hepatoadrenal fusion: case report of an unusual lesion. Hum Pathol 1978;9:234–6.
30. Dolan MF, Janovski NA. Adreno-hepatic union. Arch Pathol 1968;86:22–4.
31. Fock G. Ectopic liver in omphalocele. Acta Paediatrica 1963;52:288–92.
32. Heid J, GJ, von Haam E. Hepatic heterotopy in the splenic capsule. Arch Pathol 1948;46:377–79.
33. Honma K. Adreno-hepatic fusion. An autopsy study. Zentralbl Pathol 1991;137:117–22.
34. Lacerda MA, Ludwig J, Ward EM. Intrahepatic spleen presenting as a mass lesion. Am J Gastroenterol 1993;88:2116–7.
35. Le Bail B, Carles J, Saric J, et al. Ectopic liver and hepatocarcinogenesis [letter]. Hepatology 1999;30:284–5.
36. Mendoza A, Voland J, Wolf P, Benirschke K. Supradiaphragmatic liver in the lung. Arch Pathol Lab Med 1986;110:1085–6.
37. Mobini J, Krouse TB, Cooper DR. Intrahepatic pancreatic heterotopia. Review and report of a case presenting as an abdominal mass. Am J Digest Dis 1974;19:64–70.
38. Naganuma H, Ishida H, Niizawa M, Morikawa P, Masamune O, Kato T. Intrathoracic accessory lobe of the liver. J Clin Ultrasound 1993;21:143–6.
39. Nebel OT, Farrell RL, Kirchner JP, Macionus RF. Aberrant pancreas—an endoscopic diagnosis. Am J Gastroenterol 1973;60:295–300.

40. Nickels J, Laasonen EM. Pancreatic heterotopia. Scand J Gastroenterol 1970;5:639–40.

41. Rendina EA, Ventura F, Pescarmona EO, et al. Intrathoracic lobe of the liver. Case report and review of the literature. Eur J Cardiothorac Surg 1989;3:75–8.

42. Schaefer B, Meyer G, Arnholdt H, Hohlbach G. Heterotope Pankreaspseudocyste in der leber. Chirurg 1989;60:556–8.

43. Shah KD, Beck AR, Jhaveri MK, et al. Infantile hemangioendothelioma of heterotopic intrathoracic liver associated with diaphragmatic hernia. Hum Pathol 1987;18:754–6.

44. Shapiro JL, Metlay LA. Heterotopic supradiaphragmatic liver formation in association with congenital cardiac anomalies. Arch Pathol Lab Med 1991;115:238–40.

45. Tejada E, Danielson C. Ectopic or heterotopic liver (choristoma) associated with the gallbladder. Arch Pathol Lab Med 1989;113:950–2.

46. Vercelli-Retta J. Fetal supradiaphragmatic accessory liver lobe. Report of a case and review of the literature. Virchows Arch [A] 1978;378:259–63.

47. Weller CV. Heterotopia of adrenal in liver and kidney. Am J Med Sci 1925;169:696–712.

48. Wheeler DA, Edmondson HA. Coelomic fat ectopia in the liver. Arch Pathol Lab Med 1985;109:783–5.

49. Willis RA. Some unusual developmental heterotopias. Br Med J 1968;3:267–72.

50. Wolf HK, Burshette JL Jr, Garcia JA, Michalopoulos G. Exocrine pancreatic tissue in human liver: a metaplastic process? Am J Surg Pathol 1990;14:590–5.

Adrenal Rest Tumors

51. Contreras P, Altieri E, Liberman C, et al. Adrenal rest tumor of the liver causing Cushing's syndrome: treatment with ketoconazole preceding an apparent surgical cure. J Clin Endocrinol Metab 1985;60:21–8.

52. Edmondson HA. Tumors of the liver and intrahepatic bile ducts. Atlas of Tumor Pathology. 1st Series, Fascicle 25. Washington, D.C.: Armed Forces Institute of Pathology, 1958:195–211.

53. Mason JB, Speese J. Tumor of liver of adrenal origin. Ann Surg 1933;97:150–3.

54. Miyazaki I, Shimizu K. Adrenal rest tumor of the liver. Ryoikibetsu Shokogun Shirizu 1995;7:285–7.

55. Wallace EZ, Leonidas JR, Stanek AE, Avramides A. Endocrine studies in a patient with functioning adrenal rest tumor of the liver. Am J Med 1981;70:1122–5.

Accessory Lobes

56. Battle WM, Laufer I, Moldofsky PJ, Trotman BW. Anomalous liver lobulations as a cause of perigastric masses. Am J Dig Dis 1979;24:65-9.

57. Cullen TS. Accessory lobes of the liver. Arch Surg 1925;11:718–64.

58. Johnstone G. Accessory lobe of liver presenting through a congenital deficiency of anterior abdominal wall. Arch Dis Child 1965;40:541–4.

59. Hansbrough ET, Lipin RJ. Intrathoracic accessory lobe of the liver. Ann Surg 1957;145:564-7.

60. Naganuma H, Ishida H, Niizawa M, Morikawa P, Masamune O, Kato T. Intrathoracic accessory lobes of the liver. J Clin Ultrasound 1993;21:143–6.

61. Peter H, Strohm WD. Torquierter akzessorischer Leberlappen als Ursache eines akuten abdomens. Leber Magen Darm 1980;4:203–6.

62. Reitemeier RJ, Butt HR, Baggenstoss AH. Riedel's lobe of the liver. Gastroenterology 1958;34:1090–5.

6

HEPATOBLASTOMA

Definition. Hepatoblastoma is the most frequent liver tumor in children. It mimics the developing fetal or embryonal liver and displays a variety of cell types and histologic patterns ranging from anaplastic and embryonal cells, to cells resembling immature hepatocytes, to heterotopic differentiated tissues including osteoid, striated muscle fibers, and squamous epithelium.

Clinical Features. The annual incidence of hepatic malignancies in children 0 to 14 years of age is approximately 0.2/100,000 children in the United States; hepatoblastomas account for 47 percent of the malignancies and nearly 27 percent of all pediatric hepatic tumors (113). By age group, hepatoblastoma accounts for 1.5 percent of all malignancies in children under 5 years of age and 3.3 percent of all malignancies in white and black children under 1 year of age (95).

Nearly 90 percent of hepatoblastomas are seen in the first 5 years of life, with 68 percent presenting in the first 2 years and 4 percent present at birth. The relative frequency of hepatoblastoma in younger children is most apparent when noting that this tumor accounts for over 40 percent of all hepatic tumors (benign and malignant) in children under 2 years of age, but only 7.5 percent of liver tumors in children 5 to 20 years old (113). In Japan, Ikeda et al. (45) noted an increasing incidence of hepatoblastoma in very low birth weight infants, from 0.7 percent of patients with birth weights of less than 1,500 g in 1985 to 1989 to 8.6 percent with similar low birth weights in 1990 to 1993. In the United States, Ross and Gurney (96) have observed a similar increasing incidence: during the most recent two decades, a period corresponding with improved survival for low birth weight children, it increased 5.2 percent in children 4 years and younger. While there is no racial predilection for hepatoblastoma, there is a distinct male predominance of from 1.5:1 to 2:1 (60,113). Approximately 40 cases of hepatoblastoma have been reported in patients over 21 years of age (3,6,7,12,39,46,48,58,81), although we strongly suspect that most, if not all of these, are misdiagnoses of tumors that were actually hepatocellular carcinoma, combined hepatocellular-cholangiocarcinoma, or carcinosarcoma. At the Armed Forces Institute of Pathology, where we have the world's largest experience with liver tumors, we have never seen a case of hepatoblastoma in an adult.

Patients with hepatoblastoma usually present with an enlarging abdomen noted by a parent or observed by a physician on routine physical examination. Weight loss or anorexia are seen less frequently, as are nausea, vomiting, and abdominal pain. Jaundice is seen in only 5 percent of cases (113). On physical examination, a firm, irregular mass is noted in the right upper quadrant of the abdomen which may extend across the midline or down to the pelvic brim.

Associated Conditions and Diseases. Hepatoblastoma is associated with a variety of congenital anomalies, syndromes, and clinical presentations (Table 6-1). Congenital anomalies are present in 5 to 6 percent of patients with hepatoblastoma and include such disparate features as horseshoe kidney, cleft palate, heterotopic lung tissue, and umbilical hernia (110–112). Beckwith-Wiedemann syndrome (macrosomia, macroglossia, visceromegaly, abdominal wall defects, hemihypertrophy) is associated with hepatoblastoma and a variety of other pediatric tumors including Wilms' tumor, adrenal carcinoma, and gonadoblastoma (53,60,66,71,84,124,136). Hepatoblastoma has been described in association with trisomy 18 including some cases with abdominal wall defects (13,79,120,122). Syndromes associated with other gastrointestinal lesions include familial adenomatous polyposis and the adenomatous polyposis coli gene (*APC*) (see below) and Gardner's syndrome (30,57,59,82). Less commonly occurring syndromes include Aicardi's syndrome (agenesis of the corpus callosum, lacunar chorioretinopathy, vertebral anomalies, electroencephalographic abnormalities), Goldenhar's syndrome (oculoauriculovertebral sequence, epibulbar dermoids, preauricular skin tags), and Prader-Willi syndrome (obesity, hypotonia, hypogonadism) (40,121).

A striking presentation of hepatoblastoma is seen in children (particularly young boys) whose

Table 6-1

CLINICAL SYNDROMES, CONGENITAL MALFORMATIONS, AND OTHER CONDITIONS ASSOCIATED WITH HEPATOBLASTOMA

Absence of left adrenal gland

Aicardi's syndrome

Alcohol embryopathy

Beckwith-Wiedemann syndrome

Beckwith-Wiedemann syndrome with opsoclonus, myoclonus

Bilateral talipes

Budd-Chiari syndrome

Cleft palate, macroglossia, dysplasia of ear lobes

Cystothioninuria

Down's syndrome, malrotation of colon, Meckel's diverticulum, pectum excavatum, intrathoracic kidney, single coronary artery

Duplicated ureters

Fetal hydrops

Familial polyposis coli

Gardner's syndrome

Goldenhar's syndrome (oculoauriculovertebral dysplasia, absence of portal vein)

Hemihypertrophy

Heterotopic lung tissue

Heterozygous alpha-1-antitrypsin deficiency

HIV* or HBV infection

Horseshoe kidney

Hypoglycemia

Inguinal hernia

Isosexual precocity

Maternal use of clomiphene citrate and Pergonal

Meckel's diverticulum

Oral contraceptive, mother

Oral contraceptive, patient

Osteoporosis

Persistent ductus arteriosus

Prader-Willi syndrome

Renal dysplasia

Right-sided diaphragmatic hernia

Schinzel-Geidion syndrome

Synchronous Wilms' tumor

Trisomy 18

Type 1a glycogen storage disease

Umbilical hernia

Very low birth weight

*HIV = human immunodeficiency virus; HBV = hepatitis B virus.

tumors produce human chorionic gonadotropin (HCG) leading to precocious puberty with genital enlargement, the appearance of pubic hair, and a deepening voice. The elevated levels of HCG are accompanied by increases in levels of serum luteinizing hormone and plasma testosterone (43,44,72,74,75,77,135).

In addition to the occurrence in familial conditions such as familial adenomatous polyposis, hepatoblastoma has been noted in a number of siblings pairs including identical male twins and two siblings with type 1a glycogen storage disease (47,76,92,116).

The association between hepatoblastoma and familial adenomatous polyposis (FAP) due to the germline mutation of the adenomatous polyposis coli (*APC*) gene (16,30,59,61,62,82) merits further consideration. Giardiello et al. (82) identified an *APC* mutation at the 5' end of the gene in all eight patients with hepatoblastoma from seven FAP kindreds. Oda et al. (82) have also noted genetic alterations in the *APC* gene (loss of heterozygosity or somatic mutations) in 9 of 13 cases of hepatoblastoma in nonfamilial adenomatous polyposis patients. A distinct male predominance (nearly 75 percent) is seen in *APC* gene–related hepatoblastomas.

Laboratory Findings. Anemia is common (70 percent) in patients with hepatoblastoma and is associated with thrombocytosis in 50 percent of cases. Platelet counts greater than 500 x 10^9/L were noted in 35 percent of 99 cases by Shafford and Pritchard, with 29 percent over 800 x 10^9/L (105). Along with alpha-fetoprotein, thrombocytosis has been used as a measure of disease activity (28,137).

Alpha-fetoprotein (AFP) is elevated at the time of diagnosis in up to 90 percent of patients with hepatoblastoma and parallels the course of the disease, with a return to normal levels after complete resection and a re-elevation with recurrence of the tumor (112). The "least" well-differentiated hepatoblastomas, e.g., small cell undifferentiated, may in some cases show little or no elevation of AFP (125). Van Tornout et al. (128) have noted that for unresectable or metastatic hepatoblastoma, AFP levels can reliably predict outcome and identify poor responders to treatment. In studying patients who had undergone initial surgery and chemotherapy, those patients whose AFP failed to decrease by at least two logs had a much poorer prognosis. In contrast, a large early decrease in AFP levels was a strong independent predictor of favorable outcome. Von Schweinitz et al. (130) also noted that normal or low levels of AFP were often associated with a small cell undifferentiated hepatoblastoma that did not produce AFP, and very high levels (over 1,000,000 ng/ml) were associated with extensive or metastatic tumor, both indicating an unfavorable outcome. It is important to remember, however, that AFP is present at levels of 25 to 50,000 ng/ml at birth and does not fall to "adult" levels of less than 25 ng/ml until 5 to 6 months of age (78). AFP levels in infants with tumors resected in the first 6 months of life may therefore be "appropriately" elevated even though the tumor has been completely resected.

Serum cholesterol levels were elevated in 10 of 59 patients with hepatoblastoma (73,112). Bilirubin is mildly elevated in 20 to 25 percent of cases, although jaundice is seen in only 6 percent (89). In approximately 60 percent of cases a mild elevation of alkaline phosphatase and aspartate aminotransferase is present (1).

Radiologic Findings. These are helpful in the preoperative diagnosis of hepatoblastoma and for differentiating it from the other solid, cystic, and vascular tumors and congenital and infectious lesions of the liver. Computed tomography (CT) can demonstrate the solitary or multifocal mass of a hepatoblastoma with attenuation values between those of water and normal liver parenchyma. Calcification may also be seen by CT in more than 50 percent of cases (69). Spiral (helical) CT with three-dimensional reconstruction has proven useful in the preoperative evaluation of children with hepatoblastoma (88). King et al. (51), however, recognized the limitations of CT in predicting the resectability of hepatoblastomas before and after preoperative chemotherapy, because CT occasionally overestimated the amount of tumor present. Ultrasonography displays a mass with increased heterogenous echogenicity, punctate or amorphous calcification, and occasional cystic areas. With Doppler ultrasonography, the neovascularity of the hepatoblastoma can be detected by peak systolic Doppler frequency shifts equal to or greater than 4 kHz (10).

Differentiation of hepatoblastoma from other childhood hepatic solid, cystic, or vascular lesions such as mesenchymal hamartoma, infantile

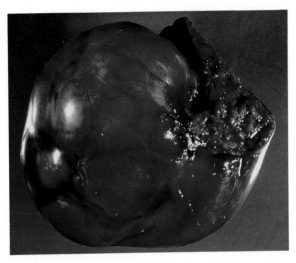

Figure 6-1
HEPATOBLASTOMA
The external surface shows a bulging, red-tan mass resected from the right lobe, which displays an intact smooth capsule traversed by many blood vessels.

hemangioendothelioma, and hepatocellular carcinoma can be aided by magnetic resonance imaging (MRI) with standard spin-echo T1- and T2-weighted imaging enhanced by the application of advanced sequences such as gradient-echo, fast spin-echo, and fat suppression techniques (90). The histologic features of the tumor can be differentiated by MRI as well, with the homogenous character of an "epithelial" lesion contrasting with the heterogeneous character of a "mixed" hepatoblastoma with its fibrotic bands. Decreased signal intensity compared to normal liver is noted on T1-weighted images, while increased signal intensity is seen on T2-weighted images. Hypointense bands on MRI identify fibrotic bands and the presence of vascular invasion may be detected by gradient-echo MRI imaging (90).

Gross Findings. Hepatoblastomas present as a single mass in 80 percent of cases. The right lobe is involved in 57 percent of cases, the left lobe in 15 percent, and both lobes in 27 percent, either as an extension of a single mass across the midline or as multiple tumor nodules. The diameter of single masses varies from 5 to 22 cm and the weight from 150 to over 1,400 g (89). The tumors are nodular with prominent surface vessels (fig. 6-1). In sections, they are well-circumscribed and bulge from the surface of the liver (figs. 6-2, 6-3). The color and consistency of the tumor depends

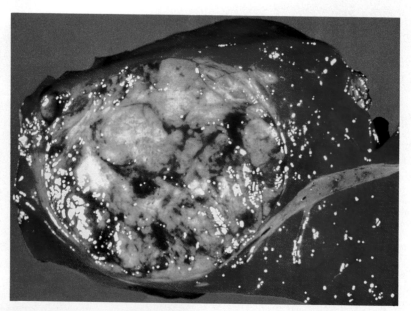

Figure 6-2
EPITHELIAL
HEPATOBLASTOMA
This tumor, composed of light tan tissue, is separated from the normal liver by a "capsule," although small areas of light tan tumor can be seen in the normal liver (right).

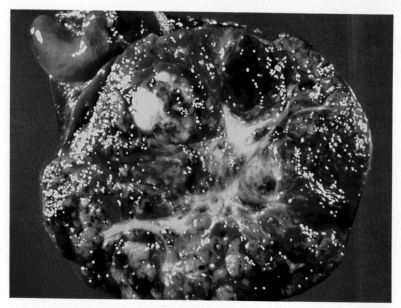

Figure 6-3
MIXED EPITHELIAL
AND MESENCHYMAL
HEPATOBLASTOMA
The cut surface shows hemorrhagic and tan nodules along with areas of dense white tissue.

on the type and amount of epithelial and mesenchymal tissues present (see later). Pure fetal epithelial lesions are coarsely lobulated with tan to brown nodules that are often similar in color to the normal liver (fig. 6-2). Areas of hemorrhage and necrosis may be present throughout the lesion, particularly in patients who have received preoperative chemotherapy. Mixed epithelial and mesenchymal lesions display a more variegated cut surface with areas of dense white tissue (mesenchymal and fibrous septa) separating tan, brown, or green nodules of epithelial cells and osteoid-like

material (figs. 6-3, 6-4) (109). Foci of necrosis and hemorrhage are also usually present.

Sectioning should focus on examination of the resection margins for the presence of tumor. This may be facilitated by inking the surgical margin, allowing it to dry, and then making sections perpendicular to the surgical surface at 1-cm intervals. Sections may then be taken from the inked margin, from the junction of tumor with uninvolved liver, and from random portions of the tumor or areas of unusual color or consistency (fig. 6-5). In general, one section of tumor should be taken for

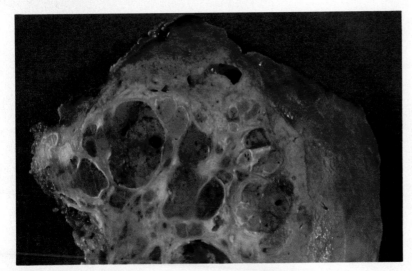

Figure 6-4
MIXED EPITHELIAL
AND MESENCHYMAL
HEPATOBLASTOMA
The section is variegated tan and green with thin to broad septa of dense yellow to white tissue.

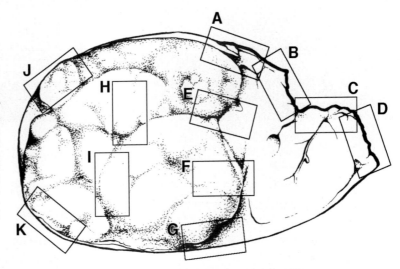

Figure 6-5
SELECTION OF SECTIONS FOR MICROSCOPIC EXAMINATION
These should include the surgical resection margins (A-D), the junction of tumor with uninvolved liver (A,E-G), and random sections of tumor (H-K). The total number of sections of tumor taken should equal or exceed the largest diameter of the tumor in centimeters, in this case eight sections for a tumor of 7 to 8 cm in greatest diameter. (Fig. 4 from Stocker J. An approach to handling pediatric liver tumors. Am J Clin Pathol 1998;109(Suppl 1):S68–73.)

microscopic study for each centimeter of the largest diameter of the tumor, e.g., 14 sections for a tumor that is 14.3 x 8.5 x 6.5 cm (109).

Microscopic Findings. Histologically, hepatoblastoma has been subdivided into six patterns based on the types and combinations of cells present (Table 6-2). Two patterns, pure fetal epithelial and mixed epithelial and mesenchymal without teratoid features, account for nearly two thirds of the tumors (19). The macrotrabecular and small cell undifferentiated patterns account for only 3 percent each.

The *pure fetal epithelial pattern,* seen in 31 percent of cases, is composed of sheets of small,

Table 6-2

**HISTOLOGIC CLASSIFICATION
OF HEPATOBLASTOMA WITH
RELATIVE FREQUENCY**

Epithelial type	56%
Fetal pattern	31%
Embryonal and fetal pattern	19%
Macrotrabecular pattern	3%
Small cell undifferentiated pattern	3%
Mixed epithelial and mesenchymal type	44%
Without teratoid features	34%
With teratoid features	10%

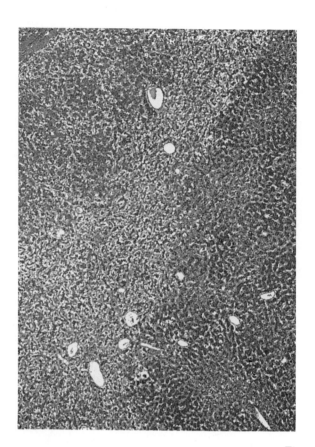 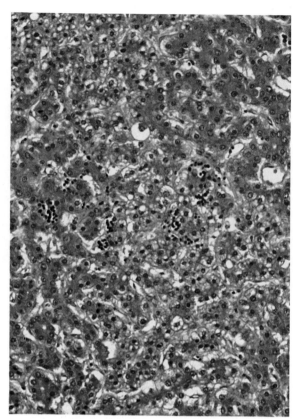

Figure 6-6
FETAL EPITHELIAL HEPATOBLASTOMA
Left: Low-power view shows a "light and dark" pattern.
Right: Higher magnification shows thin trabeculae of two to three cells in thickness; note the hematopoietic cells in the tumor sinusoids.

uniform, round to cuboidal cells resembling fetal hepatocytes (fig. 6-6) (46a). The cells contain abundant clear to finely granular cytoplasm with distinct cellular membranes, a small round nucleus with fine nuclear chromatin, and an indistinct nucleolus (fig. 6-7). Variable amounts of cytoplasmic glycogen and lipid within clusters of fetal epithelial cells impart a "light and dark" pattern to the tumor when viewed at low-power magnification (figs. 6-6, 6-8–6-10). The cells are arranged in thin trabeculae, one to three cells in thickness (figs. 6-6, 6-7), separated by narrow sinusoids lined by endothelial cells and Kupffer cells (98). In children who have not received preoperative chemotherapy, the sinusoids frequently contain clusters of erythroid and myeloid precursor cells and megakaryocytes (extramedullary hematopoiesis) (figs. 6-6, 6-10, 6-11). Canaliculi may occasionally be demonstrated between hepatocytes, but

bile is rarely present (fig. 6-12). Staining of the sinusoidal endothelial cell lining with *Ulex europeaus* antigen 1 (UEA-1) and anti-CD34 is much more diffuse in fetal hepatoblastoma than in normal liver where the staining is focal and confined to a few sinusoids near the portal areas. Ruck et al. (100) suggest that this feature may help in the differentiation of normal liver (focal staining) from well-differentiated fetal epithelial hepatoblastoma (diffuse staining).

The *embryonal pattern* consists of a combination of fetal epithelial cells and sheets or clusters of small, angulated cells with a high nuclear/cytoplasmic ratio, increased nuclear chromatin, and indistinct cytoplasmic membranes (figs. 6-13–6-18) (46a). These cells may occur singly with little cohesion with other cells or cluster into pseudorosette, glandular, or acinar formations (figs. 6-15–6-18). The embryonal cells resemble the blastemal cells

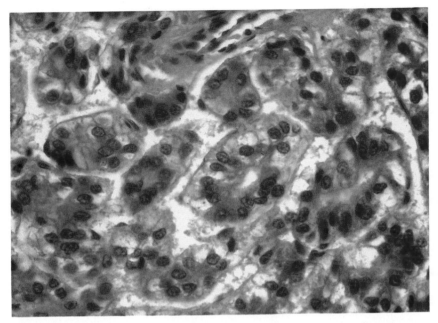

Figure 6-7
FETAL EPITHELIAL
HEPATOBLASTOMA
Cells within trabeculae are cuboidal to polyhedral with round, central nuclei that contain finely granular chromatin. The cytoplasm is clear, granular or smooth, and is delimited by a distinct cell membrane.

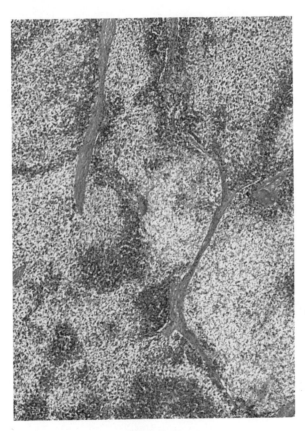

Figure 6-8
FETAL EPITHELIAL HEPATOBLASTOMA
Variable concentrations of glycogen and lipid within the cells impart a "light and dark" pattern to this tumor. Note the fibrous septa subdividing portions of the tumor.

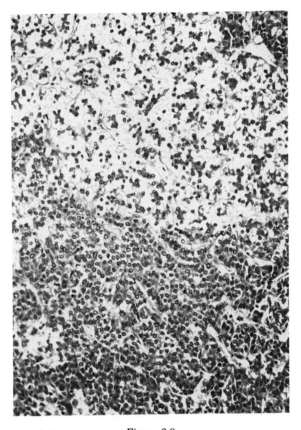

Figure 6-9
FETAL EPITHELIAL HEPATOBLASTOMA
The cytoplasm of the hepatoblastoma cells (top) is filled with lipid material which more widely separates the nuclei of these cells than those below. The size of the nuclei, however, is similar in all of the cells.

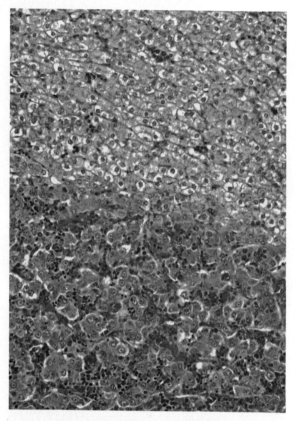

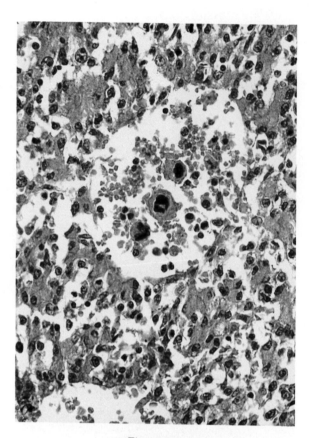

Figure 6-10
FETAL EPITHELIAL HEPATOBLASTOMA
Clusters of hematopoietic cells are scattered throughout the sinusoids between trabeculae of light (top) and dark (bottom) cells.

Figure 6-11
FETAL EPITHELIAL HEPATOBLASTOMA
A vein within the tumor contains megakaryocytes and other hematopoietic precursor cells.

Figure 6-12
FETAL EPITHELIAL
HEPATOBLASTOMA
Canaliculi containing bile are visible in the center of this field. The nucleoli in some of the cells are more prominent than usually seen in fetal epithelial hepatoblastoma cells.

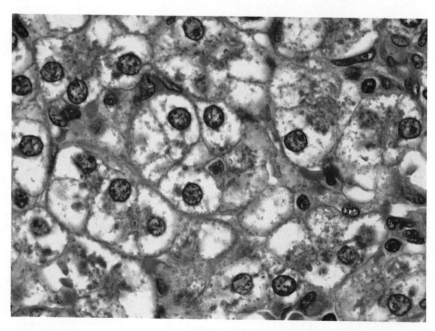

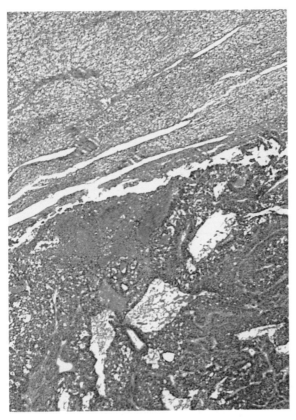

Figure 6-13
FETAL AND EMBRYONAL
EPITHELIAL HEPATOBLASTOMA
Sheets composed of trabeculae of fetal epithelial cells (top) lie adjacent to a mass of blastemal-like cells, some forming irregular glandular structures.

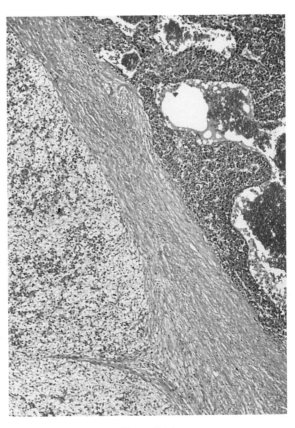

Figure 6-14
FETAL AND EMBRYONAL
EPITHELIAL HEPATOBLASTOMA
Fetal epithelial cells with a high cytoplasmic lipid concentration (bottom left) are separated by a band of fibrous connective tissue from a vascular mass of more "immature" appearing embryonal cells (top right).

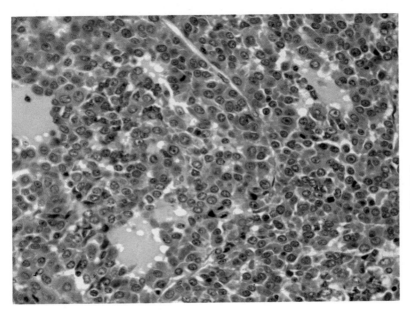

Figure 6-15
FETAL AND EMBRYONAL
EPITHELIAL HEPATOBLASTOMA
The embryonal epithelial cells appear cuboidal and display little cohesiveness. Note the gland-like structures formed of cells loosely organized around a space filled with lightly stained fluid.

167

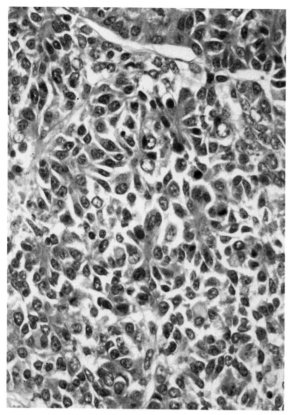

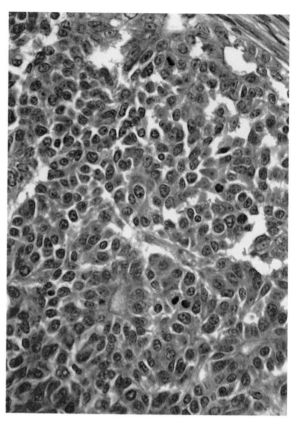

Figure 6-16
FETAL AND EMBRYONAL
EPITHELIAL HEPATOBLASTOMA
The embryonal cells are very poorly cohesive and consist of round to ovoid cells with scant cytoplasm and tapered ends.

Figure 6-17
FETAL AND EMBRYONAL
EPITHELIAL HEPATOBLASTOMA
The embryonal cells may resemble other blastemal cells (e.g., nephroblastoma or neuroblastoma), with hyperchromatic nuclei and increased mitotic activity.

Figure 6-18
FETAL AND EMBRYONAL
EPITHELIAL
HEPATOBLASTOMA
A cluster of embryonal cells form a rosette with a small indistinct lumen. Note the hematopoietic precursor cells (left).

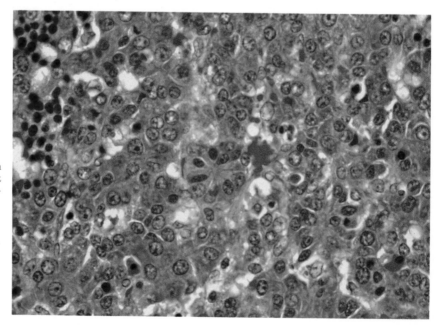

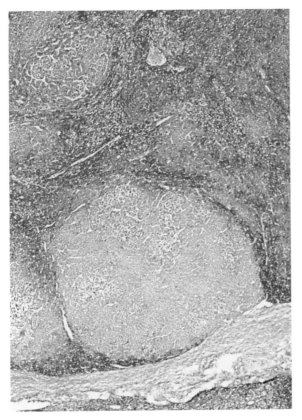

Figure 6-19
FETAL AND EMBRYONAL
EPITHELIAL HEPATOBLASTOMA
The pale foci of embryonal cells are readily distinguished from the surrounding dark red fetal epithelial cells which are full of glycogen (periodic acid–Schiff stain).

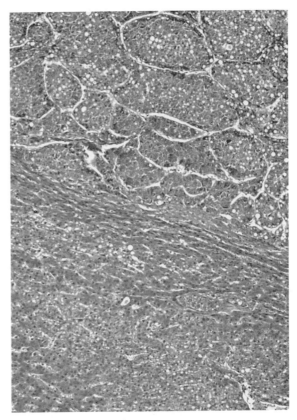

Figure 6-20
MACROTRABECULAR
HEPATOBLASTOMA
One to two cells–thick trabeculae of a "typical" fetal epithelial hepatoblastoma (bottom) lie adjacent to much broader macrotrabeculae composed of cells that are only slightly larger.

of Wilms' tumor and the "small, round, blue cells" of other "embryonal" tumors such as neuroblastoma or rhabdomyoblastoma (fig. 6-17). Individual cells may be ovoid with tapered ends, round or angular with scant cytoplasm, or cuboidal and lined up side-by-side around a central lumen. Nuclei vary somewhat in size (anisonucleosis) and in the density of chromatin (hyperchromasia), and mitotic activity is prominent, although bizarre mitoses are uncommon (fig. 6-17). Clusters of cells are divided by a delicate vascular network and foci of hematopoietic cells may be present (fig. 6-18). The foci of embryonal cells are often intermixed with clusters of fetal epithelial calls, but the virtual absence of stainable glycogen and lipid in the scant cytoplasm of the embryonal epithelial cells allows their easy identification with periodic acid–Schiff (PAS) or oil red O stain (fig. 6-19).

The *macrotrabecular pattern* refers to cases of fetal or fetal/embryonal epithelial hepatoblastoma that contain trabeculae more than 10 cells in thickness in a repetitive pattern within the tumor (figs. 6-20, 6-21). These trabeculae contain embryonal epithelial, fetal epithelial, and/or a third larger cell type with more abundant cytoplasm than seen in the fetal epithelial cells or normal hepatocytes. The trabeculae may sometimes resemble the pseudoglandular pattern of hepatocellular carcinoma (fig. 6-21). Cases with only an isolated macrotrabecular focus are classified on the basis of the epithelial (fetal, fetal/embryonal) or mixed epithelial/mesenchymal components present, and not as macrotrabecular.

The *small cell undifferentiated pattern* is composed of noncohesive sheets of small cells that resemble the group of "small blue cell" pediatric

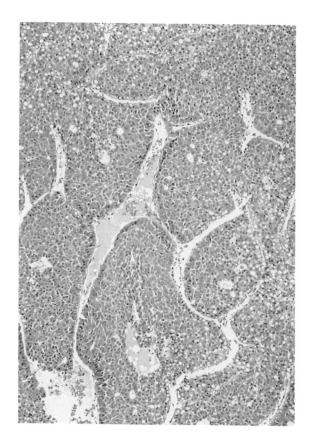
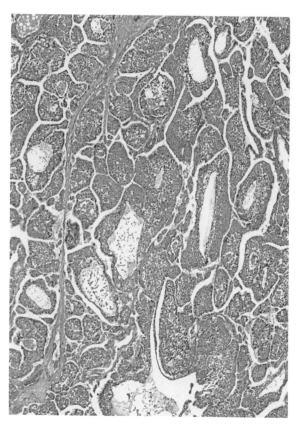

Figure 6-21
MACROTRABECULAR HEPATOBLASTOMA
Left: The macrotrabeculae are solid or display irregular central areas containing fluid.
Right: The macrotrabeculae contain pseudoglands.

neoplasms including neuroblastoma, lymphoma, Ewing's sarcoma, rhabdomyosarcoma, and desmoplastic small round cell tumor (49). The cells are arranged in solid masses with many areas of necrosis (figs. 6-22, 6-23). Nuclei are vesicular, may be pyknotic, and often display mitotic activity (fig. 6-23). The cells are difficult to identify as hepatic in origin since they contain only scant amounts of glycogen, fat droplets, or bile pigment. There are smaller numbers of sinusoids than with fetal epithelial hepatoblastoma, pronounced intracellular expression of extracellular matrix proteins, and large numbers of extracellular fibers immunoreactive for collagen type III (98). Diagnosis may require electron microscopy to establish the presence of glycogen, lipid droplets, or bile canaliculi, or immunohistochemistry to demonstrate the presence of cytoplasmic cytokeratin (31). This subtype of tumor, accounting for only 3 percent of hepatoblastomas,

is felt by Gonzales-Crussi (31) to represent the least differentiated form of hepatoblastoma.

The *mixed epithelial and mesenchymal pattern* of hepatoblastoma contains areas of fetal and embryonal epithelial cells along with primitive mesenchyme and various mesenchymally derived tissues (figs. 6-24–6-31) (46a). In the tumors without teratoid features (see below) the mesenchymal tissue is limited to immature and mature fibrous tissue, osteoid-like tissue, and cartilaginous tissue (fig. 6-26). The primitive mesenchymal tissue is often highly cellular and composed of elongated, spindle-shaped cells with scant cytoplasm and elongated, plump nuclei (fig. 6-27). The cells may be loosely arranged in a pale myxomatous stroma or may display a parallel orientation with definite collagen fibers and young fibroblasts; mature fibrous septa may also be seen (fig. 6-28). Scattered throughout the mesenchyme or within the areas of epithelial

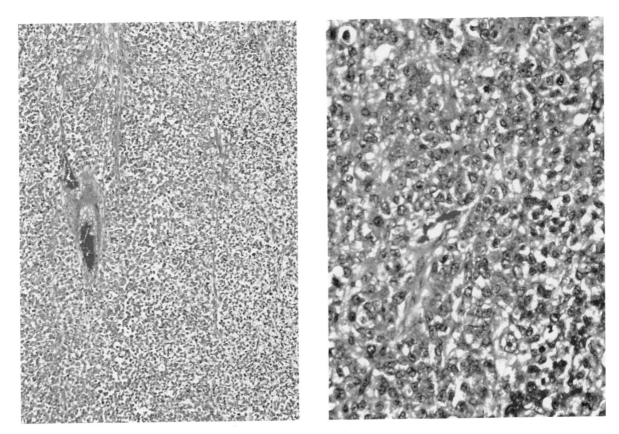

Figure 6-22
SMALL CELL UNDIFFERENTIATED HEPATOBLASTOMA

Left: Sheets of small, round, blue cells display few distinguishing features; note the rich vascular background.

Right: At higher magnification the cells lack cohesiveness, have scant cytoplasm, and contain small round nuclei with coarse chromatin granules.

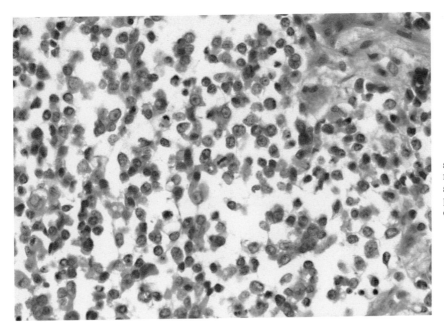

Figure 6-23
SMALL CELL
UNDIFFERENTIATED
HEPATOBLASTOMA

The cells are similar to those seen in metastatic neuroblastoma, nephroblastoma, and rhabdomyosarcoma, with a high nuclear/cytoplasmic ratio, small nuclei with indistinct nucleoli, and mitoses.

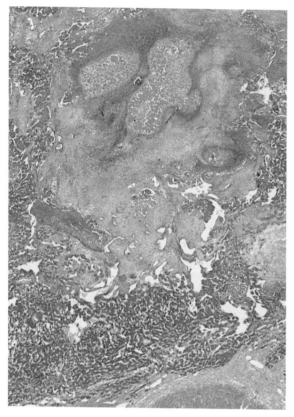

Figure 6-24
MIXED EPITHELIAL AND
MESENCHYMAL HEPATOBLASTOMA

Trabeculae of fetal epithelial cells (bottom) blend with vascular, pale, basophilic mesenchymal tissue. Note the irregular "islands" of osteoid-like material (top).

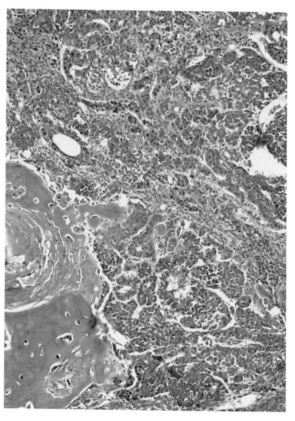

Figure 6-25
MIXED EPITHELIAL AND
MESENCHYMAL HEPATOBLASTOMA

Fetal epithelial cells (eosinophilic) are admixed with embryonal epithelial cells (basophilic). Note the osteoid focus.

Figure 6-26
MIXED EPITHELIAL AND
MESENCHYMAL
HEPATOBLASTOMA

Mature cartilaginous tissue lies adjacent to fetal epithelial hepatoblastoma cells.

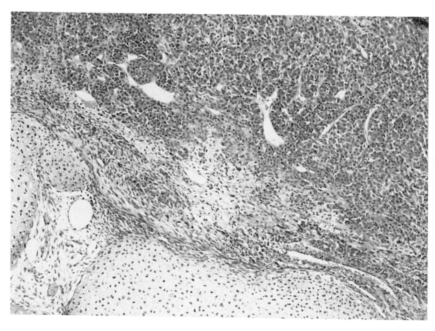

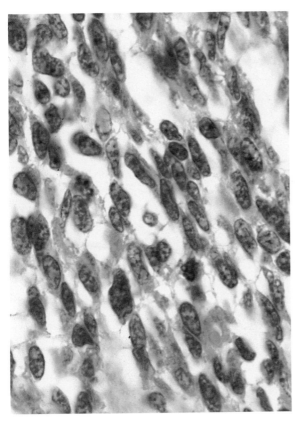

Figure 6-27
MIXED EPITHELIAL AND
MESENCHYMAL HEPATOBLASTOMA
The primitive mesenchymal tissue in this area of a mixed tumor is composed of elongated spindle-shaped cells with plump nuclei and pale cytoplasm.

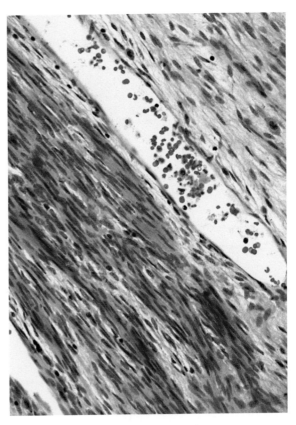

Figure 6-28
MIXED EPITHELIAL AND
MESENCHYMAL HEPATOBLASTOMA
The mesenchymal tissue in the center displays mature fibrocytes with collagen deposition.

hepatoblastoma cells are foci of osteoid-like and cartilaginous material. The osteoid-like foci are composed of a smooth, eosinophilic, fibrillary matrix with "lacunae" containing irregular, angulated cells with abundant eosinophilic cytoplasm and one or more, round to oval nuclei with vesiculated nuclear chromatin (figs. 6-29–6-31). These cells resemble osteoblasts, but are positive for alpha-1-antitrypsin, alpha-1-antichymotrypsin, alpha-fetoprotein, carcinoembryonic antigen, chromogranin A, cytokeratin, epithelial membrane antigen, vimentin, and S-100 protein; the extracellular areas are positive for collagen type I (1,98,134). The osteoblast-like cells may occasionally be seen to blend with the embryonal epithelial cells of the adjacent tumor and, along with the immunohistochemical properties, suggest an epithelial origin for the cells and surrounding material (fig. 6-31, right) (97).

In some cases of mixed epithelial and mesenchymal hepatoblastoma, the only mesenchymal component present may be one or more small foci of osteoid-like material.

In approximately 20 percent of the mixed epithelial and mesenchymal hepatoblastomas, a variety of tissue types may be present in addition to the primitive mesenchyme, fibrous tissue, and osteoid-like and cartilaginous foci usually associated with the "mixed" tumor. These *teratoid hepatoblastomas* may contain tissues of mesenchymal and epithelial derivation including striated muscle, bone, cartilage, stratified squamous epithelium, mucinous epithelium, and melanin pigment among others (figs. 6-32–6-35) (65,99).

Hepatoblastoma Combined with Other Tumors. Conrad et al. (18) reported a discrete cystic teratoma of the liver contiguous to a hepatoblastoma. The teratoma contained normal-appearing

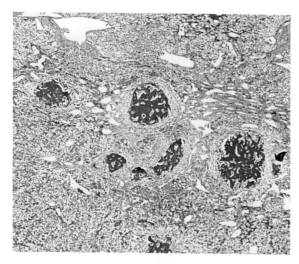

Figure 6-29
MIXED EPITHELIAL AND
MESENCHYMAL HEPATOBLASTOMA

Foci of osteoid-like material (blue) are surrounded by a collar of immature, vascular mesenchymal tissue (Masson's trichrome stain).

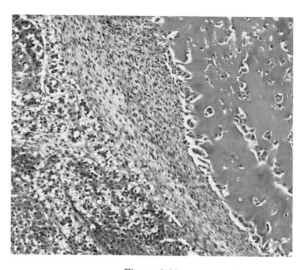

Figure 6-30
MIXED EPITHELIAL AND
MESENCHYMAL HEPATOBLASTOMA

Fetal epithelial hepatoblastoma cells, many with a clear cytoplasm, are separated by immature mesenchymal tissue from a focus of osteoid-like material whose margin blends with the cells of the mesenchymal tissue.

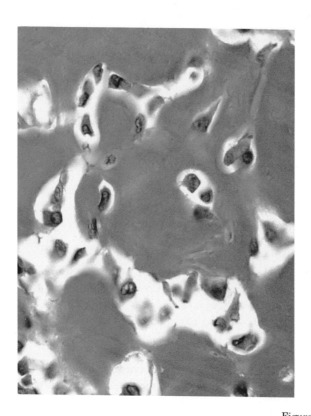

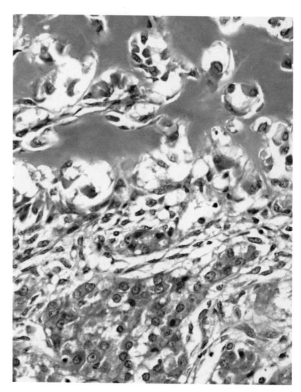

Figure 6-31
MIXED EPITHELIAL AND MESENCHYMAL HEPATOBLASTOMA

Left: The osteoid-like material contains lacunae filled with cuboidal, ovoid, or elongated cells with small to abundant amounts of eosinophilic cytoplasm.

Right: At the margin of the osteoid-like material is an irregular row of cells with nuclear and cytoplasmic characteristics midway between the fetal epithelial hepatoblastoma cells (bottom) and the lacuna cells within the osteoid-like material.

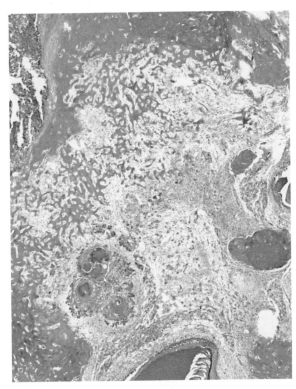

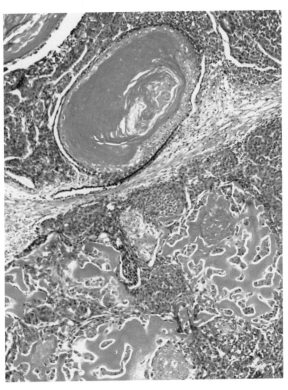

Figure 6-32
MIXED EPITHELIAL AND MESENCHYMAL
HEPATOBLASTOMA WITH TERATOID FEATURES

In addition to the fetal epithelial hepatoblastoma cells this tumor contains osteoid-like foci, loose to dense mesenchymal tissue, and a discrete focus of keratinized squamous epithelium (bottom).

Figure 6-33
MIXED EPITHELIAL AND MESENCHYMAL
HEPATOBLASTOMA WITH TERATOID FEATURES

Irregular trabeculae of osteoid-like material (bottom) and a focus of squamous epithelium (top) are surrounded by fetal and embryonal epithelial cells.

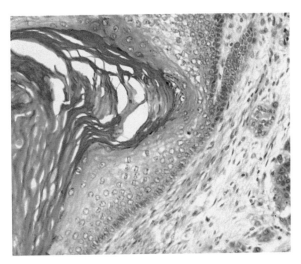

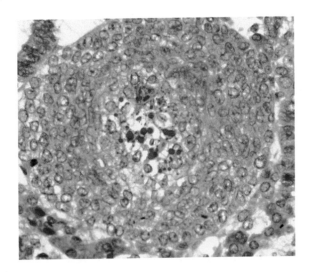

Figure 6-34
MIXED EPITHELIAL AND MESENCHYMAL HEPATOBLASTOMA WITH TERATOID FEATURES

Left: This focus of squamous epithelium displays the normal maturation of cells from the basal cell layer to the cornified material in the center.

Right: A spherical cluster of cells with regular, round, clear nuclei surrounds a core containing smooth eosinophilic droplets; note the adjacent fetal and embryonal epithelium.

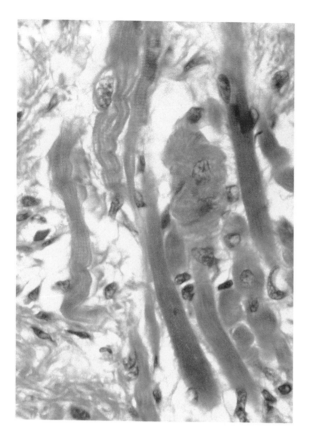 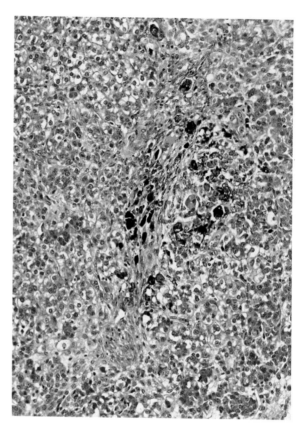

Figure 6-35
MIXED EPITHELIAL AND MESENCHYMAL HEPATOBLASTOMA WITH TERATOID FEATURES
Left: Skeletal muscle fibers, some with clear cross striations, are a component of this tumor.
Right: Some of the cells in this area of embryonal hepatoblastoma are filled with dense melanin pigment.

skin with pilosebaceous units and eccrine glands, along with adipose tissue and mature lamellar bone. The hepatoblastoma was composed of fetal and embryonal epithelial cells with no mesenchymal elements (18). Cross and Variend (20) reported a mixed epithelial and mesenchymal hepatoblastoma that contained areas of yolk sac tumor composed of rounded papillary structures with central capillaries covered by cuboidal cells, Shiller-Duval bodies, and small glandular spaces.

Diagnosis by Biopsy and Fine Needle Aspiration. The large size of many hepatoblastomas often necessitates preoperative chemotherapy (see below) before surgical resection can be attempted. In order to establish the diagnosis, needle biopsy, fine needle aspiration, or open biopsy may be performed. Open biopsy and needle biopsy often are adequate in establishing the diagnosis; fine needle aspiration may prove dif-

ficult, particularly in cases of small cell undifferentiated or embryonal epithelial lesions. Fine needle aspiration has been reported to be accurate in diagnosing hepatoblastoma in approximately 65 percent (19 of 29) of cases, primarily those of fetal epithelial and mixed type (11,21,34, 107,126,133). The diagnosis was most frequently confused with metastatic tumor including Wilms' tumor, neuroblastoma, and rhabdomyosarcoma (107,133).

Immunohistochemical Findings. The various patterns of hepatoblastoma display differing immunoreactivities probably based on their degree of differentiation. Thus, the fetal epithelial cell areas stain for a broad range of epithelial markers, while the small cell undifferentiated areas show positivity for only a few (Table 6-3) (1,15,80, 89,98,100,102,106,111,127,134). Expression of alpha-fetoprotein is illustrated in figure 6-36. Ruck et al. (102) noted a correlation between the

Table 6-3
IMMUNOHISTOCHEMICAL FINDINGS IN HEPATOBLASTOMA*

	Fetal Cell Areas	Embryonal Cell Areas	Small Cell Areas	Mesenchymal Areas	"Osteoid" Areas
Keratin	++**	++	++	+/–	+
Hepatocyte (Hep Par 1)	++	+			
α-fetoprotein	++	++	–		+
α-1-antitrypsin	++	++	+/–	+	++
α-1-antichymotrypsin	++	++	+	+	+
Ferritin	++	+	+		+
Polyclonal carcinoembryonic antigen (canaliculi)	++	++	–	–	+/–
Epithelial membrane antigen		+	–		++
Transferrin	+	++			
Human chorionic gonadotropin	+	+			
Vimentin	–	–	–	++	++
Serotonin	+/–	+/–	–	–	–
Somatostatin	+/–	+/–	–	–	–
Neuron-specific enolase	–	+/–	–	+	++
S-100 protein	+/–	+	+/–	+	++
Desmin	–	–		–	–
Chromogranin A	+/–	+/–	–	–	+

*Modified from reference 113.
**++ = Majority of cases strongly positive; + = moderately or weakly positive in some cases; +/– = positive in some reports and negative in others; – = negative in all reports.

cytokeratin staining of normal biliary epithelium and liver parenchymal cells and the types of epithelial cells in hepatoblastoma, with CK19 more prominent in small cell and embryonal epithelial cell areas (and in biliary epithelium) and CK18 more prominent in fetal epithelial areas (and in normal hepatocytes). Osteoid areas were positive for both CK18 and CK19, while spindle cells areas were not immunoreactive for any of the cytokeratins. These characteristics have suggested to Abenoza et al. (1), and Ruck et al. (102), that the primitive small cells give rise to embryonal hepatoblastoma cells and after further maturation, fetal hepatoblastoma cells. Expression of insulin-like growth factor 2 and insulin-like growth factor binding protein have been noted in 11 hepatoblastomas; the expression correlated inversely with the degree of tumor cell differentiation. Akmal et al. (4) suggest that these markers may be used to assess the degree of

differentiation of the tumor. Interestingly, hypoglycemia has been noted as a presenting sign of hepatoblastoma on rare occasion, with the hypoglycemia disappearing after removal of the tumor (35). Fetal hepatoblastoma cells stain with the newly developed anti-hepatocyte antibody, Hep Par 1, and their canaliculi stain with polyclonal antibodies to carcinoembryonic antigen, similar to the staining pattern of hepatocellular carcinoma (see chapter 8), while embryonal cells show less consistent staining (24).

Ultrastructural Findings. Ultrastructurally, fetal epithelial cells appear as primitive polygonal structures with round to ovoid nuclei, conspicuous rough endoplasmic reticulum in parallel lamellae, pools of glycogen, numerous mitochondria, and a moderate number of lysosomes. The cells are arranged in trabeculae with well-developed intercellular junctions and occasional canaliculi (1). Embryonal epithelial cells are smaller

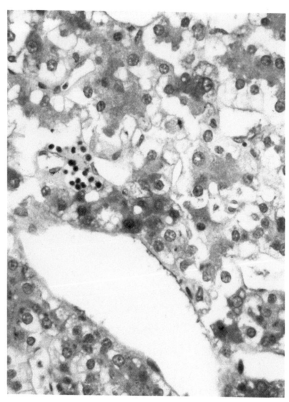

Figure 6-36
PURE FETAL EPITHELIAL HEPATOBLASTOMA
The cytoplasm of most of the cells contains alpha-fetoprotein, which is demonstrated immunohistochemically.

and have a high nuclear/cytoplasmic ratio and only a few organelles, primarily mitochondria and rough endoplasmic reticulum. Osteoid-like material consists of collagen fibrils in dense bundles which surround nests of cells with a well-developed rough endoplasmic reticulum and paranuclear, whorled, 10-nm filaments. As noted by light microscopy, the cells at the margins of the osteoid-like areas blend with epithelial hepatoblasts (1). In small cell tumors, the cells are more round than oval, vary from 7 to 14 μm in diameter, and have a relatively dense cytoplasm and nucleus. Tonofilaments, intercellular junctions, and microvilli may also be present (102). Ruck et al. (102) noted that the tonofilaments were marked by the antibody to CK7.

Other Special Studies. Chromosomal abnormalities have been found in many tumors. Trisomy 2, trisomy 20, and 4q structural rearrangements are the most common (5,8,9,14,27,37,38,55,63,68,85,94,104,108,111,112,117,123).

A derivative chromosome 4 from an unbalanced translocation between the long arms of chromosomes 1 and 4 has been noted as a recurring abnormality in hepatoblastoma while rarely seen in other types of neoplasm (104). Of 32 cases studied by Kraus et al. (55), there was loss of heterozygosity (LOH) on chromosome 1p in 7, on 1q in 7, and on both 1p and 1q in 3 more, suggesting that tumor suppressor genes at the telomeric region of chromosome arm 1p and different regions of chromosome arm 1q may be involved in the pathogenesis of hepatoblastoma. Albrecht et al. (5) noted LOH on chromosome 11p restricted to the telomeric region 11p15.5 in 6 of 18 hepatoblastomas and determined that the parental origin was exclusively maternal.

P53 expression is seen less frequently in hepatoblastoma than in other childhood tumors. In 10 cases of hepatoblastoma, Chen et al. (17) noted only 1 case of overexpression of p53 protein in a macrotrabecular type at stage IV. Ruck et al. (102) noted p53 protein immunoreactivity in two small cell hepatoblastomas and in the embryonal areas of two fetal/embryonal epithelial hepatoblastomas, but not in the fetal areas of eight fetal or fetal/embryonal epithelial tumors, or in the mesenchymal areas of four mixed tumors (101). Somatic mutations, however, were detected in 9 of 10 hepatoblastomas by Oda et al. (83) in the 5 to 8 exons of the p53 gene. They suggested that environmental mutagens may be involved in some cases of hepatoblastoma.

DNA analysis by flow cytometry has been reported in over 70 cases: a diploid pattern was noted in the well-differentiated (fetal) portions of the tumors and an aneuploid pattern was present in embryonal portions or in small cell (anaplastic) tumors (19,42,56,103). Krober et al. (56) noted an aneuploid peak in tumors with embryonal and fetal components when the areas were analyzed together and encouraged analysis of all differing areas of a tumor if ploidy is to be used in drawing conclusions about the prognosis in individual cases. Hara et al. (42) noted an increased incidence of vascular invasion and a poorer prognosis in patients with an aneuploid tumor.

Spread and Metastasis. Metastatic spread of hepatoblastoma is seen most frequently in the lung, but may occur in bone, brain, eye, and ovaries (13,23,32,70,93). Local extension into hepatic vessels and the inferior vena cava may also be present (119). Aggressive treatment of metastatic pulmonary disease using both chemotherapy and multiple resections has been successful in increasing long-term survival. Feusner et al. (24) noted recurrent hepatoblastoma in 10 of 33 stage I patients, 6 of whom had pulmonary involvement. Three of these 6 patients were disease free from 64 to 104 months after their most recent recurrence following chemotherapy combined with surgical resection of the pulmonary disease. Passmore et al. (86) described a 12-year-old boy whose hepatoblastoma was initially resected at age 14 months, followed by resection of pulmonary metastases at ages 2 1/2, 3 1/2, 4 1/2, 5 1/2, and 9 1/2 years. Multiple surgical resections, along with chemotherapy and radiation therapy have also been successful in treating pulmonary and brain metastases 10 1/2 years after the initial resection of a hepatoblastoma in a 17-month-old girl (93).

Clinical Staging. Most patients in the United States are staged according to the Children's Cancer Study Group (CCSG) classification (Table 6-4) (36). Other classifications include the TNM system or variations of the CCSG staging classification (41,109). Based on these classifications, approximately 38 percent of hepatoblastomas are stage I at the time of initial diagnosis and prior to any chemotherapy, about 9 percent are stage II, 24 percent stage III, and 29 percent stage IV (19,26,36). With preoperative chemotherapy and liver transplantation, as noted above, the majority of the 53 percent "unresectable" (stages III and IV) cases can be rendered "resectable" (22,118).

Treatment. Surgery remains the mainstay in the treatment of hepatoblastoma, with prognosis directly related to tumor stage (i.e., resectability) (see below). Small, solitary lesions localized to a single lobe can be adequately treated by lobectomy. Larger lesions, including those requiring preoperative chemotherapy to allow resection, may require more extensive surgery including trisegmentectomy or transplantation (2,22,29, 52,119). Surgical complications, particularly hemorrhage, are noted in 14 percent of primary and 29 percent of second resections (129).

At the time of diagnosis, 40 to 60 percent of hepatoblastomas are considered to be unresectable, and 10 to 20 percent of patients are found to have pulmonary metastases (25). Preoperative chemotherapy converts nearly 85 percent of

Table 6-4

STAGING OF HEPATOBLASTOMA*

Stage I	Complete resection
Stage II	Microscopic residual Negative nodal involvement No spilled tumor
Stage III	Gross residual or Nodal involvement or Spilled tumor
Stage IV	Metastatic disease

*Table 2 from Conran RM, Hitchcock CL, Waclawiw MA, et al. Hepatoblastoma: the prognostic significance of histologic type. Pediatr Pathol 1992;12:167–83.

these "unresectable" lesions to ones that can be entirely grossly removed, i.e, to stage I or II, with subsequent long-term survival (87,91). Recently established protocols now include administration of preoperative chemotherapy to all patients with hepatoblastoma (22). Ehrlich et al. (22) noted a 91 percent response in 22 patients to preoperative chemotherapy of 3 to 6 cycles. In 19 of these 20 patients, a significant reduction in the extent of resection was attained (as calculated by CAT scan to be necessary for complete excision of the tumor at initial diagnosis). While rare cases of survival with chemotherapy alone have been reported (138), most current protocols utilize surgery and chemotherapy (33). Cisplatin and adriamycin by continuous intravenous infusion in repeated cycles have been the major agents used in the preoperative and postoperative treatment of hepatoblastoma (22,67). As noted above, preoperative chemotherapy is now used whether or not a tumor is considered resectable at the time of initial presentation (50).

Preoperative chemotherapy has increased the resectability of hepatoblastoma from 40 to 60 percent to 90 percent, with the more extensive tumors requiring transplantation to remove the involved portions of liver (114). Survival without recurrence for over 24 months has been reported in 15 of 21 patients (71 percent) with stages III and IV disease who had orthotopic liver transplantation (2,22,54,64,114,115).

Prognosis. The stage of the tumor at the time of initial resection is the key prognostic factor in determining the survival of children and adults with hepatoblastoma (19,22,36,118,130,131). Overall survival for all patients with hepatoblastoma is 65 to 70 percent; those with stage I disease may achieve a 100 percent survival rate; those with stage II, a rate of 75 to 80 percent; stage III, 65 to 68 percent; and stage IV, 0 to 27 percent (19,131,132). As noted above, preoperative and postoperative chemotherapy and aggressive treatment of pulmonary and central nervous system metastases have significantly changed the survival rate for patients with stage IV disease. While the histologic pattern was felt to influence prognosis, a variety of studies have demonstrated that survival is independent of histologic subtype when adjusted for age, sex, and disease

stage (19,32). Only small cell undifferentiated hepatoblastoma may have a worse prognosis than others, but the number of cases of this uncommon type makes analysis uncertain (19).

In a comparison of patients' disease-free survival rate with tumor characteristics and stages, von Schweinitz et al. (130) noted that prognosis was significantly (positively) related to tumor involvement of one lobe (versus both lobes), fetal epithelial growth pattern (versus embryonal), alpha-fetoprotein levels of 100 to 1,000,000 ng/ml (versus less than 100 or greater than 1,000,000 ng/ml), and multifocal dissemination (versus unifocal growth pattern in the liver with distant metastases and vascular invasion).

REFERENCES

1. Abenoza P, Manivel JC, Wick MR, Hagen K, Dehner LP. Hepatoblastoma: an immunohistochemical and ultrastructural study. Hum Pathol 1987;18:1025–35.
2. Achilleos OA, Buist LJ, Kelly DA, et al. Unresectable hepatic tumors in childhood and the role of liver transplantation. J Pediatr Surg 1996;31:1563–7.
3. Ahn HJ, Kwon KW, Choi YJ, et al. Mixed hepatoblastoma in an adult—a case report and literature review. J Korean Med Sci 1997;12:369–73.
4. Akmal SN, Yun K, MacLay J, Higami Y, Ikeda T. Insulin-like growth factor 2 and insulin-like growth factor binding protein 2 expression in hepatoblastoma. Hum Pathol 1995;26:846–51.
5. Albrecht S, von Schweinitz D, Waha A, Kraus JA, von Deimling A, Pietsch T. Loss of maternal alleles on chromosome arm 11p in hepatoblastoma. Cancer Res 1994;54:5041–4.
6. Altmann HW. Epithelial and mixed hepatoblastoma in the adult. Histological observations and general considerations. Pathol Res Pract 1992;188:16–26.
7. Babaryka I, von Bouquoy F. Hepatoblastoma in adults. Leber Magen Darm 1981;11:283–7.
8. Balogh E, Swanton S, Kiss C, Jakab Z, Seckler-Walker LM, Olah E. 2q21–qter trisomy in hepatoblastoma. Orv Hetil 1997;138:3179–83.
9. Bardi G, Johansson B, Pandis N, et al. Trisomy 2 as the sole chromosomal abnormality in a hepatoblastoma. Genes Chromosomes Cancer 1992;4:78–80.
10. Bates S, Keller M, Ramos I, Carter D, Taylor KJ. Hepatoblastoma: detection of tumor vascularity with duplex Doppler US. Radiology 1990;176:505–7.
11. Bhatia A, Mehrotra P. Fine needle aspiration cytology in a case of hepatoblastoma. Acta Cytol 1986;30:439–41.
12. Bortolasi L, Marchiori L, Dal Dosso I, Colombari R, Nicoli N. Hepatoblastoma in adult age: a report of two cases. Hepatogastroenterology 1996;43:1073–8.
13. Bove KE, Soukup S, Ballard ET, Ryckman F. Hepatoblastoma in a child with trisomy 18: cytogenetics, liver anomalies, and literature review. Pediatr Pathol Lab Med 1996;16:253–62.
14. Byrne JA, Smith PJ. The 11p15.5 ribonucleotide reductase M1 subunit locus is not imprinted in Wilms' tumour and hepatoblastoma. Hum Genet 1993;91:275–7.
15. Cangiarella J, Greco MA, Waisman J. Hepatoblastoma. Report of a case with cytologic, histologic and ultrastructural findings. Acta Cytol 1994;38;455–8.
16. Cetta F, Montalto G, Petracci M. Hepatoblastoma and APC gene mutation in familial adenomatous polyposis [Letter]. Gut 1997;41:417.
17. Chen TC, Hsieh LL, Kuo TT. Absence of p53 gene mutation and infrequent overexpression of p53 protein in hepatoblastoma. J Pathol 1995;176:243–7.
18. Conrad RJ, Gribbin D, Walker NI, Ong TH. Combined cystic teratoma and hepatoblastoma of the liver. Probable divergent differentiation of an uncommitted hepatic precursor cell. Cancer 1993;72:2910–3.
19. Conran RM, Hitchcock CL, Waclawiw MA, et al. Hepatoblastoma: the prognostic significance of histologic type. Pediatr Pathol 1992;12:167–83.
20. Cross SS, Variend S. Combined hepatoblastoma and yolk sac tumor of the liver. Cancer 1992;69:1323–6.
21. Dekmezian R, Sneige N, Popok S, Ordonez NG. Fine-needle aspiration cytology of pediatric patients with primary hepatic tumors: a comparative study of two hepatoblastomas and a liver-cell carcinoma. Diagn Cytopathol 1988;4:162–8.
22. Ehrlich PF, Greenberg ML, Filler RM. Improved long-term survival with preoperative chemotherapy for hepatoblastoma. J Pediatr Surg 1997;32:999–1003.
23. Endo EG, Walton DS, Albert DM. Neonatal hepatoblastoma metastatic to the choroid and iris. Arch Ophthalmol 1996;114:757–61.
24. Fasano M, Thiese ND, Nalesnik M, et al. Immunohistochemical evaluation of hepatoblastomas with use of the hepatocyte-specific marker, hepatocyte paraffin 1, and the polyclonal anti-carcinoembryonic antigen. Mod Pathol 1998;11:934–8.

25. Feusner JH, Krailo MD, Haas JE, et al. Treatment of pulmonary metastases of initial stage I hepatoblastoma in childhood. Report from the Childrens Cancer Group. Cancer 1993;71:859–64.

26. Finegold M. Tumors of the liver. Semin Liver Dis 1994;14:270–81.

27. Fletcher JA, Kozakewich HP, Pavelka K, et al. Consistent cytogenetic aberrations in hepatoblastoma: a common pathway of genetic alterations in embryonal liver and skeletal muscle malignancies? Genes Chromosomes Cancer 1991;3:37–43.

28. Forouhar FA, Quinn JJ, Cooke R, Foster JH. The effect of chemotherapy on hepatoblastoma. Arch Pathol Lab Med 1984;108:311–4.

29. Geiger JD. Surgery for hepatoblastoma in children. Curr Opin Pediatr 1996;8:276–82.

30. Giardiello FM, Petersen GM, Brensinger JD, et al. Hepatoblastoma and APC gene mutation in familial adenomatous polyposis. Gut 1996;39:867–9.

31. Gonzalez-Crussi F. Undifferentiated small cell ("anaplastic") hepatoblastoma. Pediatr Pathol 1991;11:155–61.

32. Green LK, Silva EG. Hepatoblastoma in an adult with metastasis to the ovaries. Am J Clin Pathol 1989;92:110–5.

33. Guglielmi M, Perilongo G, Cecchetto G. Rationale and results of the International Society of Pediatric Oncology (SIOP) Italian pilot study on childhood hepatoma: surgical resection d'emblee or after primary chemotherapy. L Surg Oncol 1993;3(Suppl):122–6.

34. Gupta RK, Naran S, Alansari AG. Fine needle aspiration cytodiagnosis in a case of hepatoblastoma. Cytopathology 1994;5:114–7.

35. Ha K, Ikeda T, Okada S, et al. Hypoglycemia in a child with hepatoblastoma. Med Pediatr Oncol 1980;8:335–41.

36. Haas JE, Muczynski KA, Krailo M, et al. Histopathology and prognosis in childhood hepatoblastoma and hepatocarcinoma. Cancer 1989;64:1082–95.

37. Haas OA, Zoubek A, Grumayer ER, Gadner H. Constitutional interstitial deletion of 11p11 and pericentric inversion of chromosome 9 in a patient with Wiedemann-Beckwith syndrome and hepatoblastoma. Cancer Genet Cytogenet 1986;23:95–104.

38. Hansen K, Bagtas J, Mark HF, Homans A, Singer DB. Undifferentiated small cell hepatoblastoma with a unique chromosomal translocation: a case report. Pediatr Pathol 1992;12:457–62.

39. Harada T, Matsuo K, Kodama S, Higashihara H, Nakayama Y, Ikeda S. Adult hepatoblastoma: case report and review of the literature. Aust N Z J Surg 1995;65:686–8.

40. Hashizume K, Nakajo T, Kawarasaki H, et al. Prader-Willi syndrome with del(15)(q11,q13) associated with hepatoblastoma. Acta Paediatr Jpn 1991;33:718–22.

41. Hata Y. The clinical features and prognosis of hepatoblastoma: follow-up studies done on pediatric tumors enrolled in the Japanese Pediatric Tumor Registry between 1971 and 1980. Part I. Committee of Malignant Tumors, Japanese Society of Pediatric Surgeons. Jpn J Surg 1990;20:498–502.

42. Hata Y, Ishizu H, Ohmori K, et al. Flow cytometric analysis of the nuclear DNA content of hepatoblastoma. Cancer 1991;68:2566–70.

43. Heimann A, White PF, Riely CA, Ritchey AK, Flye MW, Barwick KW. Hepatoblastoma presenting as isosexual precocity. The clinical importance of histologic and serologic parameters. J Clin Gastroenterol 1987;9:105–10.

44. Heinrich UE, Bolkenius M, Daum R, Oppermann HC, Mehls O, Brandeis WE. Virilizing hepatoblastoma—significance of alpha fetoprotein and human chorionic gonadotropin as tumor markers in diagnosis and follow-up. Eur J Pediatr 1981;135:313–7.

45. Ikeda H, Matsuyama S, Tanimura M. Association between hepatoblastoma and very low birth weight: a trend or a chance? J Pediatr 1997;130:557–60.

46. Inoue S, Nagao T, Ishida Y, et al. Successful resection of a large hepatoblastoma in a young adult: report of a case. Surg Today 1995;25:974–7.

46a. Ishak KG, Glunz PR. Hepatoblastoma and hepatocarcinoma: a report of 47 cases. Cancer 1967;20:396–422.

47. Ito E, Sato Y, Kawauchi K, et al. Type 1a glycogen storage disease with hepatoblastoma in siblings [published erratum appears in Cancer 1987 Aug 15;60(4):723]. Cancer 1987;59:1776–80.

48. Kacker LK, Khan EM, Gupta R, et al. Hepatoblastoma in an adult with biliary obstruction and associated portal venous thrombosis. HPB Surg 1995;9:47–9.

49. Kaw YT, Hansen K. Fine needle aspiration cytology of undifferentiated small cell ("anaplastic") hepatoblastoma. A case report. Acta Cytol 1993;37:216–20.

50. King D, Ortega J, Campbell J. The surgical management of children with incompletely resected hepatic cancer is facilitated by intensive chemotherapy. J Pediatr Surg 1991;26:1074–81.

51. King SJ, Babyn PS, Greenberg ML, Phillips MJ, Filler RM. Value of CT in determining the resectability of hepatoblastoma before and after chemotherapy. Am J Roentgenol 1993;160:793–8.

52. Kitahara S, Makuuchi M, Ishizone S, et al. Successful left trisegmentectomy for ruptured hepatoblastoma using intraoperative transarterial embolization. J Pediatr Surg 1995;30:1709–12.

53. Koishi S, Kubota M, Taniguchi Y, et al. Myelodysplasia in a child with Beckwith-Wiedemann syndrome previously treated for hepatoblastoma with multi-agent chemotherapy [Letter]. J Pediatr Hematol Oncol 1996;18:419–20.

54. Koneru B, Flye MW, Busuttil RW, et al. Liver transplantation for hepatoblastoma. The American experience. Ann Surg 1991;213:118–21.

55. Kraus JA, Albrecht S, Wiestler OD, von Schweinitz D, Pietsch T. Loss of heterozygosity on chromosome 1 in human hepatoblastoma. Int J Cancer 1996;67:467–71.

56. Krober S, Ruck P, Xiao JC, Kaiserling E. Flow cytometric evaluation of nuclear DNA content in hepatoblastoma: further evidence for the inhomogeneity of the different subtypes. Pathol Int 1995;45:501–5.

57. Krush AJ, Traboulsi EI, Offerhaus JA, Maumenee IH, Yardley JH, Levin LS. Hepatoblastoma, pigmented ocular fundus lesions and jaw lesions in Gardner syndrome. Am J Med Genet 1988;29:323–32.

58. Kuniyasu H, Yasui W, Shimamoto F, et al. Hepatoblastoma in an adult associated with c-met protooncogene imbalance. Pathol Int 1996;46:1005–10.

59. Kurahashi H, Takami K, Oue T, et al. Biallelic inactivation of the APC gene in hepatoblastoma. Cancer Res 1995;55:5007–11.

60. Lack EE, Neave C, Vawter GF. Hepatoblastoma. A clinical and pathologic study of 54 cases. Am J Surg Pathol 1982;6:693–705.

61. Le Sher AR, Castronuovo JJ Jr, Filippone AL Jr. Hepatoblastoma in a patient with familial polyposis coli. Surgery 1989;105:668–70.

62. Li FP, Thurber WA, Seddon J, Holmes GE. Hepatoblastoma in families with polyposis coli. JAMA 1987;257:2475–7.

63. Little MH, Thomson DB, Hayward NK, Smith PJ. Loss of alleles on the short arm of chromosome 11 in a hepatoblastoma from a child with Beckwith-Wiedemann syndrome. Hum Genet 1988;79:186–9.

64. Lockwood L, Heney D, Giles GR, Lewis IJ, Bailey CC. Cisplatin-resistant metastatic hepatoblastoma: complete response to carboplatin, etoposide, and liver transplantation. Med Pediatr Oncol 1993;21:517–20.

65. Manivel C, Wick MR, Abenoza P, Dehner LP. Teratoid hepatoblastoma. The nosologic dilemma of solid embryonic neoplasms of childhood. Cancer 1986;57:2168–74.

66. Martelli C, Blandamura S, Massaro S, Zulian M, Altavilla G, Piazza M. A case study of Beckwith-Wiedemann syndrome associated with hepatoblastoma. Clin Exp Obstet Gynecol 1993;20:82–7.

67. Martinez Ibanez V, Marques Gubern A, de Diego M, et al. Hepatoblastoma today. Our experience. Cir Pediatr 1996;9:10–2.

68. Mascarello JT, Jones MC, Kadota RP, Krous HF. Hepatoblastoma characterized by trisomy 20 and double minutes. Cancer Genet Cytogenet 1990;47:243–7.

69. Miller J, Greenspan B. Integrated imaging of hepatic tumors in children. Part I. Malignant lesions (primary and metastatic). Radiology 1985;145:83–90.

70. Miyagi J, Kobayashi S, Kojo N, et al. Brain metastasis of hepatoblastoma—a case report and review of literature. No Shinkei Geka 1984;12:753–8.

71. Molina J, Munoz M, De Miguel C, Martinez-Penuela JM, Villanueva A, Delgado A. Wiedemann-Beckwith syndrome with hepatoblastoma [author's transl]. An Esp Pediatr 1981;15:365–70.

72. Morinaga S, Yamaguchi M, Watanabe I, et al. An immunohistochemical study of hepatoblastoma producing human chorionic gonadotropin. Cancer 1983;51:1647–52.

73. Muraji T, Woolley MM, Sinatra F, et al. The prognostic implication of hypercholesterolemia in infants and children with hepatoblastoma. J Pediatr Surg 1985;20:228–30.

74. Nakagawara A, Ikeda K, Hayashida Y, Tsuneyoshi M, Enjoji M, Kawaaoi A. Immunocytochemical identification of human chorionic gonadotropin- and alpha-fetoprotein-producing cells of hepatoblastoma associated with precocious puberty. Virchows Arch [A] 1982;398:45–51.

75. Nakagawara A, Ikeda K, Tsuneyoshi M, et al. Hepatoblastoma producing both alpha-fetoprotein and human chorionic gonadotropin. Clinicopathologic analysis of four cases and a review of the literature. Cancer 1985;56:1636–42.

76. Napoli VM, Campbell WG Jr. Hepatoblastoma in infant sister and brother. Cancer 1977;39:2647–50.

77. Navarro C, Corretger JM, Sancho A, et al. Paraneoplasic precocious puberty. Report of a new case with hepatoblastoma and review of the literature. Cancer 1985;56:1725–9.

78. Novak D, Suchy F, Balistreri W. Disorders of the liver and biliary system relevant to clinical practice. In: Oski F, ed. Principles and practice of pediatrics. Philadelphia: JB Lippincott, 1990:1746–77.

79. Nyberg DA, Fitzsimmons J, Mack LA, et al. Chromosomal abnormalities in fetuses with omphalocele. Significance of omphalocele contents. J Ultrasound Med 1989;8:299–308.

80. O'Brien W, Finlay JL, Gilbert-Barness EF. Patterns of antigen expression in hepatoblastoma and hepatocellular carcinoma in childhood. Pediatr Hematol Oncol 1989;6:361–5.

81. Oda H, Honda K, Hara M, et al. Hepatoblastoma in an 82-year-old man. An autopsy case report. Acta Pathol Jpn 1990;40:212–8.

82. Oda H, Imai Y, Nakatsuru Y, et al. Somatic mutations of the APC gene in sporadic hepatoblastomas. Cancer Res 1996;56:3320–3.

83. Oda H, Nakatsuru Y, Imai Y, et al. A mutational hot spot in the p53 gene is associated with hepatoblastomas. Int J Cancer 1995;60:786–90.

84. Orozco-Florian R, McBride JA, Favara BE, et al. Congenital hepatoblastoma and Beckwith-Wiedemann syndrome: a case study including DNA ploidy profiles of tumor and adrenal cytomegaly. Pediatr Pathol 1991;11:131–42.

85. Parada LA, Bardi G, Hallen M, et al. Cytogenetic abnormalities and clonal evolution in an adult hepatoblastoma. Am J Surg Pathol 1997;21:1381–6.

86. Passmore SJ, Noblett HR, Wisheart JD, Mott MG. Prolonged survival following multiple thoracotomies for metastatic hepatoblastoma. Med Pediatr Oncol 1995;24:58–60.

87. Pierro A, Langevin AM, Filler RM, et al. Preoperative chemotherapy in "unresectable" hepatoblastoma. J Pediatr Surg 1989;24:24–8;discussion 29.

88. Plumley DA, Grosfeld JL, Kopecky KK, et al. The role of spiral (helical) computerized tomography with three-dimensional reconstruction in pediatric solid tumors. J Pediatr Surg 1995;30:317–21.

89. Pollice L, Zito FA, Troia M. Hepatoblastoma: a clinicopathologic review. Pathologica 1992;84:25–32.

90. Powers C, Ros PR, Stoupis C, et al. Primary liver neoplasms: MR imaging with pathologic correlation. Radiographics 1994;14:459–82.

91. Reynolds M. Conversion of unresectable to resectable hepatoblastoma and long-term follow-up study. World J Surg 1995;19:814–6.

92. Riikonen P, Tuominen L, Seppa A, Perkkio M. Simultaneous hepatoblastoma in identical male twins. Cancer 1990;66:2429–31.

93. Robertson PL, Muraszko KM, Axtell RA. Hepatoblastoma metastatic to brain: prolonged survival after multiple surgical resections of a solitary brain lesion. J Pediatr Hematol Oncol 1997;19:168–71.

94. Rodriguez E, Reuter VE, Mies C, et al. Abnormalities of 2q: a common genetic link between rhabdomyosarcoma and hepatoblastoma? Genes Chromosomes Cancer 1991;3:122–7.

95. Ross JA. Hepatoblastoma and birth weight: too little, too big, or just right? [editorial; comment]. J Pediatr 1997;130:516–7.

96. Ross JA, Gurney JG. Hepatoblastoma incidence in the United States from 1973 to 1992. Med Pediatr Oncol 1998;30:141–2.

97. Ruck P, Harms D, Kaiserling E. Neuroendocrine differentiation in hepatoblastoma. An immunohistochemical investigation. Am J Surg Pathol 1990;14:847–55.

98. Ruck P, Kaiserling E. Extracellular matrix in hepatoblastoma: an immunohistochemical investigation. Histopathology 1992;21:115–26.

99. Ruck P, Kaiserling E. Melanin-containing hepatoblastoma with endocrine differentiation. An immunohistochemical and ultrastructural study. Cancer 1993;72:361–8.

100. Ruck P, Xiao JC, Kaiserling E. Immunoreactivity of sinusoids in hepatoblastoma: an immunohistochemical study using lectin UEA-1 and antibodies against endothelium-associated antigens, including CD34. Histopathology 1995;26:451–5.

101. Ruck P, Xiao JC, Kaiserling E. p53 protein expression in hepatoblastoma: an immunohistochemical investigation. Pediatr Pathol 1994;14:79–85.

102. Ruck P, Xiao JC, Kaiserling E. Small epithelial cells and the histogenesis of hepatoblastoma. Electron microscopic, immunoelectron microscopic, and immunohistochemical findings. Am J Pathol 1996;148:321–9.

103. Schmidt D, Wischmeyer P, Leuschner I, et al. DNA analysis in hepatoblastoma by flow and image cytometry. Cancer 1993;72:2914–9.

104. Schneider NR, Cooley LD, Finegold MJ, et al. The first recurring chromosome translocation in hepatoblastoma: der(4)t(1;4)(q12;q34). Genes Chromosomes Cancer 1997;19:291–4.

105. Shafford EA, Pritchard J. Extreme thrombocytosis as a diagnostic clue to hepatoblastoma [Letter]. Arch Dis Child 1993;69:171.

106. Slugen I, Fiala P, Pauer M, Majercik M, Ondrias F, Cernak P. Mixed hepatoblastoma in the adult: morphological and immunohistochemical findings. Bratisl Lek Listy 1990;91:507–15.

107. Sola Perez J, Perez-Guillermo M, Bas Bernal AB, Mercader JM. Hepatoblastoma. An attempt to apply histologic classification to aspirates obtained by fine needle aspiration cytology. Acta Cytol 1994;38:175–82.

108. Soukup SW, Lampkin BL. Trisomy 2 and 20 in two hepatoblastomas. Genes Chromosomes Cancer 1991;3:231–4.

109. Stocker JT. An approach to handling pediatric liver tumors. Am J Clin Pathol 1998;109(Suppl 1):S68–73.

110. Stocker JT. Hepatic tumors in children. In: Suchy FS, ed. Liver disease in children. St. Louis: Mosby, 1994:901–29.

111. Stocker JT. Hepatoblastoma. Semin Diagn Pathol 1994;11:136–43.

112. Stocker JT, Conran R. Hepatoblastoma. In: Okuda K, Tabor E, eds. Liver cancer. New York: Churchill Livingstone, 1997:263–78.

113. Stocker JT, Conran R, Selby D. Tumor and pseudotumors of the liver. In: Stocker J, Askin F, eds. Pathology of solid tumors in children. London: Chapman & Hall, 1998:83–110.

114. Stringer MD, Hennayake S, Howard ER, et al. Improved outcome for children with hepatoblastoma. Br J Surg 1995;82:386–91.

115. Superina R, Bilik R. Results of liver transplantation in children with unresectable liver tumors. J Pediatr Surg 1996;31:835–9.

116. Surendran N, Radhakrishna K, Chellam VG. Hepatoblastoma in siblings. J Pediatr Surg 1989;24:1169–71.

117. Swarts S, Wisecarver J, Bridge JA. Significance of extra copies of chromosome 20 and the long arm of chromosome 2 in hepatoblastoma. Cancer Genet Cytogenet 1996;91:65–7.

118. Tagge E, Tagge D, Reyes J, et al. Resection, including transplantation, for hepatoblastoma and hepatocellular carcinoma: impact on survival. J Pediatr Surg 1992;27:292–7.

119. Takayama T, Makuuchi M, Kosuge T, et al. A hepatoblastoma originating in the caudate lobe radically resected with the inferior vena cava. Surgery 1991;109:208–13.

120. Tanaka K, Uemoto S, Asonuma K, et al. Hepatoblastoma in a 2-year-old girl with trisomy 18. Eur J Pediatr Surg 1992;2:298–300.

121. Tanaka T, Takakura H, Takashima S, et al. A rare case of Aicardi syndrome with severe brain malformation and hepatoblastoma. Brain Dev 1985;7:507–12.

122. Teraguchi M, Nogi S, Ikemoto Y, et al. Multiple hepatoblastomas associated with trisomy 18 in a 3-year-old girl. Pediatr Hematol Oncol 1997;14:463–7.

123. Tonk VS, Wilson KS, Timmons CF, Schneider NR. Trisomy 2, trisomy 20, and del(17p) as sole chromosomal abnormalities in three cases of hepatoblastoma. Genes Chromosomes Cancer 1994;11:199–202.

124. Tsai SY, Jeng YM, Hwu WL, Ni YH, Chang MH, Wang TR. Hepatoblastoma in an infant with Beckwith-Wiedemann syndrome. J Formos Med Assoc 1996;95:180–3.

125. Tsunoda Y, Okamatsu T, Iijima T, Shibusawa M, Yatsuzuka M. Non-alpha-fetoprotein-producing anaplastic hepatoblastoma cell line [letter]. In Vitro Cell Dev Biol Anim 1996;32:194–6.

126. Us-Krasovec M, Pohar-Marinsek Z, Golouh R, Jereb B, Ferlan-Marolt V, Cerar A. Hepatoblastoma in fine needle aspirates. Acta Cytol 1996;40:450–6.

127. Van Eyken P, Sciot R, Callea F, Ramaekers F, Schaart G, Desmet VJ. A cytokeratin-immunohistochemical study of hepatoblastoma. Hum Pathol 1990;21:302–8.

128. Van Tornout JM, Buckley JD, Quinn JJ, et al. Timing and magnitude of decline in alpha-fetoprotein levels in treated children with unresectable or metastatic hepatoblastoma are predictors of outcome: a report from the Children's Cancer Group. J Clin Oncol 1997;15:1190–7.

129. von Schweinitz D, Burger D, Mildenberger H. Is laparotomy the first step in treatment of childhood liver tumors? The experience from the German Cooperative Pediatric Liver Tumor Study HB-89. Eur J Pediatr Surg 1994;4:82–6.

130. von Schweinitz D, Hecker H, Schmidt von Arndt G, Harms D. Prognostic factors and staging systems in childhood hepatoblastoma. Int J Cancer 1997;74:593–9.

131. von Schweinitz D, Wischmeyer P, Leuschner I, et al. Clinicopathological criteria with prognostic relevance in hepatoblastoma. Eur J Cancer 1994;30A:1052–8.

132. Vos A. Primary liver tumours in children. Eur J Surg Oncol 1995;21:101–5.

133. Wakely PE Jr, Silverman JF, Geisinger KR, Frable WJ. Fine needle aspiration biopsy cytology of hepatoblastoma. Mod Pathol 1990;3:688–93.

134. Warfel KA, Hull MT. Hepatoblastomas: an ultrastructural and immunohistochemical study. Ultrastruct Pathol 1992;16:451–61.

135. Watanabe I, Yamaguchi M, Kasai M. Histologic characteristics of gonadotropin-producing hepatoblastoma: a survey of seven cases from Japan. J Pediatr Surg 1987;22:406–11.

136. Wilfong AA, Parke JT, McCrary JA. Opsoclonus-myoclonus with Beckwith-Wiedemann syndrome and hepatoblastoma. Pediatr Neurol 1992;8:77–9.

137. Yamaguchi H, Ishii E, Hayashida Y, Hirata Y, Sakai R, Miyazaki S. Mechanism of thrombocytosis in hepatoblastoma: a case report. Pediatr Hematol Oncol 1996;13:539–44.

138. Yokomori K, Hori T, Asoh S, Tuji A, Takemura T. Complete disappearance of unresectable hepatoblastoma by continuous infusion therapy through hepatic artery. J Pediatr Surg 1991;26:844–6.

7
PUTATIVE PRECANCEROUS LESIONS

This chapter deals with lesions that are suspected precursors of hepatocellular carcinoma (HCC). Diseases that antedate and are considered to predispose to HCC, e.g., hepatocellular adenoma and cirrhosis of diverse etiology, are considered in various other chapters. The precancerous lesions described in this chapter arise mainly though not exclusively in the cirrhotic liver, the major risk factor for HCC. They include regenerative nodules, dysplastic foci, dysplastic nodules, iron-free foci in genetic hemochromatosis, foci of altered hepatocytes, and proliferation of hepatic stem cells. The terminology used in this chapter for dysplastic foci and nodules follows that proposed by the International Working Party (IWP) in 1995 (30), with some exceptions.

REGENERATIVE NODULES

In the IWP terminology, *multiacinar regenerative nodules* are defined as hepatocellular nodules containing more than one portal tract, that are located in a liver that is otherwise abnormal either with cirrhosis or with severe disease of portal veins, hepatic veins, or sinusoids (30). These nodules are generally at least 5 mm in diameter. This definition includes large regenerative nodules of acute or subacute liver injury, as well as large regenerative (macroregenerative) nodules of an established cirrhosis. To further complicate matters the latter are separately referred to as *multiacinar cirrhotic nodules* (containing more than one portal tract) as opposed to *monoacinar cirrhotic nodules* (containing no more than one portal tract). The small, monoacinar cirrhotic nodules are surrounded by fibrous tissue in contrast to monoacinar regenerative nodules (diffuse nodular hyperplasia or nodular regenerative hyperplasia). *Nodular regenerative hyperplasia* typically consists of small nodules (monoacinar regenerative nodules) but may have large nodules (multiacinar regenerative nodules), as found in so-called partial nodular transformation. The profusion of terms, particularly in reference to large hepatocellular nodules, leads us to avoid using such terms as multiacinar regenerative nodules, multiacinar

cirrhotic nodules, macroregenerative nodules, and adenomatous hyperplasia. Instead, we prefer using the established descriptive terms, *micronodule* and *macronodule* if the liver is cirrhotic, and *regenerative nodule* (small or large) if the liver is not cirrhotic. Our terminology for all benign hepatocellular proliferations is outlined in chapter 2 (Table 2-1).

LIVER CELL DYSPLASIA (LARGE AND SMALL CELL CHANGE)

The term liver cell dysplasia (LCD) was first coined by Anthony et al. (5) to describe a change characterized by cellular enlargement, nuclear pleomorphism, and multinucleation of liver cells occurring in groups or occupying whole cirrhotic nodules (fig. 7-1). The change was found in only 1 percent of patients with normal livers, in 6.9 percent of patients with cirrhosis, and in 64.5 percent of patients with cirrhosis and HCC. There was a strong relationship between LCD and hepatitis B surface antigen (HBsAg) seropositivity. Anthony (5) concluded that the presence of LCD identified a group of patients at high risk for the development of HCC, and that such patients should be followed by serial alpha-fetoprotein determinations. The term LCD is used in this section since it is the term used in the studies that are summarized. However, as noted later, this term has now been superceded by *large cell change* for *large cell dysplasia* and *small cell change* for *small cell dysplasia*. A long-term prospective study by Borzio et al. (10) has confirmed that LCD in patients with cirrhosis is independently associated with an increased risk of HCC, a view supported by the more recent studies of Genne-Carie et al. (23) and LeBail et al. (35). The association of LCD with HCC has been confirmed in many (2,40–43) but not all (11,13,26) studies. Age over 60 years and HBsAg positivity have also been found to be independent risk factors by one group of investigators (10).

While LCD was originally linked to hepatitis B infection, it was later reported in 42.5 percent of patients with non-A, non-B hepatitis, being most often associated with cirrhosis (37). Indeed, it is

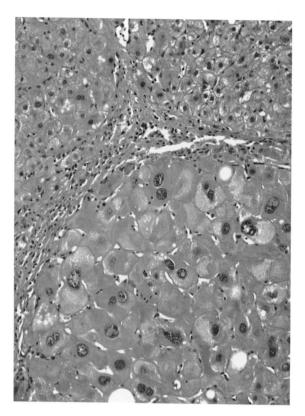 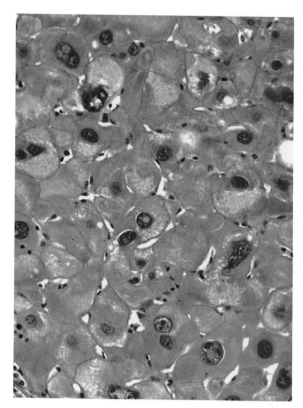

Figure 7-1
LARGE CELL CHANGE (LARGE CELL DYSPLASIA)
Left: In this cirrhotic liver, the hepatocyte nuclei are large, pleomorphic, and hyperchromatic.
Right: Higher magnification shows the markedly abnormal hepatocyte nuclei, but the cells have abundant cytoplasm.

a change that can occur in cirrhosis of diverse etiology, although about half the cases are found in cirrhosis associated with viral hepatitis (35).

In the report of Anthony et al. (5), the nuclear/cytoplasmic ratio of the dysplastic liver cells was considered to be normal. A morphometric study by Watanabe et al. (74) supported that view. However, in a subsequent study, Roncalli et al. (50) found the nuclear/cytoplasmic ratio was increased in cells in LCD. Several flow cytometric studies have failed to support the precancerous nature of LCD (26,31,51). Thomas et al. (69) and An et al. (4) found that LCD contains DNA aneuploid cells, which, in their opinion, supports its role in the evolution of HCC. In the study of An et al., 92 percent of dysplastic cases were aneuploid compared to 60 percent of HCC cases.

Several groups of investigators have attempted to identify histochemical and immunohistochemical differences between the hepatocytes in LCD and non-neoplastic liver cells. Omata et al. (43),

using immunohistochemical methods, found that dysplastic cells did not harbor HBsAg any more frequently than did nondysplastic cells. Roncalli et al. (48) also were unable to detect HBsAg or HBcAg in dysplastic liver cells. In another study, Roncalli et al. (49) found no differences in the immunohistochemical expression of carcinoembryonic antigen, alpha-1-antitrypsin, and alpha-fetoprotein between normal and dysplastic hepatocytes. One histochemical study has shown a pattern of enzyme deviation in HCC that could not be demonstrated in hepatitis B-positive or dysplastic liver cells (71). Cells of HCC gave an intensely positive reaction for gamma-glutamyl transpeptidase activity but were deficient in glucose-6-phosphatase, alkaline phosphatase, and nonspecific esterase activities. Cohen and De Rosa (14) found expression of p53 in 48 percent of their cases of HCC, but in only 3 percent of those of LCD. Zhao and colleagues (76) noted expression of bcl-2 protein in 5 of 37 (13.5 percent) HCCs but not in

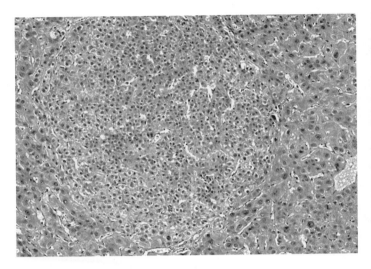

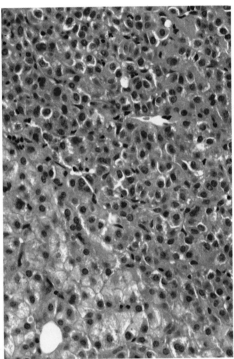

Figure 7-2
SMALL CELL CHANGE (SMALL CELL DYSPLASIA)
Above: The dysplastic focus (which borders on well-differentiated HCC) has minimal nuclear pleomorphism but very high nuclear/cytoplasmic ratios and thickened liver cell plates with cytoplasmic basophilia.

Right: Higher magnification, showing very high nuclear/cytoplasmic ratios but minimal nuclear irregularity.

liver cell dysplasia. In addition to the lack of a morphologic transition of LCD to HCC, Lee at al. (36) found that LCD hepatocytes had a low proliferation rate (Ki-67 and proliferative cell nuclear antigen [PCNA]) but a greater degree of apoptosis than normal hepatocytes. They proposed that LCD derives from derangements of the hepatocyte's normal process of polyploidization, a view suggested earlier by Kagawa et al. (31). Such derangements, possibly caused by chronic inflammation-induced DNA damage, could yield a population of enlarged liver cells with nuclear atypia and pleomorphism, frequent binucleation, and minimal proliferation. According to that hypothesis, LCD could be a habitual feature of cirrhosis and a regular accompaniment of HCC, but would not represent a direct malignant precursor.

Watanabe et al. (74) have expanded the original definition of LCD to include a "small cell" variant. Small cell dysplasia, now referred to as small cell change, is characterized by an increased nuclear/cytoplasmic ratio (figs. 7-2, 7-3), in contrast to large cell dysplasia or large cell change which has a normal ratio. Also, multinucleation and large nucleoli are characteristic of large cell change but not small cell change. The nuclei of small cell change are larger than those of normal

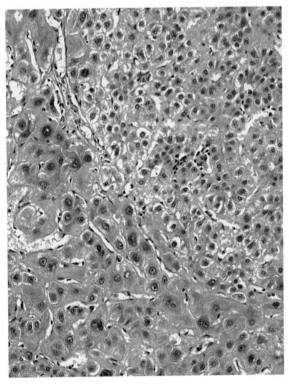

Figure 7-3
SMALL CELL CHANGE (SMALL CELL DYSPLASIA)
This field shows small cell change (top) adjacent to large cell change (bottom).

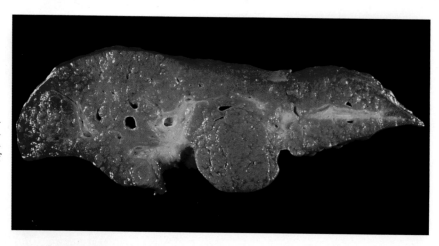

Figure 7-4
LARGE REGENERATIVE
(MACROREGENERATIVE)
NODULE

In this pretransplant hepatectomy specimen, there is a large nodule that bulges from the undersur-
face of the liver. The remainder of
the liver is cirrhotic.

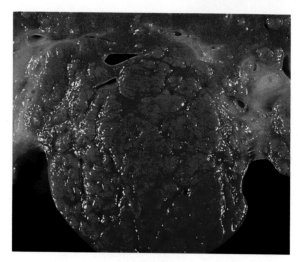

Figure 7-5
LARGE REGENERATIVE
(MACROREGENERATIVE) NODULE
Higher magnification of the nodule in figure 7-4.

hepatocytes but smaller than those of HCC; nucleolar size is intermediate between normal and
HCC cells (74). Morphometric studies by
Watanabe et al. (74). have suggested that small
cell change, rather than large cell change, is the
precancerous lesion in man.

Dysplastic Foci

The term dysplastic focus is defined in the
IWP terminology as a "cluster of hepatocytes less
than 1 mm in diameter with dysplasia but without
definite histologic criteria of malignancy" (30).
Either large or small cell changes (as described
above) may be present in dysplastic foci, which are

usually found in cirrhosis of any type. These foci
have distinct but irregular margins but do not
have a pushing margin. Portal areas are not present in the foci but may be seen at the margin.

Dysplastic Nodules

Adenomatous hyperplasia is a term that has
been used for nodular lesions in the cirrhotic liver
considered premalignant by many investigators (7,
17,21,34,41,42,53,59,65,68,73,75). The nodules vary
from small foci of a few millimeters to larger nodules
10 mm or more in diameter; the latter have been
termed *macroregenerative nodules* (large regenerative nodules) by some authors (figs. 7-4–7-6);
however, it is important to emphasize that the
latter may or may not be "dysplastic." The reported
incidence in cirrhotic livers has varied from 14 to
25 percent (73). They are found in cirrhosis associated with viral hepatitis B or C but also in cirrhosis
of other etiologies, e.g., primary biliary cirrhosis
(61). Dysplastic nodules may be of any size, have a
soft texture, and often bulge from the cut surface
(fig. 7-5). They may be paler than the rest of the
liver and can be bile-stained; necrosis and hemorrhage are not present. The surrounding liver is
usually but not invariably (67) cirrhotic (fig. 7-4).
Dysplastic nodules have further been subclassified
into low- and high-grade types (30).

Low-Grade Dysplastic Nodules. These are
composed of liver cells that are minimally abnormal, and are arranged in two cell–thick plates
(figs. 7-6–7-8). Portal areas are present (fig. 7-8).
The nuclear/cytoplasmic ratio is normal or
slightly increased. Nuclear atypia is minimal
and there are no mitoses. Steatosis and Mallory

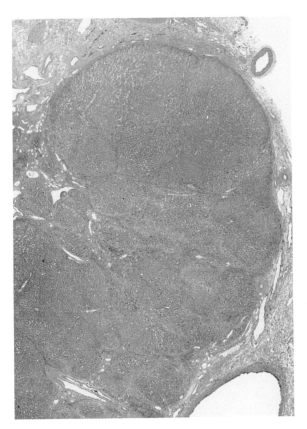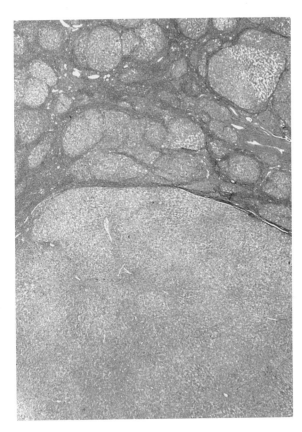

Figure 7-6
MACROREGENERATIVE NODULE

Left: Low-power view of a nodule.
Right: In this hepatitis B-related cirrhosis, there is a segment of a large nodule adjacent to many smaller nodules.

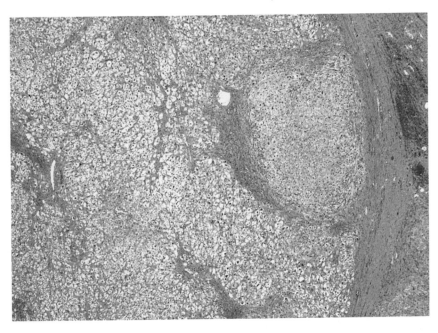

Figure 7-7
MACROREGENERATIVE
NODULE

In this case of hepatitis C-related cirrhosis, there is a large nodule, but there are no atypical features to the liver cells.

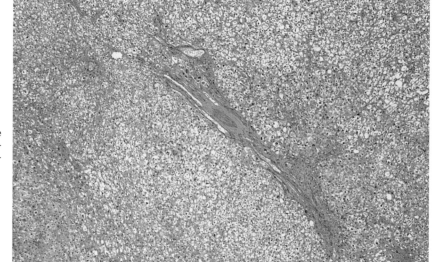

Figure 7-8
MACROREGENERATIVE
NODULE
Higher magnification of the nodule in figure 7-7 shows a relatively quiescent area with a pre-existing portal area.

bodies may be seen (40,60,64). Dysplastic foci, large cell type, may be present.

High-Grade Dysplastic Nodules. These are characterized by one or more additional features: plates more than two cells thick with areas of pseudogland formation (fig. 7-9), cytoplasmic basophilia, a high nuclear/cytoplasmic ratio (fig. 7-10), nuclear hyperchromasia, an irregular nuclear contour, rare mitoses, and resistance to iron accumulation. There is no invasion of stroma or portal areas in the nodules. These features may be confined to one or more foci within the nodule, giving the appearance of subpopulations (subcomponents or "nodule-in-nodule" formation) (fig. 7-11). The differences between low-grade and high-grade dysplastic nodules are listed in Table 7-1; they include some features that are referenced but not discussed further.

High-Grade Dysplastic Nodules and Hepatocellular Carcinoma (HCC). There is general agreement that high-grade dysplastic nodules can evolve into HCC. According to a study by Eguchi et al. (17) approximately 40 percent of cases of adenomatous hyperplasia undergo malignant change. These investigators found that the mean size of the hyperplastic lesion containing cancerous foci (15.8 +/- 2.2 mm) was significantly larger than that of adenomatous hyperplasia without such foci (10.1 +/- 2.6 mm). In another study, all nodules larger than 1.5 cm in diameter were

found to be HCC (53). In that study, a degree of cellularity more than twice that of a regenerative nodule was an indicator of HCC.

Malignant transformation of adenomatous hyperplasia has been documented in a study of Takayama et al. (59). These investigators followed patients for 1 to 5 years after a biopsy-proven diagnosis of adenomatous hyperplasia. The criteria for diagnosis were a doubling of nodular volume and changes in imaging studies. Between 6 and 50 months after biopsy, 9 of 18 nodules met the criteria for malignant transformation; histologic proof of HCC was obtained later in 7 of the 9 nodules.

Morphologic criteria favoring malignancy include distinct trabeculae or plates more than two cells thick, focal absence of reticulin fibers, marked nuclear atypia, a high nuclear/cytoplasmic ratio, moderate or marked mitotic activity, and invasion of portal areas or the stroma (Table 7-1; fig. 7-12) (33,34,39). Differences in the number and distribution of intranodular arteries and the expression of CD34 (capillarization) have been found between cirrhotic nodules, dysplastic nodules, and HCC (46). Unpaired arteries are more numerous and the expression of CD34 greater in HCC than in dysplastic nodules, but the practical utility of these differences in a given needle biopsy specimen is questionable. As mentioned in the IWP paper (30) the diagnosis of

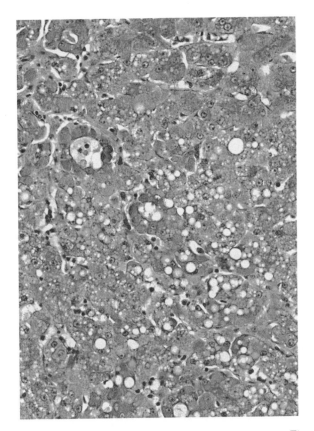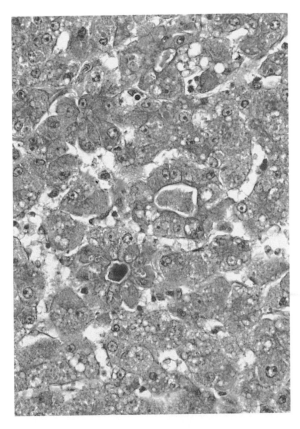

Figure 7-9
HIGH-GRADE DYSPLASTIC NODULE
Left: This cirrhotic nodule has atypical hepatocytes with multinucleation and pseudogland formation.
Right: Higher magnification shows pseudoglands that contain bile.

HCC cannot be excluded in any dysplastic lesion that is sampled only with a biopsy. When insufficient criteria are present to arrive at a diagnosis, a term such as *hepatocellular nodule of uncertain type* or *hepatocellular nodule of uncertain malignant potential* may be used.

Readers interested in further information on the relationship between dysplastic nodules and HCC are referred to several excellent reviews (20,21,29,41,65).

HEPATIC IRON-FREE FOCI

Hepatic iron-free foci (IFF) are "sublobular" nodules of hepatocytes found in genetic hemochromatosis which contain much less iron than the surrounding parenchyma (15). They may be single or multiple, and are found in livers with fibrosis or cirrhosis (fig. 7-13). The foci typically develop near portal areas, and silver stains may

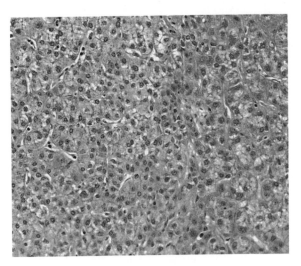

Figure 7-10
HIGH-GRADE DYSPLASTIC NODULE
An area of cells with a high nuclear/cytoplasmic ratio (left) within a high-grade dysplastic nodule.

191

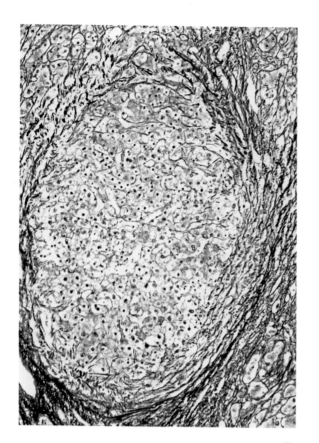
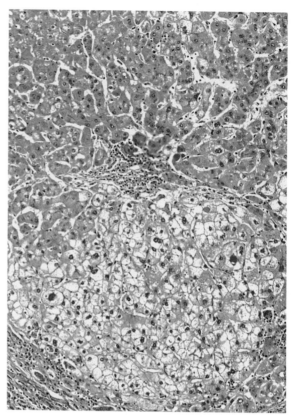

Figure 7-11
HIGH-GRADE DYSPLASTIC NODULE

Left: Reticulin stain shows a focus of small cell dysplasia with reduced reticulin fibers within a preexisting cirrhotic nodule.
Right: Another nodule shows a focus of "nodule-in-nodule" with clear cell change.

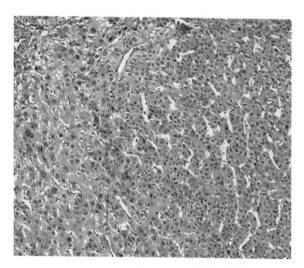

Figure 7-12
HEPATOCELLULAR CARCINOMA ARISING
IN HIGH-GRADE DYSPLASTIC NODULE

Note the microtrabecular pattern and the high nuclear/cytoplasmic ratio of the carcinoma cells.

reveal an expanding lesion. Deugnier et al. (15) followed 12 patients with IFF for 0.9 to 15 years (7 +/- 6 years). HCC developed in 6 (50 percent) compared to 2 (8 percent) from a control group of 24 patients without IFF, matched according to age, sex, degree of fibrosis, liver iron content, and duration of follow-up. The mean number of IFF (per IFF-positive specimen) was 3.2 +/- 2.1. Ten patients had dysplastic foci (half large and half small cell types) in the IFF, but no correlation was found between the type of dysplastic focus and the subsequent development of HCC (15). Proliferative cell nuclear antigen (PCNA) was positive in 75 percent of IFF and in 24 +/- 21 percent of hepatocyte nuclei in IFF. The study of Deugnier and colleagues clearly demonstrates the preneoplastic nature of IFF. They recommended that the finding of IFF in a liver biopsy specimen from a patient with genetic hemochromatosis should lead to regular screening for HCC.

Table 7-1

COMPARISON OF LOW-GRADE AND HIGH-GRADE DYSPLASTIC NODULES WITH HEPATOCELLULAR CARCINOMA

Criterion	Low-Grade Nodule	High-Grade Nodule	Hepatocellular Carcinoma, Well Differentiated
Synonyms and related terms	Adenomatous hyperplasia Macroregenerative nodule, ordinary Macroregenerative, type I	Adenomatous hyperplasia, atypical Macroregenerative nodule, atypical Macroregenerative nodule type II	
Portal areas	Present	Present or absent (focally)	Absent
Plates	Two cells thick	Two cells thick	>Two cells thick
Trabeculae	Absent	Absent	Present
Pseudoglands	Absent	Absent or present	Present or absent
"Nodule-in-nodule" change	Absent or present	Present or absent	Present or absent
Reticulin network	Present	Usually present	Usually absent
Internodular arteries (46)*	Present, few	Present, many	Present
Steatosis (64)	Present or absent	Present or absent	Present or absent
Mallory bodies (40,60)	Present or absent	Present or absent	Present or absent
Stainable Cu/Cu-binding protein (63)	Present, uneven	Unknown	Present or absent
Stainable iron (63)	Present or absent	Absent in "iron-free foci" in genetic hemochromatosis (15)	Absent
Liver cell "atypia"	Minimal or absent	Present, focal (cytoplasmic basophilia, high N/C ratio, hyperchromasia, nuclear irregularities, other)	Same as high-grade nodule
Mitoses	Absent	Absent or few	Variable (0–5/10 HPF)
Clear cell change	Absent	Present or absent	Present or absent
Dysplastic foci	Large cell, present or absent	Large or small cell, present or absent	Present or absent in in adjacent liver
Proliferative activity	Normal	Increased (34,75)	Increased
Invasion of stroma of portal tracts (33,39)	Absent	Absent	Present or absent
Alpha-fetoprotein (66)	Not expressed	Present or absent	Present or absent
Aneuploidy	6% (44)	58% (44)	50.0% (21a) to 78% (7a)
Clonality	Monoclonal or polyclonal (45)	Polyclonal (47); monoclonal (4); monoclonal or polyclonal (45)	Monoclonal

*Numbers in parentheses indicate references. N/C = nuclear/cytoplasmic; HPF = high-power field.

FOCI OF ALTERED HEPATOCYTES

Foci of altered hepatocytes are preneoplastic lesions that have been identified in various animal models of hepatocarcinogenesis (8). Their occurrence and significance in the human liver was recently investigated by Su et al. (58). These investigators studied 163 explanted and resected human livers with or without HCC. Foci of altered hepatocytes, including *glycogen storing foci, mixed cell foci,* and *basophilic foci,* were found in 84 of 111 (75.7 percent) cirrhotic livers. They also were more prevalent in livers with HCC (29 of 32 [90.6 percent]) than in those without HCC (55 of 79 [44.3 percent]). The glycogen storing foci were typically periportal and consisted of "clear" cells

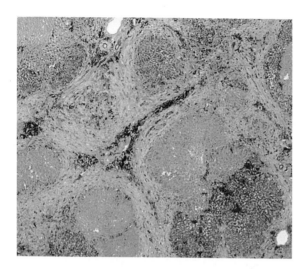
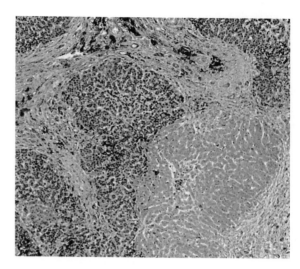

Figure 7-13
IRON-FREE FOCI
Left: Several small iron-free foci are present in this low-power field (Perl's iron stain).
Right: Higher magnification of one of the iron-free foci.

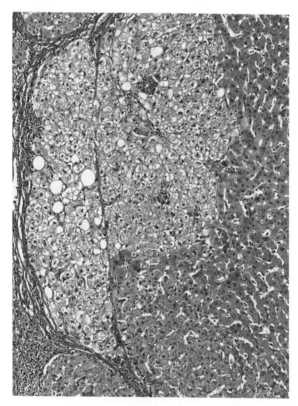

Figure 7-14
FOCUS OF ALTERED HEPATOCYTES
Although there are no atypical cytologic or nuclear features, the "clear cell" appearance of this focus within a cirrhotic nodule indicates it is glycogen-rich and may be analogous to animal models of carcinogenesis.

larger than normal hepatocytes; their cytoplasm was full of glycogen (+/- fat) and the nuclei were small (figs. 7-11, 7-14). The mixed cell foci consisted of an admixture of clear cells and amphophilic (or less often basophilic) cells.

Foci of altered hepatocytes were observed by Su et al. (58) more frequently (78.7 percent) in patients with cirrhosis associated with hepatitis B or C or chronic alcohol abuse (high-risk groups) than in that due to other causes (50 percent). Mixed cell foci, predominantly in cirrhotic livers of the high-risk group, were more proliferative, larger, and more often involved in the formation of nodules of altered hepatocytes (39.3 percent) than were glycogen storing foci (8.5 percent). The results of the study of Su et al. (58) suggested that foci of altered hepatocytes are preneoplastic lesions, the mixed cell foci being more advanced than the glycogen storing foci. Oncocytic and amphophilic cell foci were also observed, but their significance remains to be clarified. Two types of small cell change, diffuse and intrafocal, were identified but only the intrafocal change was related to increased proliferative activity (PCNA) and a more frequent nodular change of the affected focus of altered hepatocytes, thus suggesting a close association with progression from the altered focus to HCC. The findings are of considerable interest to students of hepatocarcinogenesis but await confirmation by other investigators.

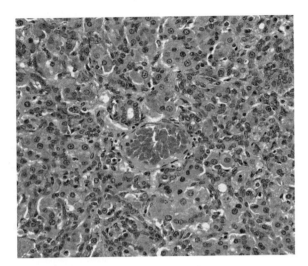 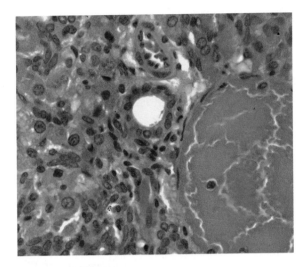

Figure 7-15
OVAL CELLS

Left: Experimental carcinogenesis, rat liver. The oval cells are ill-defined, have small dark nuclei, and are located between hepatocytes in the periportal area.
Right: Higher magnification of the oval cells.

LIVER STEM CELLS

The traditional view of the pathogenesis of experimentally induced liver cancer is the development, after months or years of exposure to a carcinogen, of foci of altered hepatocytes (basophilic, amphophilic, acidophilic, or mixed foci) that then evolve into nodules (hyperplastic, neoplastic, or preneoplastic). These nodules show progressive morphologic or enzymatic changes that antedate the development of liver cancer. The number of nodules progressively decreases such that, at the time that unequivocal carcinoma develops, only one to three persistent nodules remain (8,18). The sequence of foci to nodules to HCC implies "dedifferentiation" of mature hepatocytes. Since the early 1970s, however, it has been known that hepatocarcinogens can stimulate the proliferation of bile duct–like cells (initially termed *oval cells*) in experimental animals (fig. 7-15). These cells were subsequently found to express liver cell markers (albumin and alpha-fetoprotein); the antigenic and enzymatic characteristics of these cells are compared to those of hepatocytes and bile duct cells in Table 7-2.

These cells are derived from bipolar liver stem cells, and can differentiate into normal duct cells or hepatocytes. They can also migrate into persistent nodules to give rise to HCC (55). Cells thought to be oval cells have been identified in

Table 7-2

MARKERS OF PUTATIVE LIVER STEM CELLS (OVAL CELLS)*

Marker	Liver Cells	Duct Cells	Oval Cells
Albumin	+	–	+
Alpha-fetoprotein	–	–	+
OV-6**	–	+	+
Cytokeratin 19	–	+	+
Enzymes			
ATPase	+	–	–
γ-glutamyl transpeptidase	–	+	+
β-glucuronidase	+	–	–
Epoxide hydrolase	+	–	–
Glucose-6-phosphatase	+	+/–	+/–
Phase I metabolizing enzymes	+	–	–
Phase II metabolizing enzymes	+	++	
Isoenzymes			
Aldolase	B	A	A,B,C
Pyruvate kinase	L	K	K,K-L
Hematopoietic stem cell markers**			
C-kit	–	+	+
CD33	–	+	+
CD34	–	+	+

*Modified from reference 55.
**Blakolmer et al. (9).

195

human hepatitis B virus (HBV)–associated HCC (27,28) although this awaits independent confirmation; the expression of TGF-alpha and HBV markers in these oval cells has been suggested as a possible mechanism of hepatocarcinogenesis (28). The origin and characteristics of liver stem cells and their role in normal development of the liver, regeneration, and hepatocarcinogenesis are detailed in numerous reviews from which the discussion in this section is derived (16,18,19, 24,25,38,54–57,70). The liver stem cells may derive from a transition duct cell or from a small nondescript periportal cell. There is also sound evidence for the existence of a precursor *hepatobiliary stem cell* along the biliary tract, and even a *gastrointestinal determined stem cell* retained in the bile ducts (55). In considering the cellular origin and differentiation of liver neoplasia, Sell (55) postulates that mutations causing arrest at the stem cell level of differentiation result in hepatoblastoma;

arrest of the transition duct cell results in mixed hepatocellular and cholangiocarcinoma; arrest of the liver cell results in hepatocellular carcinoma; while arrest at the bile duct cell level results in cholangiocarcinoma.

It should be clear from the preceding sections that much remains to be resolved in the field of hepatic preneoplasia in humans. What is the relationship between the currently accepted putative precancerous lesions in man (dysplastic foci, small cell type; dysplastic nodules, low and high grade; iron-free foci in hemochromatosis) and the liver stem cell? Are the so-called foci and nodules of altered hepatocytes described in human livers (58) comparable to similarly named lesions in experimental hepatocarcinogenesis? Are the foci of altered hepatocytes in the human liver the result of dedifferentiation, and does a liver stem cell play a role in the subsequent development of HCC?

REFERENCES

1. Aihara T, Noguchi S, Sasaki Y, et al. Clonal analysis of precancerous lesion of hepatocellular carcinoma. Gastroenterology 1996;111:455–61.

2. Akagi G, Furuya K, Kanamura A, Chihara T, Osuka H. Liver cell dysplasia and hepatitis B surface antigen in liver cirrhosis and hepatocellular carcinoma. Cancer 1984;54:315–8.

3. Alpini G, Aragona E, Dabeva M, Salvi R, Shatritz DA, Tavoloni N. Distribution of albumin and alpha-fetoprotein in mRNAs in normal, hyperplastic, and preneoplastic rat liver. Am J Pathol 1992;141:623–32.

4. An CS, Petrovic LM, Reyter I, et al. The application of image analysis and neural network technology to the study of large-cell liver-cell dysplasia and hepatocellular carcinoma. Hepatology 1997;26:1224–31.

5. Anthony PP, Vogel CL, Barker LF. Liver cell dysplasia: a premalignant condition. J Clin Pathol 1973;26:217–23.

6. Arakawa M, Kage M, Sugihara S, Nakashima T, Suenaga M, Okuda K. Emergence of malignant lesions within an adenomatous hyperplastic nodule in a cirrhotic liver. Observations in five cases. Gastroenterology 1986;91:198–208.

7. Arakawa M, Sugihara S, Kenmochi K, et al. Small mass lesions in cirrhosis: transition from benign adenomatous hyperplasia to hepatocellular carcinoma? J Gastroenterol Hepatol 1986;1:3–14.

7a. Attallah AM, Tabll AA, Salem SF, et al. DNA ploidy of liver biopsies from patients with liver cirrhosis and hepatocellular carcinoma: a flow cytometric analysis. Cancer Lett 1999;142:65–9.

8. Bannasch P, Zerban H. Experimental chemical hepatocarcinogenesis. In: Okuda K, Tabor E, eds. Liver cancer. New York: Churchill Livingstone, 1997:213–53.

9. Blakolmer K, Jaskiewicz K, Dunsford HA, Robson SC. Hematopoietic stem cell markers are expressed by ductal plate and bile duct cells in developing human liver. Hepatology 1995;21:1510–6.

10. Borzio M, Bruno S, Roncalli M, et al. Liver cells dysplasia is a major factor for risk of hepatocellular carcinoma in cirrhosis: a prospective study. Gastroenterology 1995;108:812–7.

11. Chen M, Gerber MA, Thung SN, Thorton JC, Chung WK. Morphometric studies of hepatocytes containing hepatitis B surface antigen. Am J Pathol 1984;114:217–21.

12. Cohen C, Berson SD. Liver cell dysplasia in normal, cirrhotic, and hepatocellular carcinoma patients. Cancer 1986;57:1535–8.

13. Cohen C, Berson SD, Geddis EW. Liver cell dysplasia. Association with hepatocellular carcinoma, cirrhosis and hepatitis B antigen carrier status. Cancer 1979;44:1671–6.

14. Cohen C, DeRosa PB. Immunohistochemical p53 in hepatocellular carcinoma and liver cell dysplasia. Mod Pathol 1994;7:536–9.
15. Deugnier YM, Charalambous P, Le Quilleuc D, et al. Preneoplastic significance of hepatic iron-free foci in genetic hemochromatosis: a study of 185 patients. Hepatology 1993;18:1363–9.
16. Divan BA, Ward JM, Rice JM. Origin and pathology of hepatoblastoma in mice. In: Sirica AE, ed. The role of cell types in hepatocarcinogenesis. Boca Raton: CRC Press, 1992:71–120.
17. Eguchi A, Nakashima O, Okudaira S, Sugihara S, Kojiro M. Adenomatous hyperplasia in the vicinity of small hepatocellular carcinoma. Hepatology 1992;15:843–8.
18. Farber E. On cells of origin of liver cell cancer. In: Sirica AE, ed. The role of cell types in hepatocarcinogenesis. Boca Raton: CRC Press, 1992:1–28.
19. Fausto N, Lemire JM, Shiojiri N. Oval cells in liver carcinogenesis. In Sirica AE, ed. The role of cell types in hepatocarcinogenesis. Boca Raton: CRC Press, 1992:89–108.
20. Ferrell LD, Crawford JM, Dhillon AP, et al. Proposal for standardized criteria for the diagnosis of benign, borderline, and malignant hepatocellular lesions arising in chronic advanced liver disease. Am J Surg Pathol 1993;17:1113–23.
21. Ferrell LD, Wright T, Lake J, et al. Incidence and diagnostic features of macroregenerative nodules vs. small hepatocellular carcinoma in cirrhotic livers. Hepatology 1992;16:1372–81.
21a. Fujimoto J, Okamoto E, Yamanaka N, Scheuer PJ, Nakanuma Y. Flow cytometric DNA analysis of hepatocellular carcinoma. Cancer 1991;67:939–44.
22. Furuya K, Nakamura M, Yamamoto Y, et al. Macroregenerative nodule of the liver. A clinicopathologic study of 345 autopsy cases of chronic liver disease. Cancer 1988;61:99–105.
23. Ganne-Carrie, N, Chastang C, Chapel F, et al. Predictive score for the development of hepatocellular carcinoma and additional value of liver large cell dysplasia in Western patients with cirrhosis. Hepatology 1996;23:112–8.
24. Grisham JW. Hepatic epithelial stem-like cells. Verch Dtsch Ges Pathol 1995;79:47–54.
25. Grisham JW, Coleman WB. Neoformation of liver epithelial cells: progenitor cells, stem cells, and phenotypic transitions. Gastroenterology 1996;110:1311–3.
26. Henmi A, Uchida T, Shikata T. Karyometric analysis of liver cell dysplasia and hepatocellular carcinoma. Evidence against precancerous nature of liver cell dysplasia. Cancer 1985;55:2594–9.
27. Hsia CC, Evarts RP, Nakatsukasa H, Marsden ER, Thorgeirsson SS. Occurrence of oval-type cells in hepatitis B virus-associated human hepatocarcinogenesis. Hepatology 1992;16:1327–33.
28. Hsia CC, Thorgeirsson SS, Tabor E. Expression of hepatitis B surface and core antigens and transforming growth factor-alpha in "oval cells" of the liver in patients with hepatocellular carcinoma. J M Viral 1994;43:216–21.
29. Hytiroglou P, Theise ND. Differential diagnosis of hepatocellular nodular lesions. Semin Diagn Pathol 1998;15:285–99.
30. International Working Party. Terminology of nodular hepatocellular lesions. Hepatology 1995;22:983–93.
31. Kagawa K, Deguchi T, Tomimasu H, et al. Feulgen-DNA cytofluorimetry of the liver cell dysplasia (LCD) in the liver cirrhosis. Jpn J Gastroenterol 1984;81:82–91.
32. Kondo F, Ebara M, Sugiura N, et al. Histological features and clinical course of large regenerative nodules: evaluation of their precancerous potentiality. Hepatology 1990;12:592–8.
33. Kondo F, Kondo Y, Nagato Y, Tomizawa M, Wada K. Interstitial tumor cell invasion in small hepatocellular carcinoma: evaluation in microscopic and low magnification views. J Gastroenterol Hepatol 1994;9:604–12.
34. Le Bail B, Belleannée G, Bernard PH, Saric J, Balabaud C, Bioulac-Sage P. Adenomatous hyperplasia in cirrhotic liver: histological evaluation, cellular density, and proliferative activity of 35 macronodular lesions in the cirrhotic explants of 10 adult French patients. Hum Pathol 1995;26:897–906.
35. Le Bail B, Bernard PH, Carles J, et al. Prevalence of liver cell dysplasia and association with HCC in a series of 100 cirrhotic liver explants. J Hepatol 1997;27:835–42.
36. Lee R, Tsamandas AC, Demetris AJ. Large cell change (liver cell dysplasia) and hepatocellular carcinoma in cirrhosis: matched case-control study, pathological analysis, and pathogenetic hypothesis. Hepatology 1997;26:1415–22.
37. Lefkowitch JH, Apfelbaum TF. Liver cell dysplasia and hepatocellular carcinoma in non-A, non-B hepatitis. Arch Pathol Lab Med 1987;111:170–3.
38. Marceau N, Blouin MJ, Noël M, Török N, Loranger A. The role of bipotential progenitor cells in liver ontogenesis and neoplasia. In: Sirica AE, ed. The role of cell types in hepatocarcinogenesis. Boca Raton: CRC Press, 1992:121–49.
39. Nakano M, Saito A, Takasaki K, et al. A histopathology study of early hepatocellular carcinoma: portal tract invasion and progression to advanced hepatocellular carcinoma. Acta Pathol Jpn 1990;31:754–62.
40. Nakanuma Y, Ohta G. Is Mallory body formation a preneoplastic change? A study of 101 cases of liver bearing hepatocellular carcinoma and 82 cases of cirrhosis. Cancer 1985;55:2400–4.
41. Nakanuma Y, Terada T, Ueda K, Tersaki S, Nonomura A, Matsui O. Adenomatous hyperplasia of the liver as a precancerous lesion. Liver 1993;13:1–9.
42. Nakashima T, Okuda K, Kojiro M, et al. Pathology of hepatocellular carcinoma in Japan: 232 consecutive cases autopsied in ten years. Cancer 1983;51:863–77.
43. Omata M, Mori J, Yokosuka O, et al. Hepatitis B virus antigens in liver tissue in hepatocellular carcinoma and advanced chronic liver disease—relationship to liver cell dysplasia. Liver 1992;2:125–32.
44. Orsatti G, Theise ND, Thung SN, Paronetto F. DNA image cytometric analysis of macroregenerative nodules (adenomatous hyperplasia) of the liver: evidence in support of their preneoplastic nature. Hepatology 1993;17:621–7.
45. Paradis V, Laurnedeau I, Vidaud M, Bedossa P. Clonal analysis of macronodules in cirrhosis. Hepatology 1998;28:953–8.
46. Park YN, Yang CP, Fernandez GJ, et al. Neoangiogenesis and sinusoidal capillarization in dysplastic nodules of the liver. Am J Surg Pathol 1998;22:656–62.

47. Piao Z, Park YN, Kim H, Park C. Clonality of large regenerative nodules in liver cirrhosis. Liver 1997;17: 251–6.

48. Roncalli M, Borzio M, De Biagi G, et al. Liver cell dysplasia and hepatocellular carcinoma: a histological and immunohistochemical study. Histopathology 1985;9:209–21.

49. Roncalli M, Borzio M, De Biagi G, et al. Liver cell dysplasia in cirrhosis. A serologic and immunohisto-chemical study. Cancer 1986;57:1515–21.

50. Roncalli M, Borzio M, Tombesi MV, Ferrari A, Servida E. A morphometric study of liver cell dysplasia. Hum Pathol 1988;19:471–4.

51. Rubin EM, De Rose PB, Cohen C. Comparative image cytometric DNA ploidy of liver cell dysplasia and hepatocellular carcinoma. Mod Pathol 1994;7:677–80.

52. Sakurai M. Liver cell dysplasia and hepatitis B surface and core antigens in cirrhosis and hepatocellular carci-noma of autopsy cases. Acta Pathol Jap 1978;28:705–19.

53. Sakamoto M, Hirohashi S, Shimosato Y. Early stages of multistep hepatocarcinogenesis: adenomatous hy-perplasia and early hepatocellular carcinoma. Hum Pathol 1991;22:172–8.

54. Sell S. Comparison of liver progenitor cells in human atypical ductular reactions with those seen in experimen-tal models of liver injury. Hepatology 1998;27:317–31.

55. Sell S. Liver stem cells. Mod Pathol 1994;7:105–12.

56. Sell S. The role of determined stem-cells in the cellular lineage of hepatocellular carcinoma. Int J Dev Biol 1993;37:189–201.

57. Sell S, Dunsford HA. Evidence for the stem cell origin of hepatocellular carcinoma and cholangiocarcinoma. Am J Pathol 1989;134:1347–63.

58. Su Q, Benner A, Hofmann WJ, et al. Human hepatic preneoplasia: phenotypes and proliferation kinetics of foci and nodules of altered hepatocytes and their relationship to liver cell dysplasia. Virchows Arch 1997;431:391–406.

59. Takayama T, Makuuchi M, Hirohashi S, et al. Malig-nant transformation of adenomatous hyperplasia to hepatocellular carcinoma. Lancet 1990;336:1150–3.

60. Terada T, Hoso M, Nakanuma Y. Mallory body clustering in adenomatous hyperplasia in human cirrhotic livers: report of four cases. Hum Pathol 1989;20:886–90.

61. Terada T, Kurumaya H, Nakanuma Y, Hayakawa Y, Matsuda H. Macroregenerative nodules of the liver in primary biliary cirrhosis: report of two autopsies. Am J Gastroenterol 1989;84:418–21.

62. Terada T, Nakanuma Y. Expression of ABH blood group antigens, receptors of Ulex europaeus' agglutinin 1, and factor VIII-related antigen on sinusoidal endothe-lial cells in adenomatous hyperplasia in human cir-rhotic liver. Hum Pathol 1991;22:486–93.

63. Terada T, Nakanuma Y. Survey of iron-accumulative macroregenerative nodules in cirrhotic livers. Hepatology 1989;10:851–4.

64. Terada T, Nakanuma Y, Hoso M, Saito K, Sasaki M, Nonomura A. Fatty macroregenerative nodule in non-steatotic liver cirrhosis. A morphologic study. Virchows Arch [A] 1988;415:131–6.

65. Theise ND. Macroregenerative (dysplastic) nodules and hepatocarcinogenesis: theoretical and clinical con-siderations. Semin Liver Dis 1995;15:360–71.

66. Theise ND, Fiel IM, Hytiroglou P, et al. Macroregenera-tive nodules in cirrhosis are not associated with ele-vated serum or stainable tissue alpha-fetoprotein. Liver 1995;15:30–4.

67. Theise ND, Lapook JD, Thung SN. A macroregenerative nodule containing multiple foci of hepatocellular carci-noma in a noncirrhotic liver. Hepatology 1993;17:993–6.

68. Theise ND, Schwartz M, Miller C, Thung SN. Macroregenerative nodules and hepatocellular carci-noma in forty-four sequential adult liver explants with cirrhosis. Hepatology 1992;16:949–55.

69. Thomas RM, Berman JJ, Yetter RA, et al. Liver cell dysplasia: a DNA aneuploid lesion with distinct morphologic features. Hum Pathol 1992;23:496–503.

70. Thorgeirsson SS. Hepatic stem cells. Am J Pathol 1993; 142:1331–3.

71. Uchida T, Miyata H, Shikata T. Human hepatocellular carcinoma and putative precancerous disorders: their enzyme histochemical study. Arch Pathol Lab Med 1981;105:180–6.

72. Ueda K, Matsui O, Nakanuma Y, et al. Deposition of copper and copper-binding protein (CBP) in adenoma-tous hyperplasia of the liver: relevance to magnetic resonance imaging. Int Hepatol Comm 1993;1:326–30.

73. Wada K, Kondo F, Kondo Y. Large regenerative nodules and dysplastic nodules in cirrhotic livers: a histopath-ologic study. Hepatology 1988;8:1684–8.

74. Watanabe S, Okita K, Harada T, et al. Morphologic studies of the liver cell dysplasia. Cancer 1983;51:2197–205.

75. Yamashita A. Comparison of the proliferative capacity of adenomatous hyperplasia and well differentiated hepat-ocellular carcinoma. J Gastroenterol 1996;31:373–8.

76. Zhao M, Zhang NX, Economou M, Blaha I, Laissue JA, Zimmermann A. Immunohistochemical detection of bcl-2 protein in liver cell lesions: bcl-2 protein is ex-pressed in hepatocellular carcinomas but not in liver cell dysplasia. Histopathology 1994;25:237–45.

❖❖❖

8

HEPATOCELLULAR CARCINOMA

This chapter deals with the most common primary hepatic malignancy of adults. Hepatocellular carcinoma (HCC) is the preferred name for this neoplasm, and while "hepatoma" is widely used, it lacks precision and should be discouraged. Similarly, the term "primary liver cancer" is used in many reports of vital statistics, and while HCC accounts for over 90 percent of this, it still causes confusion that can be avoided with precise terminology. There are a number of histologic variants of HCC, but only one of these, fibrolamellar carcinoma, differs significantly in its clinicopathologic features and natural history, and so it will be considered in the next chapter.

HCC has many intriguing aspects that have made it the subject of intense study by investigators in many fields. For internists, surgeons, and oncologists, the association of HCC with chronic liver diseases, the difficulties that surround its detection and diagnosis, and its frequent late presentation, dismal prognosis, and typically poor response to therapy provide continual challenge. For epidemiologists and students of human carcinogenesis, the striking geographic variation in the incidence of HCC, and its association with viral infections and exposure to chemical agents, have made it a paradigm for the study of the pathogenesis of human cancer. For basic scientists, the ability to propagate cell lines from HCC in tissue culture has provided the means for the study of many biochemical and physiologic processes, as there are often similarities between normal hepatocytes and the cells of well-differentiated tumors. For pathologists, the histologic diagnosis of HCC can be difficult at times, and investigators have concentrated on recognition of early lesions and techniques to aid in the differential diagnosis of well-differentiated and poorly differentiated tumors.

Definition. HCC is a malignant neoplasm composed of cells that differentiate in some way in the manner of hepatocytes.

Etiology and Epidemiology. HCC has long been of interest to students of human carcinogenesis because of its geographic variability and its association with chronic liver diseases. Recent advances in molecular biology and the discovery of the hepatitis B and C viruses have explained many of the unusual features of this neoplasm and promise to increase further our understanding of the mechanisms of hepatic carcinogenesis.

Geographic Pathology. Among the most striking features of HCC is the wide variation in its incidence in different parts of the world (fig. 8-1) (68). East Asia and southern Africa have the greatest number of cases, and in the countries of those regions HCC is among the leading causes of death from cancer, whereas in areas of low incidence, such as the United States, HCC accounts for less than 2 percent of cancer deaths and ranks 22nd in frequency with an annual incidence of approximately 4 per 100,000 (11). In general, regions with a high incidence of HCC are those that have a high prevalence of chronic hepatitis B infection (such as the Alaskan Arctic), although there are exceptions. Hepatitis C infection is associated with many cases in countries such as Japan, where the prevalence of hepatitis B is intermediate but the incidence of HCC is relatively high. Furthermore, within areas of high incidence, some regions, such as Jiangsu and Guangxi provinces in China, and Mozambique in southern Africa, have extremely high death rates from HCC, more than 10 times those in other high incidence areas.

Cirrhosis. It has been recognized since the 19th century that HCC often arises in a diseased liver, particularly in the setting of longstanding cirrhosis. Macronodular cirrhosis has always been more strongly associated with HCC than micronodular cirrhosis, and cirrhosis of virtually any cause may be complicated by the development of HCC (28). Controversy remains over whether cirrhosis itself is a premalignant condition, whether cirrhosis and HCC can be caused independently by the same agents, or whether the continuous stimulus to regeneration that exists in cirrhosis makes the liver more susceptible to environmental carcinogens. There is evidence to support all three possibilities but not enough to establish the pathogenetic relationship.

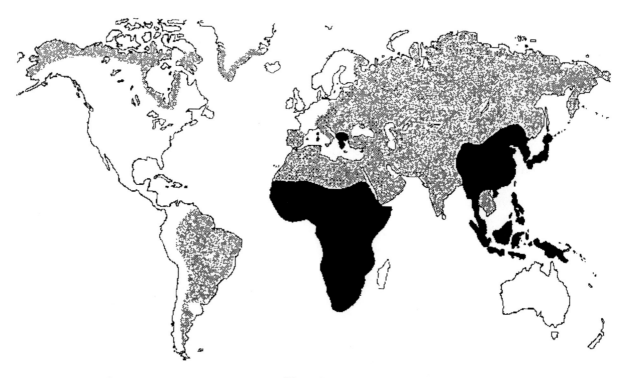

Figure 8-1
GEOGRAPHIC DISTRIBUTION OF HEPATOCELLULAR CARCINOMA
Areas with a high annual incidence (20 or more per 100,000 population) are black. Areas with an intermediate incidence (5 to 20 per 100,000) are gray. Areas with a low incidence (less than 5 per 100,000) are white.

Although most studies from different parts of the world have found a strong association of HCC with cirrhosis (75 to 90 percent of tumors arise in cirrhotic livers), there appears to be some geographic variation. In Japan and other Asian countries, approximately 90 percent of patients have underlying cirrhosis (58), whereas in some parts of Africa cirrhosis is present in only 50 to 63 percent of patients (30), although most have precirrhotic forms of chronic viral hepatitis. At the Armed Forces Institute of Pathology (AFIP), among patients from North America reviewed since 1980, the prevalence of cirrhosis in HCC was 57 percent, while in other North American series it has ranged from 46 to 91 percent (53). In the experience of the authors, HCC in a noncirrhotic liver is quite common, and North America is more like Africa than Asia or Europe in this regard. Indeed, a large number of our cases had no evidence of any underlying liver disease, although the exact proportion could not be determined as many of the diagnoses were made on small biopsy specimens in which only tissue adjacent to the tumor was available for evaluation.

Gender and Age. In every country of the world, HCC is more frequent in men than women, with male to female ratios that range from 2:1 to 5:1. In our experience at the AFIP with North American patients, the male to female ratio has been 4:1 (54). The reason for this is not known but male predominance in other risk factors, such as chronic hepatitis B infection, alcoholism, and smoking may be partly to blame, and a high percentage of tumors have androgen receptors (46), raising the possibility that androgens may promote tumor development and growth.

The incidence of HCC generally increases with age, presumably related to an increasing likelihood of exposure to causative agents. There are striking geographic differences, however. In South Africa, the average age of patients with HCC is 35 years, and 40 percent are 30 or younger, whereas in Taiwan (another area of high incidence), the majority of patients are 40 to 60 years old with a peak age-adjusted incidence in the 8th decade (3). In our series of North American cases from 1980 to 1993 reviewed at the AFIP, the mean age was 60.5 years and the peak incidence was in the 7th decade. However, HCC can occur in young adults, adolescents, and children. The youngest reported patient (of whom we are aware) was an 8-month-old with hepatitis B (78).

Hepatitis B. After the discovery of the hepatitis B virus, it soon became apparent that the parts of the world with a high prevalence of chronic hepatitis B were the same areas with a high rate of death from primary cancer of the liver, primarily HCC (fig. 8-1). Although there are other etiologic factors, hepatitis B infection has the strongest association with the development of HCC (3). The pathogenetic mechanism is still uncertain, and despite extensive investigation a direct oncogenic role, although strongly suspected, remains unproven. Evidence for an oncogenic role lies in the fact that in chronic infection, hepatitis B viral DNA sequences become integrated at random into the host genome, raising the possibility that these may serve as insertional mutagens through activation of oncogenes, inactivation of tumor suppressor genes, or mutations in p53 or other tumor suppressor genes that result in oncogene activation (45). It also seems likely that the inflammation and hepatocellular regeneration associated with chronic infection provides an increased opportunity for other carcinogens to affect the cell cycle.

Hepatitis C. Hepatitis C rivals hepatitis B in importance as an etiologic factor in HCC (56). Chronic hepatitis C infection shows much less geographic variation than hepatitis B, with a prevalence in blood donors varying from 0.3 to 1.5 percent in different countries. Serologic surveys, however, have shown dramatic geographic variation in the prevalence of hepatitis C in patients with HCC. In some countries, such as Japan, Spain, and Italy, hepatitis C infection appears to be a far more important etiologic factor than hepatitis B in the development of HCC, being found in 60 to 80 percent of patients in most series. In South Africa, Greece, and most of Asia, however, hepatitis B remains the most important cause, with only 10 to 20 percent of patients positive for hepatitis C. Nevertheless, it has been found that coinfection with hepatitis B and C produces a much greater risk of HCC than either virus alone. There have been few studies from the United States, and these have had somewhat contradictory findings: one found hepatitis C in only 13 percent, hepatitis B in 6.7 percent, and the majority of patients negative for both (10); another found hepatitis C in 43 percent, hepatitis B in 13 percent, and coinfection with both viruses in 15 percent (39), and so the role of viral hepatitis in this country is still unclear. Since hepatitis C is an RNA virus that does not integrate into the host genome, it is thought to be even less likely than hepatitis B to be directly oncogenic. Most cases of HCC associated with hepatitis C have occurred after the development of cirrhosis, but there are documented cases in precirrhotic patients, and so the mechanism whereby hepatitis C causes HCC remains unknown and an area of ongoing investigation.

Aflatoxin B1. Aflatoxins, a family of mycotoxins produced by fungi of the *Aspergillus* genus, are powerful carcinogens in experimental animals. Contamination of food, particularly grains and peanuts, by these toxins is common in the very same parts of the world where HCC is most common, namely China and southern Africa, and indeed, before the association with hepatitis B was recognized, aflatoxin B1 was thought to be a principal cause of HCC (76). It is now known that the binding of aflatoxin B1 to guanine residues of DNA can produce G to T mutations. Such mutations in codon 249 of the p53 tumor suppressor gene are thought to play an important role in carcinogenesis in areas of high endemicity (72).

Metabolic Diseases. HCC has occurred in association with a number of metabolic diseases (9,23), although the mechanisms remain obscure. Occurrence of HCC is a frequent terminal event following the development of cirrhosis in genetic hemochromatosis (approximately 25 percent), hereditary tyrosinemia (20 percent), and alpha-1-antitrypsin deficiency (15 percent). There is an increased incidence of HCC in patients with porphyria cutanea tarda, but since that disease is frequently associated with alcohol use and chronic hepatitis C infection, the role of the porphyria is unclear. A few cases of HCC have been reported in patients with glycogen storage diseases, types I and III, in association with hepatocellular adenomas and presumably representing malignant degeneration of an adenoma. HCC has also been reported in patients with other forms of porphyria, hypercitrullinemia, fructosemia, Wilson's disease, Byler's disease, and Alagille's syndrome, but such cases are all extremely rare.

Other Possible Etiologic Factors. As many chemicals are known hepatocarcinogens in experimental animals, it is often suspected but seldom if ever proven that chemical exposure may play a role in humans. Anabolic steroid use (9,25) and Thorotrast exposure (26) have been associated with a number of cases of HCC, and both are generally accepted as etiologic agents because of their rarity in the general population. Oral contraceptive steroids have been purported to play an etiologic role based on case control studies, although the number of cases is extremely small compared to the number of oral contraceptive users (9,25). Smoking has been shown to have an increased prevalence in patients with HCC, and alcohol use is also increased, although it has not been shown to be carcinogenic in the liver except through the production of cirrhosis (2).

Clinical Features. As noted above, HCC is most frequent in men and increases in incidence with advancing age. The mode of presentation is changing with changes in medical practice and the recognition that patients with chronic liver disease are at increased risk for the development of malignancy. Surveillance of patients with chronic hepatitis and cirrhosis of other causes has led to early detection of many tumors, but most patients with HCC still come to clinical attention when the tumor is at an advanced stage.

HCC is usually painful, probably due to stretching of Glisson's capsule as the tumor grows. Signs and symptoms usually point to a malignancy in the liver. Over half of patients present with malaise, weight loss, abdominal enlargement, hepatomegaly (often with a palpable mass), and various other signs of decompensated liver disease, such as jaundice or ascites; these form a constellation of findings that characterize the *frank type* of liver cancer (55). Approximately one fourth of patients present only with features of decompensated cirrhosis, the *cirrhotic type*. Rapidly accumulating ascites or variceal hemorrhage, with or without abdominal pain, in a patient with previously stable cirrhosis should prompt a clinical evaluation for the presence of HCC, since tumor-related portal vein or hepatic vein thrombosis may be the underlying cause. Occasional patients present with fever, leukocytosis, and a liver mass, mimicking hepatic abscess (*febrile type*); with rapidly progres-

sive liver failure, mimicking fulminant hepatitis (*hepatitis type*); with rupture of the tumor and hemoperitoneum (*acute abdominal type*); with sudden onset of obstructive jaundice due to invasion of the common hepatic duct (*cholestatic type*); or distant metastases, especially to lung, bone, or brain (*metastatic type*), but these are all relatively uncommon (55). The tumor may invade the hepatic veins, producing a Budd-Chiari syndrome or obstruction of the inferior vena cava, or it may even grow up the vena cava into the right atrium, producing signs and symptoms of right heart failure as the major presenting feature.

Paraneoplastic syndromes associated with HCC are uncommon but are well recognized (6,29). Hypoglycemia, erythrocytosis, and hypercholesterolemia are the most frequent, while hypercalcemia, isosexual precocious puberty, gynecomastia (in the absence of cirrhosis), carcinoid syndrome, porphyria cutanea tarda, hypertrophic pulmonary osteoarthropathy, osteoporosis, hypertension, hyperthyroidism, dysfibrinogenemias, and a variety of cutaneous changes have been reported on rare occasions (6,29).

Laboratory tests of liver function are frequently abnormal, and a sudden change, such as a rapidly rising serum alkaline phosphatase, in a patient with chronic liver disease may be a clue to the appearance of HCC. Serum alpha-fetoprotein (AFP), an oncofetal antigen, is frequently used for screening and surveillance in high-risk individuals (31). AFP is normally produced by the fetal liver (as an analog of albumin) and decreases rapidly after birth. It is reported to be elevated in 70 to 90 percent of patients with HCC, although in our experience, it often seems to be negative in difficult cases where its presence would be diagnostically useful. AFP may be elevated in other tumors and in various non-neoplastic diseases, but a very high or rising concentration in a patient with known chronic liver disease virtually always indicates the development of HCC. Many other potential tumor markers have been studied over the years, but none has proven consistently superior to AFP in tumor surveillance.

Radiographic imaging is virtually always used in the evaluation of a patient with a suspected liver tumor, and in symptomatic or advanced cases the tumors are easily detected by ultrasound, computed tomography (CT), magnetic resonance imaging (MRI), or angiography (15). For surveillance

Table 8-1

GROSS CLASSIFICATIONS OF HEPATOCELLULAR CARCINOMA

Authors	Type	Definition	Subtype
Eggel (13)	Massive	Single large mass replacing an entire lobe	–
	Nodular	Multiple discrete nodules	–
	Diffuse	Numerous cirrhosis-like nodules	–

Okuda, Peters, Simson (60)	Expanding	Well-demarcated from surrounding liver, with or without capsule formation	Cirrhotomimetic
			  With capsule
			  Nonencapsulated
			Pseudoadenomatous
			  With capsule
			  Nonencapsulated
			Sclerosing
			Diffuse
			Septate

	Spreading	Poorly demarcated from surrounding liver	Cirrhotomimetic
			Infiltrative
			  With fibrosis
			  Without fibrosis

	Multifocal	Small, uniformly sized tumors	Nondiffuse Diffuse
	Indeterminate	Large, necrotic, unclassifiable	–
Nakashima, Kojiro (50)	Expansive	Pushing aside the surrounding liver; well-demarcated, often encapsulated	Single nodular Multinodular
	Infiltrative	Invading the surrounding liver; poorly demarcated, unencapsulated	–
	Mixed infiltrative and expansive	Features of both	Mixed infiltrative and single nodular Mixed infiltrative and multinodular
	Diffuse	Numerous cirrhosis-like nodules	–

and detection of early, potentially curable tumors in high-risk patients, however, ultrasonography has become the method of choice. Skilled sonographers using specialized techniques, such as carbon dioxide–enhanced ultrasonography, can sometimes detect tumors as small as 8 mm in diameter (21), although these cannot be reliably distinguished from benign macroregenerative nodules in a cirrhotic liver. Tumors measuring 2 to 3 cm, however, are generally detected in over 80 percent of cases. CT and MRI may improve on this in cases where HCC is highly suspect, and tumors measuring 1 cm are routinely detected. Lipiodol, an oily, iodine-containing substance, accumulates in HCC after intraarterial injection and further enhances the ability of CT to detect small lesions (15).

Gross Findings. Classifications of hepatocellular carcinoma based on gross features have been proposed by several authors (Table 8-1) (13,50,60), but all generally require examination of the entire tumor (or preferably the entire liver obtained at autopsy) for application, and none has proven particularly useful in predicting prognosis, guiding therapy, or providing reliable clues to pathogenesis. Eggel's classification (13), proposed in 1910, is still adequate for most purposes. Hepatocellular carcinoma is classified as "massive" when there is a single large mass (fig. 8-2), with or without small satellite nodules; as "nodular" when there are multiple, fairly discrete nodules throughout the liver (fig. 8-3); or as "diffuse" when there are multiple, minute, indistinct nodules throughout the liver (fig. 8-4).

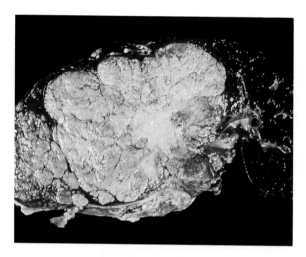

Figure 8-2
HEPATOCELLULAR CARCINOMA, MASSIVE TYPE
A single large mass replaces the right lobe, and two smaller satellite nodules are in the left lobe. On section the tumor is soft and yellow with areas that are green due to bile production.

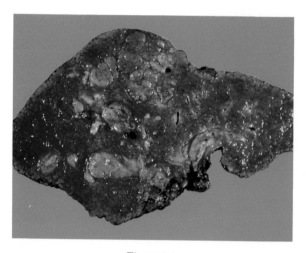

Figure 8-3
HEPATOCELLULAR CARCINOMA, NODULAR TYPE
Multiple discrete nodules are scattered throughout the liver.

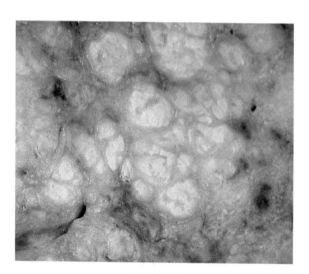

Figure 8-4
HEPATOCELLULAR CARCINOMA, DIFFUSE TYPE
There are numerous small nodules throughout the liver. A section of this cirrhotic liver shows small white tumor nodules that have replaced the tissue of the cirrhotic nodules.

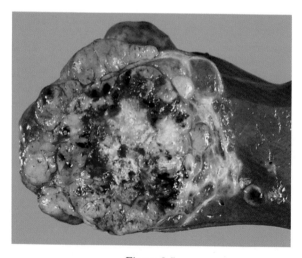

Figure 8-5
HEPATOCELLULAR CARCINOMA
This "massive" tumor is soft with necrosis and hemorrhage.

It seems reasonable that tumors grossly classified as spreading, infiltrative, or diffuse would be more rapidly progressive and would have a worse prognosis than those that are solitary and expanding ("expansive"), but this has never been proven.

HCC is almost always a soft tumor, often with areas of necrosis (fig. 8-5), except for fibrolamel-lar carcinoma (see chapter 9) and those rare tumors classified histologically as scirrhous. The color of the tumor varies from tan or yellow to grayish white or, if it produces bile, to green (figs. 8-6–8-8). Vascular invasion is common and both the portal vein and hepatic veins as well as the vena cava may be involved (fig. 8-9). Invasion of major bile ducts is an uncommon but well-recognized phenomenon that can cause biliary obstruction. A gross variant that appears to have

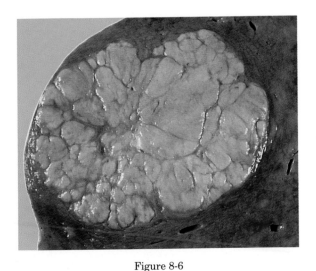

Figure 8-6
HEPATOCELLULAR CARCINOMA
This tumor is yellow compared to the normal brown of the surrounding liver, due to increased glycogen in the tumor cells.

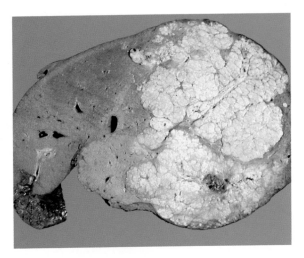

Figure 8-7
HEPATOCELLULAR CARCINOMA
The massive tumor in this specimen appears white while the surrounding liver is brown, even after fixation.

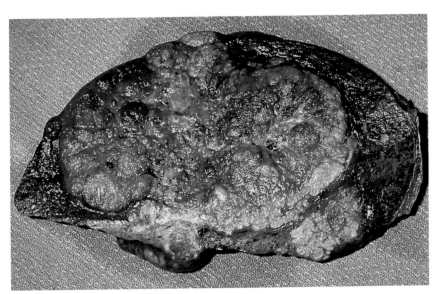

Figure 8-8
HEPATOCELLULAR
CARCINOMA
The tumor in this lobectomy specimen has green areas that represent bile production.

prognostic significance is the "encapsulated" HCC (52). These tumors, which almost always arise in a cirrhotic liver, tend to be solitary and slow growing, causing a thick fibrous capsule (fig. 8-10) to form from the cirrhotic scars. They appear to represent an early stage of disease, and since they are virtually always detected by screening they are more often resectable than other types of HCC. Pedunculated tumors, growing out from the surface of the liver (fig. 8-11), also result in a relatively good prognosis (1), due to their resectability and perhaps also to the slow expansive growth that causes the lesions to become pedunculated.

In recent years literature has developed regarding *small HCC,* defined as a tumor 2 cm or less in diameter (22), based on studies of cirrhotic livers removed at transplantation and resected tumors that were detected through surveillance of patients with chronic liver disease. Although such small tumors are usually well or moderately differentiated (49), they are often multifocal (4,66), and there is little evidence that they differ from other forms of HCC in any way other than size.

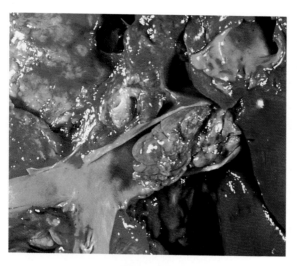

Figure 8-9
HEPATOCELLULAR CARCINOMA
In this autopsy specimen, the portal vein is opened revealing invasion by the tumor.

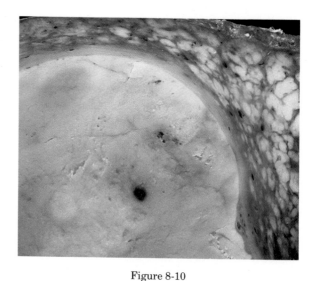

Figure 8-10
HEPATOCELLULAR CARCINOMA,
ENCAPSULATED TYPE
Resection specimen of a small tumor in a cirrhotic liver shows a thick fibrous capsule surrounding the lesion and separating it from the surrounding benign tissue.

Figure 8-11
HEPATOCELLULAR
CARCINOMA,
PEDUNCULATED TYPE
The tumor in this cirrhotic liver bulges from the inferior surface of the right lobe.

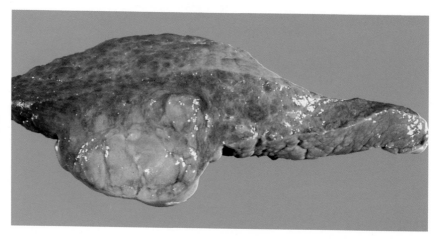

Microscopic Findings. The diagnosis of HCC requires the demonstration of evidence of hepatocellular differentiation by the tumor cells and also demonstration of features of malignancy. These may be on the basis of cytologic features, growth pattern, ultrastructure, special stains, or some combination.

Microscopically the cells of HCC resemble normal liver cells to a variable extent. Some tumors are so well differentiated that the cells are difficult to distinguish from benign liver cells, making it difficult to differentiate the tumor from hepatocellular adenoma. Other tu-

mors are anaplastic and poorly differentiated, showing only minimal evidence of liver cell origin. Most tumors, however, show definite evidence of hepatocellular differentiation, and such evidence is required for the diagnosis. Tumor cells usually have distinct cell membranes and a moderate amount of eosinophilic, finely granular cytoplasm. Bile canaliculi are nearly always present between cells and, while sometimes hard to find, can usually be seen by light microscopy (fig. 8-12). Since only hepatocytes produce true canaliculi, finding these structures is very helpful in distinguishing hepatocellular tumors from other neoplasms, particularly various metastatic poorly differentiated carcinomas. Immunostains, as discussed below, can demonstrate canaliculi when there is doubt about their presence. Bile pigment may be found in tumor cells or in dilated canaliculi (fig. 8-13, left), and when present this is the most helpful microscopic feature in establishing the diagnosis. In our experience, some bile can be found in approximately half of tumors (Table 8-2), although the quantity may be very small (fig. 8-13, right).

A variety of cellular products, mimicking normal and pathologic liver cell function, can sometimes be seen by light microscopy or found by various histochemical and immunohistochemical techniques. Fat droplets (fig. 8-14) can be seen to some degree in 68 percent of tumors (Table 8-2). Large amounts of cytoplasmic fat or glycogen can cause the cytoplasm to appear white in routine sections, producing the so-called *clear cell carcinoma* of the liver. This variant must be

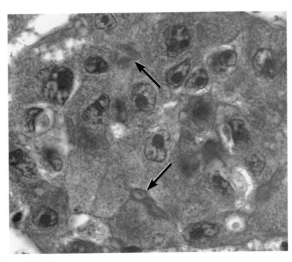

Figure 8-12
HEPATOCELLULAR CARCINOMA
The tumor cells have granular, eosinophilic cytoplasm, distinct cell borders, and prominent nuclei and nucleoli. Canaliculi (arrows) are readily apparent between tumor cells.

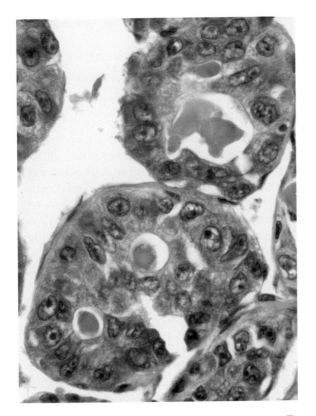

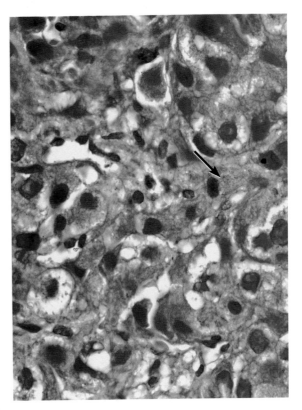

Figure 8-13
HEPATOCELLULAR CARCINOMA, BILE PRODUCTION
Left: There is abundant bile production, distending the tumor canaliculi.
Right: In this poorly differentiated tumor, bile is hard to find, but it can be seen in an occasional tumor cell (arrow).

Table 8-2

SELECTED HISTOPATHOLOGIC FEATURES IN 1,348 HEPATOCELLULAR CARCINOMAS*

Fat	68%
Bile production	48%
Cytoplasmic globules	20%
Mallory bodies	19%
Cytoplasmic "pale" bodies	8%
Extramedullary hematopoiesis	5%
Vascular invasion	74%
Bile duct invasion	3%
Inflammatory cell infiltrate	
Mild	24%
Moderate to marked	1.4%
Nuclear grade	
1	2%
2	39%
3	46%
4	13%
Growth pattern	
Trabecular	61.0%
Pseudoglandular	4.5%
Compact	17.1%
Fibrolamellar	5.5%
Scirrhous	0.2%
Mixed	11.5%

*AFIP North American cases, 1980–1993.

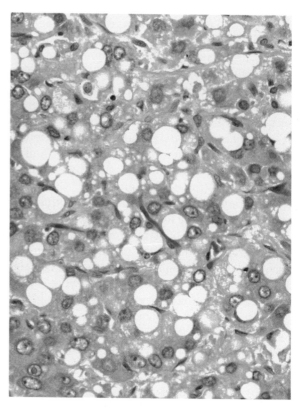

Figure 8-14
HEPATOCELLULAR CARCINOMA
Many of the cells of this well-differentiated tumor contain fat vacuoles.

differentiated from clear cell carcinoma metastatic from the kidney (45a).

Mallory bodies are present in the cytoplasm of tumor cells in approximately 20 percent of cases (Table 8-2) (48,50). These are often indistinguishable from alcoholic hyaline (fig. 8-15A,B), but sometimes appear more spherical (fig. 8-15C). Nevertheless, they have the ultrastructural and antigenic composition of Mallory bodies, and they are decorated by antibodies to ubiquitin (fig 8-15D), similar to non-neoplastic Mallory bodies. They may be few or numerous. The presence of tumor Mallory bodies is unrelated to the nature of the underlying liver disease but rather seems to be a manifestation of a metabolic error in the tumor cells, causing the cytoskeletal proteins to form the Mallory bodies.

Non-Mallory body cytoplasmic globules (fig. 8-16, left) are present in approximately 20 percent of tumors. These are often (but not always) periodic acid–Schiff (PAS) positive and diastase resistant (fig. 8-16, right) and can be shown by immunostaining to be globules of alpha-1-antitrypsin, similar to the globules that accumulate in normal liver cells in alpha-1-antitrypsin deficiency. Approximately 8 percent of tumors have lightly eosinophilic cytoplasmic inclusions (fig. 8-17) that have been called "pale bodies" (7) or "ground-glass cells" (69). Although these resemble the ground-glass cells of chronic hepatitis B infection, they actually contain fibrinogen (69). In our series (Table 8-2), pale bodies were found in 36 percent of fibrolamellar HCCs (see chapter 9) and in 6 percent of other types of HCC.

Other cytologic features that are occasionally observed in HCC include cytoplasmic Dubin-Johnson pigment (fig. 8-18) (64), copper storage (fig. 8-19) (18), clear cell change due to abundant

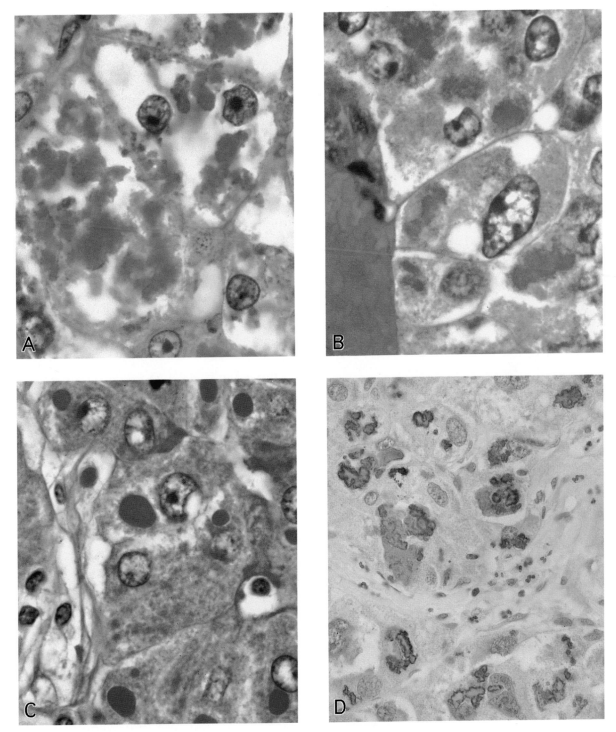

Figure 8-15
HEPATOCELLULAR CARCINOMA, MALLORY BODIES

A: In this tumor, the cells all contain large, irregular Mallory bodies, identical to those seen in severe alcoholic hepatitis.

B: In this case, the Mallory bodies are smaller and more compact, but are still similar to those of alcoholic hepatitis.

C: In this tumor, the Mallory bodies are globular and smooth, but they have the same ultrastructural and immunohisto-chemical features as more typical Mallory bodies.

D: Immunostain for ubiquitin demonstrates that the Mallory bodies of this tumor are ubiquitin-coated, just as the Mallory bodies of alcoholic hepatitis.

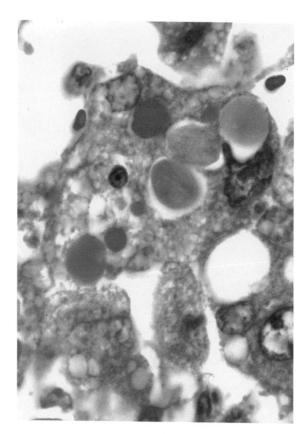
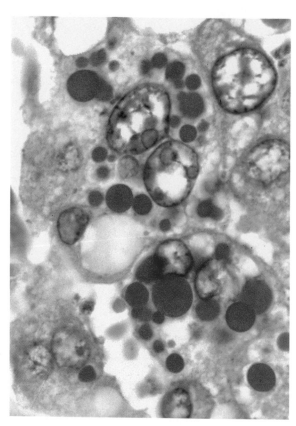

Figure 8-16
HEPATOCELLULAR CARCINOMA, ALPHA-1-ANTITRYPSIN GLOBULES
Left: Spherical cytoplasmic alpha-1-antitrypsin globules can be seen with routine H&E stain.
Right: The PAS stain after diastase digestion shows that the globules are PAS positive and diastase resistant. They also stain with antibodies to alpha-1-antitrypsin, proving their identity.

Figure 8-17
HEPATOCELLULAR
CARCINOMA
Cytoplasmic fibrinogen inclusions appear in H&E-stained sections as uniformly eosinophilic pale bodies.

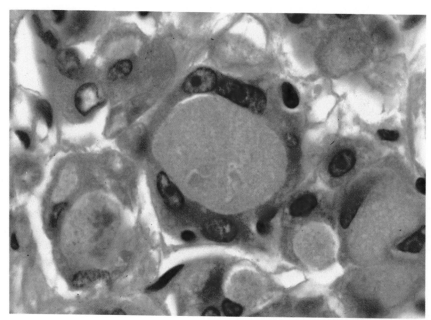

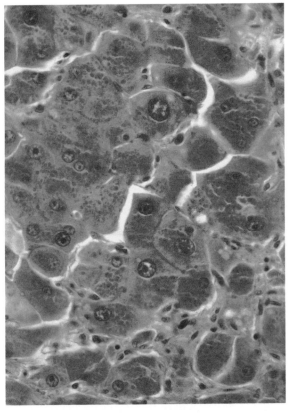

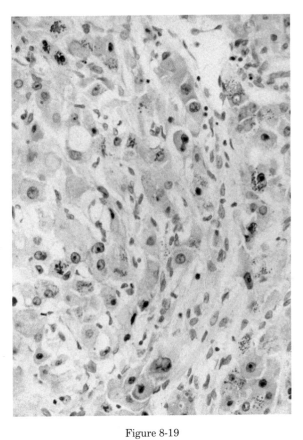

Figure 8-18
HEPATOCELLULAR CARCINOMA
The cells of this tumor contain abundant, densely brown lipofuscin-like material, identical to the pigment that accumulates in hepatocytes of patients with Dubin-Johnson syndrome.

Figure 8-19
HEPATOCELLULAR CARCINOMA
Many cells of this tumor contain lysosomal-bound granules of copper, which are stained red with rhodanine.

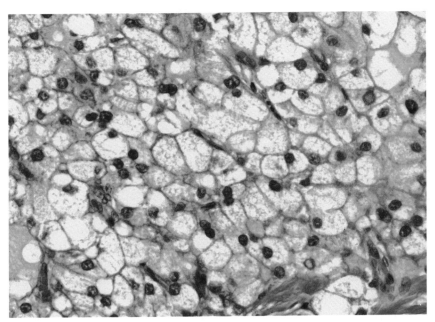

Figure 8-20
HEPATOCELLULAR
CARCINOMA,
CLEAR CELL TYPE
The cells appear clear because of abundant cytoplasmic glycogen.

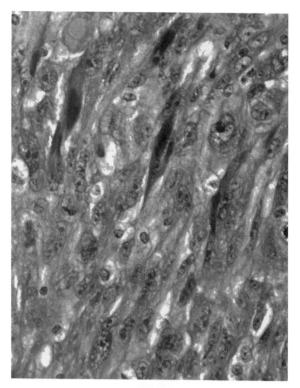

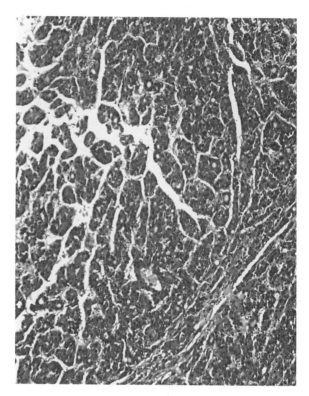

Figure 8-21
HEPATOCELLULAR CARCINOMA,
SARCOMATOID TYPE

The cells of this high-grade tumor appear spindled, but other parts of the same tumor have a typical trabecular growth pattern.

Figure 8-22
HEPATOCELLULAR CARCINOMA,
TRABECULAR TYPE

The tumor cells grow in thickened cords, called trabeculae, attempting to mimic the cell plates of normal liver. The trabeculae are lined by endothelial cells, and blood flows through the sinusoidal-like spaces between trabeculae. In this tumor the trabeculae are only a few cells thick, so it may be called microtrabecular.

glycogen (fig. 8-20) (45a,77), and spindle cell or "sarcomatoid" change (fig. 8-21) (42). In a recent study, Hasan et al. (19a) have suggested that hepatocellular tumors with Dubin-Johnson pigment are pigmented liver cell adenomas rather than hepatocellular carcinomas.

Several histologic growth patterns may be found in HCC (Table 8-2) (24). Since the cytologic features can be so variable, recognizing one of these patterns can be very helpful in arriving at a diagnosis. Most frequent is the *trabecular pattern* (figs. 8-22–8-25), in which the tumor attempts to form cell plates, as in normal liver. Rapid proliferation of the cells causes the plates to become thickened and contorted, producing the trabeculae. The trabeculae are surrounded by endothelial cells and separated by vascular spaces (sinusoid-like) with very little or no supporting connective tissue. The tumor sinusoids may contain Kupffer cells and stellate cells, but reticulin fibers are generally reduced or absent,

basement membrane components are often demonstrable beneath the endothelial cells, and the endothelial cells phenotypically resemble capillary endothelium rather than normal hepatic sinusoidal endothelium. The lack of a desmoplastic stroma is a helpful diagnostic clue and explains why, in contrast to most other malignant epithelial neoplasms, HCC is soft. The trabeculae may be only a few cells thick (microtrabecular) (figs. 8-22, 8-24) or more than 20 cells thick (macrotrabecular) (figs. 8-23, 8-24). Sometimes the centers of the trabeculae contain a very dilated canaliculus (figs. 8-26, 8-27), producing a *pseudoglandular (or acinar) pattern*. The *compact pattern* (fig. 8-28) is produced when the trabeculae grow together, compressing the sinusoids and forming sheets of tumor cells. Fibrolamellar carcinoma is an exception to the rule that HCC lacks abundant

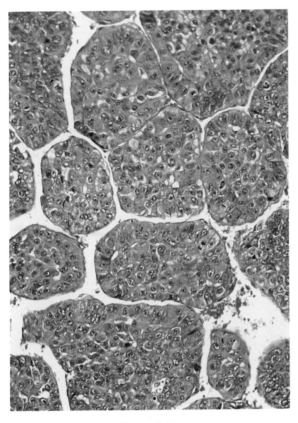

Figure 8-23
HEPATOCELLULAR CARCINOMA,
TRABECULAR TYPE

In this macrotrabecular tumor, the trabeculae are 10 to 20 cells thick.

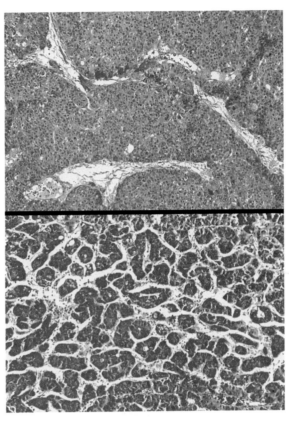

Figure 8-24
HEPATOCELLULAR CARCINOMA,
TRABECULAR TYPE

This tumor has areas that are macrotrabecular (top) and other areas that are microtrabecular (bottom).

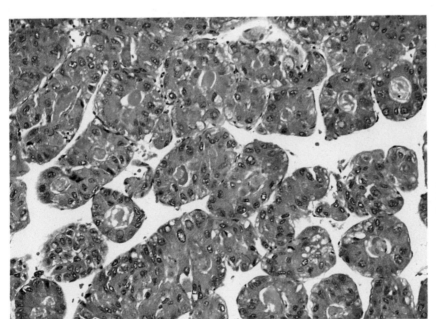

Figure 8-25
HEPATOCELLULAR
CARCINOMA,
TRABECULAR TYPE

Canaliculi in the centers of some trabeculae contain protein-aceous and sometimes bile-stained secretions.

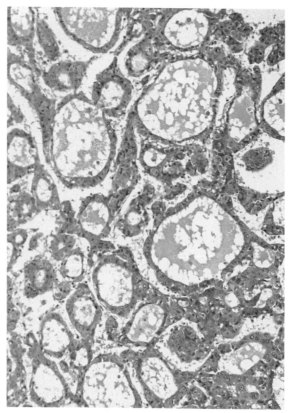

Figure 8-26
HEPATOCELLULAR CARCINOMA,
PSEUDOGLANDULAR TYPE

Canaliculi in the centers of the trabeculae are very dilated, mimicking glands.

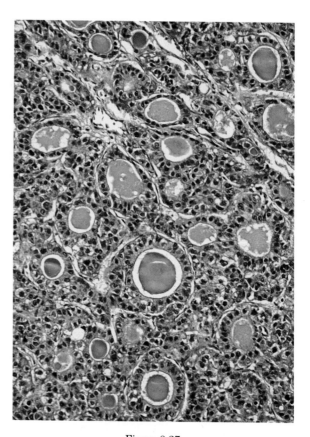

Figure 8-27
HEPATOCELLULAR CARCINOMA,
PSEUDOGLANDULAR TYPE

The dilated canaliculi contain eosinophilic material.

Figure 8-28
HEPATOCELLULAR
CARCINOMA,
COMPACT TYPE

The trabeculae have grown together, obliterating the sinusoids in between and producing a solid sheet of tumor cells.

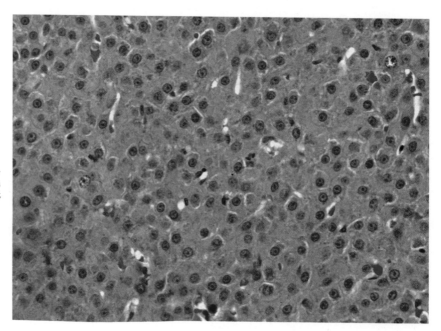

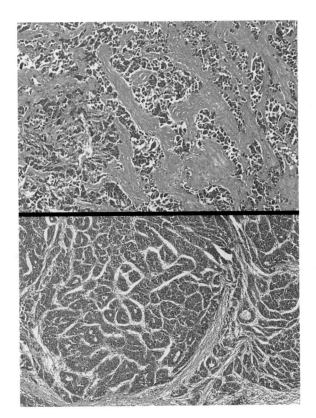

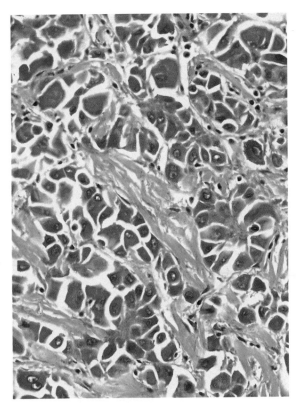

Figure 8-29
HEPATOCELLULAR CARCINOMA, SCIRRHOUS TYPE
Left: Most of this tumor has a dense fibrous stroma (top), but there are areas that are trabecular (bottom).
Right: Higher magnification shows that the tumor cells are truly hepatocyte-like.

stroma. The tumor differs cytologically from other types of HCC, and as noted above, is a sufficiently different biologic entity that it warrants separate discussion (chapter 9).

Very rarely, tumors with cytologic and phenotypic features of trabecular HCC will produce abundant stroma. These constitute the *scirrhous pattern* of HCC (fig. 8-29). The "sclerosing hepatic carcinoma" (61) may include some cases of scirrhous HCC, but in our opinion, most of these were actually intrahepatic cholangiocarcinomas, since the purported entity was proposed only on the basis of light microscopy without the benefit of immunostains or other techniques to define cellular phenotype. Mixtures of patterns, usually trabecular with compact or pseudoglandular, are frequent (fig. 8-30). Occasionally there are tumors in which part is trabecular and part resembles fibrolamellar carcinoma, but in such cases the clinical features and prognosis are those of the nonfibrolamellar HCC.

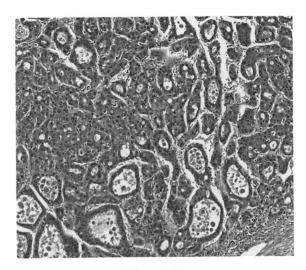

Figure 8-30
HEPATOCELLULAR CARCINOMA, MIXED
TRABECULAR AND PSEUDOGLANDULAR

215

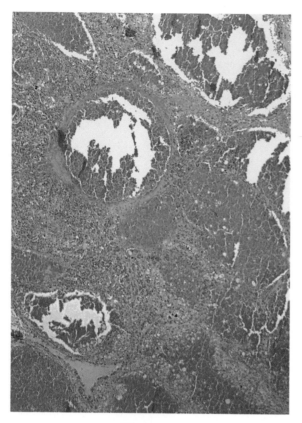

Figure 8-31
HEPATOCELLULAR CARCINOMA, PELIOID TYPE
There are blood-filled cystic spaces within the tumor, mimicking peliosis hepatis.

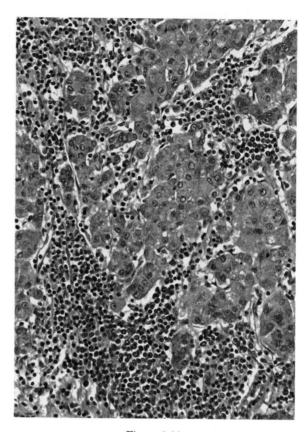

Figure 8-32
HEPATOCELLULAR CARCINOMA
This tumor has a prominent lymphoid infiltrate, suggesting a host response to the tumor.

HCC is sometimes further classified histologically based on the interaction of the tumor with the surrounding liver (50). This is analogous to the various gross classifications in that the tumors are considered to be *sinusoidal* if the malignant cells infiltrate the sinusoids; *replacing* if the tumor cells infiltrate the cell plates and displace benign liver cells; or *pseudocapsular* when fibrous tissue, usually from cirrhotic scars, is pushed ahead of the tumor mass.

Other histologic features may be seen on occasion. Vascular invasion in the surrounding liver is very frequent, being found in 74 percent of AFIP cases (Table 8-2); microscopic bile duct invasion was seen in 3 percent. Sometimes large vascular lakes will develop within the tumor, mimicking peliosis hepatis (fig. 8-31), forming the *pelioid* type of HCC (63). A lymphocytic infiltrate may be present in the tumor, usually only to a mild degree, but occasionally the inflamma-

tion is prominent (fig. 8-32). In tumors with Mallory bodies, there may be an infiltrate of neutrophils (fig. 8-33), similar to that seen in alcoholic hepatitis. Occasional tumors have foci of extramedullary hematopoiesis (fig. 8-34). Rare tumors have been reported with osteoclast-like giant cells (43) or with ossification (41).

Combined hepatocellular-cholangiocarcinoma is the term used for tumors with elements of both HCC and cholangiocarcinoma (see chapter 10). At the AFIP, tumors that fit the definition of combined hepatocellular-cholangiocarcinoma account for approximately 1 to 2 percent of HCCs and are included in the "mixed" or fibrolamellar category of growth patterns (Table 8-2). The original World Health Organization (WHO) classification (16) considered mucin production to be evidence of biliary differentiation (i.e., cholangiocarcinoma), and so a tumor with unequivocal hepatocellular differentiation (trabecular pattern,

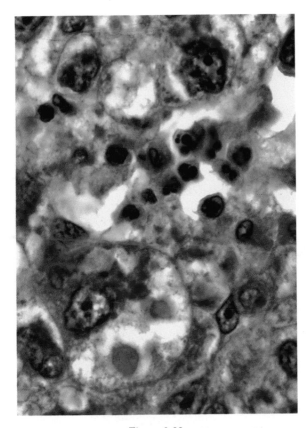

Figure 8-33
HEPATOCELLULAR CARCINOMA
This tumor has small Mallory bodies and foci with clusters of neutrophils, presumably in response to the Mallory bodies.

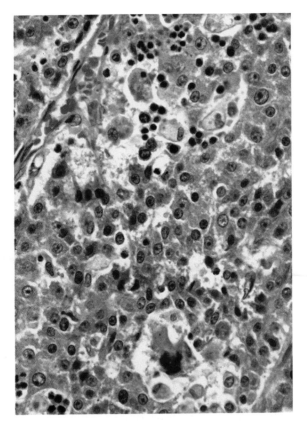

Figure 8-34
HEPATOCELLULAR CARCINOMA WITH EXTRAMEDULLARY HEMATOPOIESIS
There are hematopoietic cells including myeloid and erythroid precursors and megakaryocytes in the sinusoids of this tumor.

bile production) and either gland formation by biliary type cells or a positive mucin stain showing intracellular or intraluminal mucin is considered a combined hepatocellular-cholangiocarcinoma. HCC with a pseudoglandular pattern may be mistaken for combined hepatocellular-cholangiocarcinoma, but it can be distinguished by the fact that the cells surrounding the pseudoglands resemble hepatocytes and may produce bile but not mucin. The clinical behavior of combined hepatocellular-cholangiocarcinoma is much like that of HCC, and so these are considered a special subtype rather than a separate tumor. In the series from the AFIP (17), three types of tumors were found to fit the definition of combined hepatocellular-cholangiocarcinoma. A few (17 percent) were collision tumors in which there was a coincidental but separate HCC and cholangiocarcinoma in the same liver (fig. 8-35). Many (50 percent) were "transitional tumors" in which there were areas

of both HCC and cholangiocarcinoma, as well as areas of apparent transition from typical HCC to adenocarcinoma or to a mixed hepatocellular and glandular tumor (fig. 8-36). The remainder (33 percent) were actually fibrolamellar carcinomas (see chapter 9) with typical clinical and histologic features of that tumor, except that they produced mucin, as demonstrated by mucicarmine or Alcian blue stains.

Carcinosarcoma is an extremely rare mixed type of HCC. Most reported cases are actually HCC with spindle cell change (fig. 8-21) or a combined hepatocellular-cholangiocarcinoma with spindle cell metaplasia of the cholangiocarcinoma element rather than a true carcinosarcoma, which we regard as HCC combined with differentiated sarcomatous elements. There is a reported case of HCC combined with chondrosarcoma (32), and at the AFIP we have seen two cases of HCC with

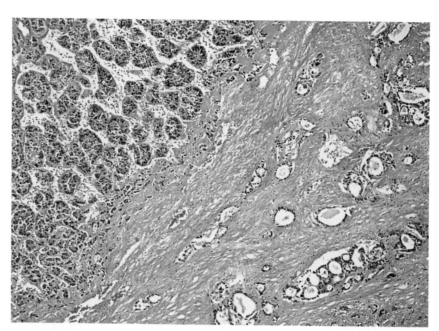

Figure 8-35
COMBINED
HEPATOCELLULAR-
CHOLANGIOCARCINOMA

This "collision tumor" has a hepatocellular carcinoma (top right) and a cholangiocarcinoma (bottom left) in the same liver.

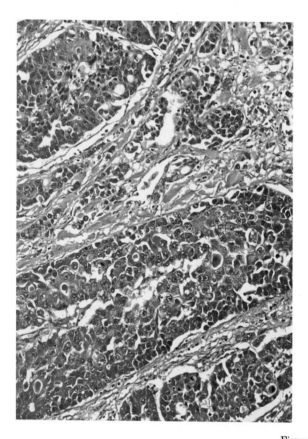

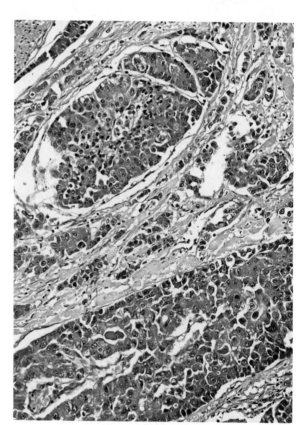

Figure 8-36
COMBINED HEPATOCELLULAR-CHOLANGIOCARCINOMA, TRANSITIONAL TYPE

Left: In this area of transition, the tumor has features of both hepatocellular carcinoma and cholangiocarcinoma. Other parts of the same tumor have areas of typical trabecular hepatocellular carcinoma and typical gland-forming, desmoplastic cholangiocarcinoma.

Right: The mucicarmine stain shows that the same cells are producing both bile and mucin, proving dual differentiation.

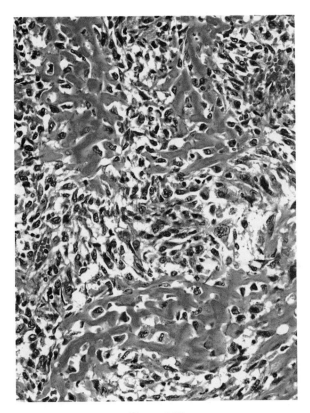

Figure 8-37
CARCINOSARCOMA
Parts of this tumor are typical hepatocellular carcinoma, but this field shows an area that resembles an osteosarcoma.

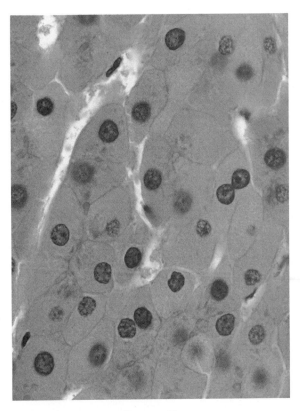

Figure 8-38
HEPATOCELLULAR CARCINOMA, GRADE 1
The tumor cells have abundant, eosinophilic cytoplasm and small, round, regular nuclei. Cytologically one cannot distinguish the cells of this tumor from normal liver or hepatocellular adenoma. However, in some areas, the tumor had invaded blood vessels.

osteosarcoma (fig. 8-37) and one of HCC with leiomyosarcoma.

Microscopic Grading. HCC can be graded on the basis of nuclear features. The nuclei are usually large, producing the high nuclear/cytoplasmic ratio characteristic of many types of malignant neoplasms. They show variable degrees of anaplasia and usually have prominent nucleoli. Edmondson and Steiner (12) proposed grading HCC on a scale of I to IV, with increasing nuclear irregularity, hyperchromatism, and nuclear/cytoplasmic ratio, associated with decreasing cytologic differentiation, for each successively higher grade. They placed great emphasis on the amount and appearance of the cytoplasm and the nuclear/cytoplasmic ratio, so that their grade IV tumors had very scant cytoplasm and often a "small cell" appearance. As Dr. Edmonson was the author of the first AFIP liver Fascicle and co-author of the second, this grading system was used in both. A correlation between the grade and

prognosis has been reported by some (19) but disputed by others (36). It is not clear that the grading system has been uniformly applied, and it has never been widely used.

For a series of 1,063 cases from the AFIP (54), we modified the Edmondson-Steiner grading system, using primarily nuclear features, and found a statistically significant correlation of survival with tumor grade. Grade 1 HCC, as in the previous system, are adenoma-like with cells that have abundant cytoplasm and minimal nuclear irregularity (fig. 8-38). A pure grade 1 tumor is impossible to distinguish from hepatocellular adenoma cytologically, and the diagnosis must be made on the basis of trabecular or pseudoglandular growth, vascular invasion, or metastasis. Sometimes areas of grade 1 HCC are seen in higher grade tumors, raising the possibility that these arose from a preexisting hepatocellular

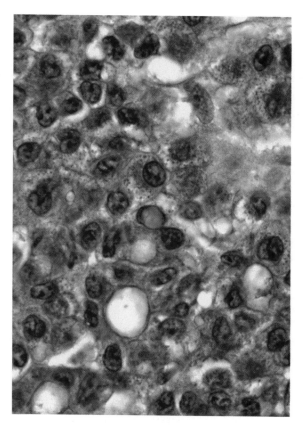

Figure 8-39
HEPATOCELLULAR CARCINOMA, GRADE 2
There is a high nuclear/cytoplasmic ratio, nuclear irregularity, hyperchromatism, and prominent nucleoli.

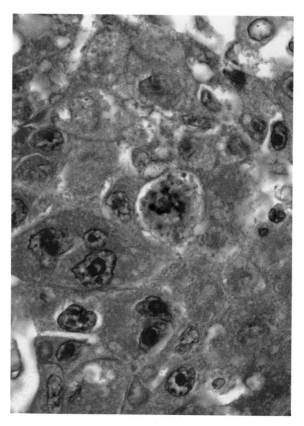

Figure 8-40
HEPATOCELLULAR CARCINOMA, GRADE 3
There is much more nuclear pleomorphism than in a grade 2 tumor.

adenoma. However, as discussed in chapter 2, we have always regarded such findings as grade 1 HCC rather than adenoma. HCCs of grades 2 to 4 generally have a higher than normal nuclear/cytoplasmic ratio in contrast to those of grade 1. Grade 2 tumors have prominent nucleoli, hyperchromatism, and some degree of irregularity of the nuclear membrane (fig. 8-39). Grade 3 has even greater nuclear pleomorphism and angulated nuclei (fig. 8-40). Grade 4 has marked pleomorphism, hyperchromatism, and usually anaplastic giant cells (fig. 8-41), some of which have been called "giant cell carcinoma" (63). It should be noted that Edmondson considered these to be grade 3, but our follow-up study (54) found them to be associated with a significantly shorter survival period. Nevertheless, since survival in general is so poor, there is little value in grading HCC except for statistical correlation in large studies. Occasional tumors may show giant

cell transformation without nuclear pleomorphism (fig. 8-42); these are graded according to the nuclear features.

Immunohistochemical Findings. Since the cells of HCC attempt to mimic normal liver cells, they may produce any of the cellular products that can be found in hepatocytes both in health and in disease, and if present, are readily demonstrated by immunostaining (Table 8-3). Unfortunately, most of these cellular products are of little use in the differential diagnosis of HCC since many can be found in tumors other than HCC, and not all are commercially available. Those that are readily available and that we and others have found most useful are listed below.

Carcinoembryonic Antigen (CEA). The liver contains a CEA-like cross-reactive substance called biliary glycoprotein I (BGP-I), located predominantly in bile canaliculi (71). Polyclonal antisera to CEA that have not been preabsorbed

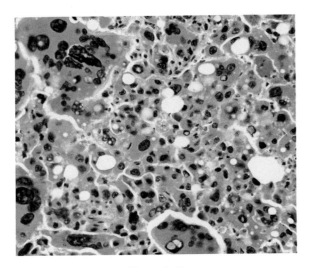

Figure 8-41
HEPATOCELLULAR CARCINOMA, GRADE 4
There is marked nuclear pleomorphism with anaplastic giant cells.

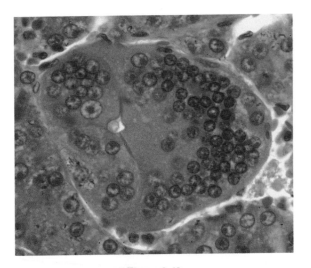

Figure 8-42
HEPATOCELLULAR CARCINOMA
WITH GIANT CELL TRANSFORMATION
Although this is a grade 2 hepatocellular carcinoma, many of the tumor cells are multinucleate.

Table 8-3

SOME OF THE NUMEROUS ANTIGENS THAT ARE SOMETIMES DEMONSTRABLE IN HCC BY IMMUNOHISTOCHEMICAL TECHNIQUES

Tumor cells
Cytokeratin
Clone AE1
Clone AE3
Clone CAM 5.2
Cytokeratin 7
Cytokeratin 8
Cytokeratin 18
Cytokeratin 19
Vimentin
Biliary glycoprotein
Carcinoembryonic antigen (CEA) (polyclonal)
Hepatocyte (Hep Par 1)
Erythropoiesis-associated antigen (ERY-1)
Ubiquitin
Epithelial membrane antigen (EMA)
α-fetoprotein
Albumin
Fibrinogen
1-antitrypsin
α-1-antichymotrypsin
α-human chorionic gonadotropin
Prothymosin
Ferritin
Transferrin receptor
Metallothionein
β-microglobulin
C-reactive protein
Factor XIIIa
Thrombospondin
CD44

Cathepsin B
Asialoglycoprotein receptor
Lewis^x blood group substance
Lewis^y blood group substance
BH blood group substance
P53 gene product
Ras oncogene p21 product
Retinoblastoma gene product
Ki-67
Proliferating cell nuclear antigen (PCNA)
Transforming growth factor-α
Transforming growth factor-1
Epidermal growth factor
Hepatitis B surface and core antigens

Endothelial cells
Factor VIII–related antigen
CD34
Ulex europaeus lectin
Fibroblast growth factor

Other mesenchymal cells
α-smooth muscle actin
CD68

Stroma
Fibronectin
Laminin
Collagen IV
Intercellular adhesion molecule-1 (ICAM-1)
Vascular endothelial growth factor

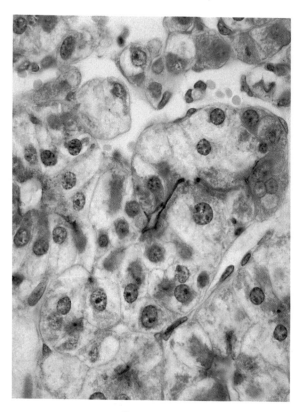

Figure 8-43
HEPATOCELLULAR CARCINOMA
The immunostain for CEA using polyclonal antibodies shows bile canaliculi between tumor cells due to cross-reacting biliary glycoprotein I.

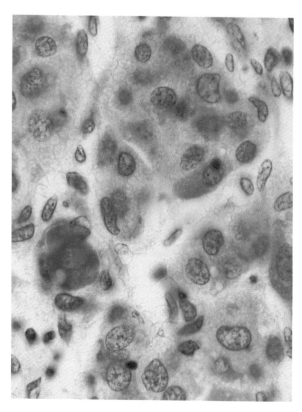

Figure 8-44
HEPATOCELLULAR CARCINOMA
The immunostain for alpha-fetoprotein is positive in this case, confirming the diagnosis.

with liver homogenate will react with BGP-I and stain the canaliculi, making them easy to see. Preabsorbed sera or highly specific monoclonal antibodies, however, are negative. Tumors that show hepatocellular differentiation frequently have a canalicular staining pattern with polyclonal anti-CEA (fig. 8-43), which is one of the most useful of all positive findings in distinguishing HCC from other malignancies.

Cytokeratin. Keratin profiles are sometimes suggested as a means of tumor classification, but there are many cases in which the tumors display aberrant keratin expression, so that immunostains for the various types of keratin must be interpreted with caution. Normal liver cells and hepatocellular tumors have relatively little keratin, predominantly types 8 and 18, while cholangiocarcinoma and most metastatic carcinomas that can be confused with HCC have a greater quantity and a richer variety of keratins (8,20,

27,74). Consequently, most HCCs are negative or stain only poorly with most antibodies to keratin, except for monoclonal antibodies, such as CAM 5.2, which react with types 8 and 18. Some HCCs, however, have biliary-type keratins (types 7 and/ or 19), and so the staining results must be interpreted in view of other histologic features. By contrast, primary and metastatic adenocarcinomas stain strongly with most antibody cocktails against a wide spectrum of cytokeratins; such strong staining is evidence against a diagnosis of HCC, while weak or negative staining supports the diagnosis.

Alpha-fetoprotein (AFP). Although serum AFP is frequently elevated in patients with HCC, the tumor is often negative with immunostain. In most published series AFP has been found in no more than 50 percent of tumors (with a wide range). It may only be focally present in tumor cell cytoplasm (fig. 8-44), and in general

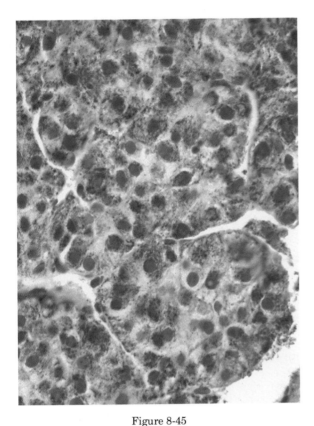

Figure 8-45
HEPATOCELLULAR CARCINOMA
Antihuman hepatocyte immunostain shows a distinctive coarse granular positivity, confirming the diagnosis.

it is less sensitive than CEA for diagnostic purposes. AFP can occur in metastatic germ cell tumors, but these seldom enter into the differential diagnosis of HCC. Other nonhepatocellular tumors only rarely produce AFP, and so its diagnostic specificity, when positive, is high.

Human Hepatocyte (Hep Par 1). This monoclonal antibody, first named hepatocyte paraffin 1 or Hep Par 1 (38,44), became commercially available while this Fascicle was nearing completion. Our experience with it is limited, and we are not yet certain of its sensitivity and specificity, but it appears very promising for distinguishing HCC from other malignancies. We have found that normal hepatocytes and most HCC cells stain in a distinctively coarse granular pattern (fig. 8-45). The degree of staining, however, varies from case to case, and some tumors have a very patchy distribution of positive cells, which could be missed in a small biopsy specimen, producing false negative results. Nearly all other benign

and malignant tumors that we have studied to date have been completely negative, with the exception of a few adenocarcinomas of the stomach and rare cholangiocarcinomas. The pattern of staining of these few exceptions, however, is different from HCC, being finer and paler. In some patients we have also observed staining in normal kidney tubules (although renal cell carcinomas have all been negative), normal intestinal epithelium, intestinal metaplasia of the stomach, and recently, in hepatoid adenocarcinomas of the gatrointestinal tract (42a). Nevertheless, this antibody appears very promising for differentiating HCC from other tumors.

Other immunostains. Alpha-1-antitrypsin can be demonstrated in the majority of HCCs, but since it is also found in numerous other tumors, it has no diagnostic value. Similarly, other plasma proteins in the cytoplasm of malignant tumor cells, whether or not made by the liver, can be demonstrated by immunostains. Hepatitis B surface and core antigens are rarely found in tumors arising in patients who are hepatitis B carriers.

Ultrastructure. Electron microscopic techniques have proven to be of limited use in diagnosis. Canaliculi and bile can sometimes be demonstrated by electron microscopy when other techniques are unsuccessful, but this is most unusual. Cytologic peculiarities can also be examined in more detail. The cells of fibrolamellar carcinoma can be shown to contain numerous mitochondria, while clear cell carcinoma can be shown to have glycogen and/or fat; cytoplasmic inclusions, such as Mallory bodies, alpha-1-antitrypsin globules, and fibrinogen inclusions can be distinguished.

Other Special Studies. Several special techniques have been reported but none has become widely used. In situ hybridization for mRNA of AFP (62), albumin (35), and several hepatocyte genes has been described and may prove useful in the future. Morphometry, flow cytometry, cytophotometry, and cytogenetics have all been applied to the study of HCC. Interesting information about the biology of these tumors has been obtained, but none of these techniques has proven useful enough to warrant use in routine diagnosis.

Differential Diagnosis. Problems in differential diagnosis generally involve distinguishing HCC from other malignancies and benign lesions. Metastases from a wide variety of primary tumors

Table 8-4

HISTOLOGIC DIFFERENTIAL DIAGNOSIS OF HEPATOCELLULAR CARCINOMA AND ADENOCARCINOMA (METASTATIC OR PRIMARY INTRAHEPATIC CHOLANGIOCARCINOMA)

	Hepatocellular Carcinoma	Adenocarcinoma
Stroma	None	Desmoplastic
Growth patterns	Trabecular Compact Pseudoglandular Scirrhous (rarely)	Tubuloglandular Papillary (rarely) Solid (rarely)
Mucin	Absent	Often present
Bile	Often present	Absent
Canaliculi	Present	Absent
Immunostains		
Carcinoembryonic antigen (CEA) (polyclonal)	Canalicular	Diffuse
Hep Par 1 (Hepatocyte)	Positive, granular (usually)	Negative or weak (rarely)
Cytokeratin (broad spectrum)	Negative or weak	Positive
Cytokeratins 7 and 19	Positive or negative	Positive (usually)
Cytokeratins 8 and 18	Positive (usually)	Positive or negative
α-fetoprotein (AFP)	Positive or negative	Negative (rare exceptions)
α-1-antitrypsin	Positive or negative	Positive or negative
Other plasma proteins	Positive or negative	Positive or negative
Hepatitis B antigens	Rarely positive	Negative

cause the majority of the diagnostic problems. Metastatic tumors usually resemble the primary one, and if this is known, comparison with the tumor in the liver usually solves the problem. When no primary is known, finding a poorly differentiated tumor with large cells that have eosinophilic cytoplasm raises the possibility of HCC, but that diagnosis should not be made without definite evidence of hepatocellular differentiation. Bile canaliculi recognizable on stains for hematoxylin and eosin (H&E) or CEA, a positive stain for AFP, a granular staining pattern with antihuman hepatocyte antibody, or a trabecular growth pattern as discussed above can allow one to make the diagnosis of HCC with more or less certainty. If no such evidence is found, the tumor is more likely to be metastatic than primary in the liver. Newer techniques and stains may increase the number of cases correctly diagnosed as HCC by a small amount, but most cases can be adequately classified by H&E stain supplemented by a few immunostains (Table 8-4).

The clear cell variant of renal cell carcinoma must be distinguished from clear cell HCC. In addition to negative CEA and anti-Hep Par 1 immunostains, metastatic renal clear cell carcinoma is positive for epithelial membrane antigen, Leu M1, and pancytokeratin, all of which are negative in clear cell HCC (45a). Cholangiocarcinoma (chapter 10) is the second most frequent primary liver malignancy, but it is still less common than metastatic adenocarcinoma. Cholangiocarcinomas and metastatic adenocarcinomas typically have a desmoplastic stromal response, in contrast to HCC, and so a tumor with abundant stroma is almost always an adenocarcinoma and not HCC. The only exceptions to this are the fibrolamellar carcinoma (see chapter 9) and the very rare scirrhous type of HCC. Before making a diagnosis of scirrhous HCC, however, one should demonstrate definite hepatocellular differentiation as noted above. Adenocarcinomas, whether metastatic or primary cholangiocarcinoma, are usually positive with

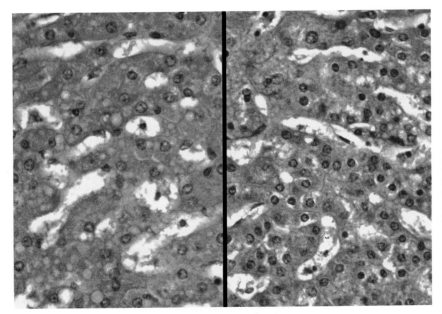

Figure 8-46
HEPATOCELLULAR
CARCINOMA
The very well-differentiated
hepatocellular carcinoma (right) can
only be distinguished from the surrounding benign cirrhotic nodules
(left) by the increased number of
nuclei, indicating a higher nuclear/
cytoplasmic ratio of the tumor.

immunostains for cytokeratin (using polyclonal and most monoclonal antibodies) and often for epithelial membrane antigen and mucin, in contrast to HCC, and immunostains for CEA tend to stain the cytoplasm diffusely, rather than in a canalicular pattern (Table 8-4).

Metastatic carcinoids and some more poorly differentiated neuroendocrine tumors may also be confused with HCC, as they typically have large tumor cells with abundant cytoplasm and a fibrous stroma. However, like adenocarcinomas, they typically have a fibrous stroma and lack features of definite hepatocellular differentiation. If the typical monotonous or organoid pattern of a carcinoid or neuroendocrine carcinoma is recognized, an immunostain for chromogranin will usually confirm the diagnosis. Some tumors are so poorly differentiated that no evidence of either hepatocellular or glandular differentiation can be found. In such cases "undifferentiated carcinoma" is an adequate diagnosis. Such tumors may be primary in the liver, but statistically they are much more likely to be metastatic.

The most difficult problem in differential diagnosis is distinguishing well-differentiated HCC from benign hepatocellular lesions. Despite suggestions to the contrary, there are no special stains or techniques that can diagnose malignancy with certainty. Hepatocellular adenomas sometimes have foci of dysplasia with some nuclear irregularity and hyperchroma-

tism, while grade 1 HCC growing in a sheet-like or solid pattern may look like an adenoma. If trabecular areas are present, or if there is more than minimal nuclear irregularity and hyperchromatism, especially if the patient has not been using contraceptive steroids, the tumor is best regarded as a well-differentiated HCC.

Macroregenerative nodules in cirrhotic livers may represent the precursor of hepatocellular carcinoma (see chapter 7), but a diagnosis of HCC should not be made without cytologic evidence of malignancy, a trabecular or pseudoglandular growth pattern, or vascular invasion. Minimal evidence of malignancy is difficult to establish, and in some cases even experts disagree (14). Features that have been found helpful in recognizing very well-differentiated HCC include crowding of nuclei (fig. 8-46) due to increased nuclear/cytoplasmic ratios, pseudogland formation, cytoplasmic basophilia, and loss of reticulin (14,34,47), although in our experience none of these is pathognomonic.

Focal nodular hyperplasia (FNH) is often confused with hepatocellular adenoma but is rarely confused with HCC. The central scar containing large arteries and the cirrhosis-like nodules of the hepatocytes, without atypia or trabecular growth, usually suggest FNH. Fibrolamellar carcinoma (chapter 9) may mimic FNH grossly, but microscopically it is quite different and the two are seldom confused.

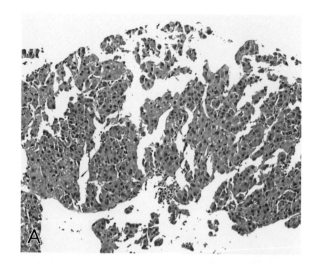

Figure 8-47
HEPATOCELLULAR CARCINOMA, CYTOLOGY

A: Sections of the cell block show typical trabecular morphology.

B: Smears with Papanicolaou stain also show trabecular arrangement of the tumor cells.

C: At high power the smears can be seen to contain fragments, with cells that have high nuclear/cytoplasmic ratios and prominent nuclei and nucleoli. Endothelial cells (arrow) can sometimes be seen at the edges of the fragments.

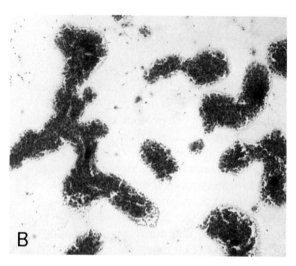

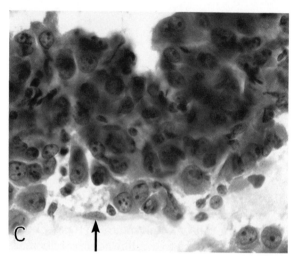

Finally, angiomyolipomas (chapter 4) may be confused with hepatocellular carcinoma, especially in small biopsies. When there is not abundant fat, the epithelioid appearance of the smooth muscle cells, with granular eosinophilic cytoplasm, pleomorphic nuclei, and irregular large nuclei, frequently leads to a misdiagnosis of HCC if the pathologist is not aware of the possibility of a primary hepatic angiomyolipoma. Some tumors may even have areas with a trabecular growth pattern while some have cytoplasmic condensations that mimic Mallory bodies. When dealing with a tumor whose appearance is not typical of HCC, when there are no definite bile canaliculi demonstrable with an immunostain for CEA, one should consider the possibility of an angiomyolipoma. Immunostains with antihuman

hepatocyte will be negative, while HMB-45 will usually be positive, confirming the diagnosis.

Cytology. Fine needle aspiration has become widespread in the diagnosis of HCC. Masses detected by the various imaging modalities can be sampled under sonographic or CT guidance. The lack of desmoplastic stroma in the typical HCC allows abundant tissue to be aspirated, and this can be used to prepare smears and cell blocks. Cell blocks, which are in fact small biopsies, are often sufficient for the diagnosis of HCC. Trabecular patterns are often apparent (fig. 8-47A), and immunostains for CEA, AFP, and cytokeratin can be performed to distinguish poorly differentiated tumors from metastases. Smears can add to the diagnostic accuracy when the cell blocks are equivocal. Features of HCC that are frequently seen in smears include the high cellularity of the specimen; dense, polygonal cells with distinct cell borders, granular cytoplasm, and sometimes bile; one or two central, round, hyperchromatic nuclei with prominent nucleoli; uniformly high nuclear/cytoplasmic ratios; trabecular fragments, often surrounded by endothelial cells (fig. 8-47B,C); and naked atypical nuclei (67).

Spread and Metastases. Studies of the gross pathology of HCC have generally emphasized the intrahepatic growth and spread of the tumor (Table 8-1). Small untreated tumors followed by imaging studies have been shown to double in volume anywhere from 27 to 398 days, with an average doubling time of 136 days (65). Based on this data it was calculated that tumors remain subclinical for an average of 3.5 years. In the early stages, most tumors appear to grow as an expanding, often encapsulated mass. Larger tumors are more likely to infiltrate the surrounding liver tissue and destroy any capsule that may have been present. Intrahepatic metastases, presumably via hematogenous spread, are common, being present in 60 percent of tumors less than 5 cm in diameter and in over 95 percent of those greater than 5 cm (80). Vascular invasion is common, and thrombosis of the portal vein or its branches occurs in 65 to 75 percent and the hepatic veins in 20 to 25 percent of patients with advanced tumors (51,63,80). Occasionally, HCC extends from the liver into the inferior vena cava, and it may grow up into the right atrium or even the right ventricle (33). Bile duct invasion occurs in approximately 5 percent of patients. Advanced tumors often invade the diaphragm and occasionally the gallbladder, and peritoneal dissemination can occur, although not commonly.

Metastasis appears to be a late event in the natural history of HCC, and most patients die of liver failure due to replacement by the tumor. Extrahepatic metastases are common at autopsy, however, and are found in over half the cases (51,63,80). The lung is the most frequent site of metastasis (approximately 50 percent), followed by the regional lymph nodes. Bone metastases are common, and patients may have a bony metastasis as the initial presentation of an occult HCC. Adrenal metastases are found in up to 15 percent of autopsies, and it has been suggested that some cases of pedunculated HCC

actually represent metastasis to the right adrenal gland from a nearby tumor (57).

Staging. HCC may be classified by TNM stage (Appendix), although this is not widely used. Since the prognosis in general is so poor, most clinical series have directed attention less toward TNM stage and more toward the nature of the underlying liver disease, the presence of cirrhosis, the functional state of the liver, and the size of the tumor in formulating an approach to treatment. Tumor resectability clearly correlates with stage, and there is evidence that overall survival and survival after therapy correlate with stage as well (37), although in multivariate analysis other clinical parameters generally have a higher predictive value (70,73). In patients with small tumors treated with orthotopic liver transplantation, TNM stage has not been found to have prognostic power (40).

Treatment. Several forms of curative and palliative therapy are available (5). A cure requires complete resection, but this is often impossible in patients with tumors larger than 5 cm or with advanced cirrhosis producing compromised hepatic function and portal hypertension. Nevertheless, this is the treatment of choice for selected patients, and long-term cure rates are approximately 50 to 75 percent for those with small tumors and adequate liver function (5,37, 75). Orthotopic liver transplantation has become available in recent years, and this has the advantage of removing the diseased liver and giving the patient a better chance of surviving the postoperative period. The long-term survival rate for patients with small tumors is approximately 75 percent (40), but inapparent pulmonary metastases or recurrent tumor in the new liver grow rapidly in the immunosuppressed transplant recipient (79) and so careful patient selection is essential. Chemotherapy, hormonal therapy, and radiotherapy have little, if any, effect on survival in HCC. Percutaneous ethanol injection directly into the HCC under ultrasound guidance causes tumor necrosis with prolongation of survival, and this can even result in apparent cures of some small (less than 3 cm) lesions. This may be used as palliation or for temporary treatment of a patient awaiting definitive therapy by resection or transplantation. Since HCC receives its blood supply from the hepatic artery rather than the portal vein, angiographic embolization of the artery has been used to produce tumor necrosis and prolong survival. The embolic material may be combined with Lipiodol and other chemotherapeutic agents, and this "chemoembolization" may provide further therapeutic efficacy.

Prognosis. Despite efforts at early diagnosis and improved therapy, the prognosis of patients with HCC remains dismal. There are cases with prolonged survival and even spontaneous cure, but these are in the realm of medical curiosities. Most patients who present with advanced, untreatable tumors are dead within a few months (29,36,44,53,55,59,70). Patients whose tumors are surgically resectable have the best prognosis, with median survival of 20 to 45 months. Recent series from the United States have found 5-year survival rates in the range of 30 to 40 percent,

with up to 75 percent for those whose tumors were smaller than 5 cm (70,75). Patients with underlying cirrhosis, however, remain at risk for the development of new tumors. Tumor encapsulation, lack of vascular invasion, and lack of underlying cirrhosis are associated with improved postsurgical survival.

Patients with the fibrolamellar variant of HCC (see chapter 9) have a distinctly better prognosis than with other types. Other histopathologic features, including tumor grade (figs. 8-34–8-37), mitotic index, and proliferative markers (Ki-67, proliferative cell nuclear antigen [PCNA], argyrophilic nucleolar organizer region) have statistically significant relationships to survival, but the overall prognosis is so poor that these are rarely used in an individual case.

REFERENCES

1. Anthony PP, James K. Pedunculated hepatocellular carcinoma. Is it an entity? Histopathology 1987;11:403–14.
2. Austin H. The role of tobacco use and alcohol consumption in the etiology of hepatocellular carcinoma. In: Tabor E, DiBisceglie AM, Purcell RH, eds. Etiology, pathology, and treatment of hepatocellular carcinoma in North America. Houston: Gulf Publishing, 1991:57–76.
3. Beasley RP. Hepatitis B virus. The major etiology of hepatocellular carcinoma. Cancer 1988;61:1942–56.
4. Bhattacharya S, Dhillon AP, Rees J, et al. Small hepatocellular carcinomas in cirrhotic explant livers: identification by macroscopic examination and lipiodol localization. Hepatology 1997;25:613–8.
5. Bruix J. Treatment of hepatocellular carcinoma. Hepatology 1997;25:259–62.
6. Cochrane M, Williams R. Humoral effects of hepatocellular carcinoma. In: Okuda K, Peters RL, eds. Hepatocellular carcinoma. New York: John Wiley & Sons, 1976:333–52.
7. Craig JR, Peters RL, Edmondson HA, Omata M. Fibrolamellar carcinoma of the liver: a tumor of adolescents and young adults with distinctive clinicopathologic features. Cancer 1980;46:372–9.
8. D'Errico AD, Baccarini P, Fiorentino M, et al. Histogenesis of primary liver carcinomas: strengths and weaknesses of cytokeratin profile and albumin mRNA detection. Hum Pathol 1996;27:599–604.
9. Deugnier Y, Turlin B. Other causes of hepatocellular carcinoma. In: Okuda K, Tabor E, eds. Liver cancer. New York: Churchill Livingstone, 1997:97–110.
10. DiBisceglie AM, Order SE, Klein JL, et al. The role of chronic viral hepatitis in hepatocellular carcinoma in the United States. Am J Gastroenterology 1991;86:335–8.
11. DiBisceglie AM, Rustgi VK, Hoofnagle JH, Dusheiko GM, Lotze MT. Hepatocellular carcinoma. Ann Intern Med 1988;108:1741–4.
12. Edmondson HA, Steiner PE. Primary carcinoma of the liver: a study of 100 cases among 48,900 necropsies. Cancer 1954;7:462–503.
13. Eggel H. Über das primäre Carcinom der Leber. Beitr z path Anat z allg Path 1910;30:506–604.
14. Ferrell LD, Crawford JM, Dhillon AP, Scheuer PJ, Nakanuma Y. Proposed standardized criteria for the diagnosis of benign, borderline, and malignant hepatocellular lesions arising in chronic advanced liver disease. Am J Surg Pathol 1993;17:1113–23.
15. Friedman AC, Frazier S, Hendrix TM, Ros PR. Focal diseases. In: Friedman AC, Dachman AH, eds. Radiology of the liver, biliary tract, and pancreas. St Louis: Mosby, 1994:169–327.
16. Gibson JB. Histological typing of tumours of the liver, biliary tract and pancreas. Geneva: World Health Organization, 1978.
17. Goodman ZD, Ishak KG, Langloss JM, Sesterhenn IA, Rabin L. Combined hepatocellular-cholangiocarcinoma: a histologic and immunohistochemical study. Cancer 1985;55:124–35.
18. Guigui B, Mavier P, Lescs MC, Pinaudeau Y, Dhumeaux D, Zafrani ES. Copper and copper binding protein in liver tumors. Cancer 1988;61:1155–8.
19. Haratake J, Takeda S, Kasai T, Nakano S, Tokui N. Predictable factors for estimating prognosis of patients after resection of hepatocellular carcinoma. Cancer 1993;72:1178–83.
19a. Hasan A, Coutts M, Portmann B. Pigmented liver cell adenoma in two male patients. Am J Surg Pathol 2000;24:1429–32.
20. Hurliman J, Gardiol D. Immunohistochemistry in the differential diagnosis of liver carcinomas. Am J Surg Pathol 1991;15:280–8.
21. Ikeda K, Saitoh S, Koida I, et al. Imaging diagnosis of small hepatocellular carcinoma. Hepatology 1994;20:82–7.

22. International Working Party. Terminology of nodular hepatocellular lesions. Hepatology 1995;22:983–93.

23. Ishak KG. Hepatocellular carcinoma associated with the inherited metabolic diseases. In: Tabor E, DiBisceglie AM, Purcell RH, eds. Etiology, pathology, and treatment of hepatocellular carcinoma in North America. Houston: Gulf Publishing Co, 1991:91–106.

24. Ishak KG, Anthony PP, Sobin LH. Histological typing of tumours of the liver, 2nd ed. Berlin: Springer-Verlag, 1994.

25. Ishak KG, Zimmerman HJ. Hepatotoxic effects of the anabolic/androgenic steroids. Sem Liver Dis 1987;7:230–6.

26. Ito Y, Kojiro M, Nakashima T, Mori T. Pathomorphologic characteristics of 102 cases of Thorotrast-related hepatocellular carcinoma, cholangiocarcinoma and hepatic angiosarcoma. Cancer 1988;62:1153–62.

27. Johnson DE, Powers CN, Rupp G, Frable WJ. Immunocytochemical staining of fine-needle aspiration biopsies of liver as a diagnostic tool for hepatocellular carcinoma. Mod Pathol 1992;5:117–23.

28. Johnson PJ, Williams R. Cirrhosis and the aetiology of hepatocellular carcinoma. J Hepatology 1987;4:140–7.

29. Kassianides C, Kew MC. The clinical manifestations and natural history of hepatocellular carcinoma. Gastroenterol Clin N Am 1987;16:553–62.

30. Kew MC. Hepatocellular carcinoma with and without cirrhosis. A comparison of South African blacks. Gastroenterology 1989;97:136–9.

31. Kew MC. Tumor markers in hepatocellular carcinoma. J Gastroenterol Hepatol 1989;4:373–84.

32. Kishimoto Y, Hijiya S, Nagasako R. Malignant mixed tumor of the liver in adults. Am J Gastroenterol 1984;79:229–35.

33. Kojiro M, Nakahara H, Sugihara S, Murakami T, Nakashima T, Kawasaki H. Hepatocellular carcinoma with intra-atrial tumor growth. A clinicopathologic study of 18 cases. Arch Pathol Lab Med 1984;108:989–92.

34. Kondo F, Wada K, Nagato Y, et al. Biopsy diagnosis of well-differentiated hepatocellular carcinoma based on new morphologic criteria. Hepatology 1989;9:751–5.

35. Krishna M, Lloyd RV, Batts KP. Detection of albumin messenger RNA in hepatic and extrahepatic neoplasms. A marker of hepatocellular differentiation. Am J Surg Pathol 1997;21:147–52.

36. Lai CL, Wu PC, Lam KC, Todd D. Histologic prognostic indicators in hepatocellular carcinoma. Cancer 1979;44:1677–83.

37. Lau H, Fan ST, Ng IO, Wong J. Long term prognosis after hepatectomy for hepatocellular carcinoma: a survival analysis of 204 consecutive patients. Cancer 1998;83:2302–11.

38. Leong AS, Sormunen RT, Tsui WM, Liew CT. Hep Par 1 and selected antibodies in the immunohistological distinction of hepatocellular carcinoma from cholangiocarcinoma, combined tumours and metastatic carcinoma. Histopathology 1998;33:318–24.

39. Liang TJ, Jeffers LJ, Reddy KR, et al. Viral pathogenesis of hepatocellular carcinoma in the United States. Hepatology 1993;18:1326–33.

40. Llovet JM, Bruix J, Fuster J, et al. Liver transplantation for small hepatocellular carcinoma: the tumor-node-metastasis classification does not have prognostic power. Hepatology 1998;27:1572–7.

41. Maeda M, Kanayama M, Uchida T, Hasumura Y, Takeuchi J. A case of hepatocellular carcinoma associated with ossification. Cancer 1986;57:134–7.

42. Maeda T, Adachi E, Kajiyama K, Takenaka K, Sugimachi K, Tsuneyoshi M. Spindle cell hepatocellular carcinoma. A clinicopathologic and immunohistochemical analysis of 15 cases. Cancer 1996;77:51–7.

42a. Maitra A, Murakata LA, Albores-Saavedra J. Immunoreactivity for hepatocyte paraffin 1 antibody in hepatoid adenocarcinomas of the gastrointestinal tract. Am J Clin Pathol 2001;115:689–94.

43. McCluggage WG, Toner PG. Hepatocellular carcinoma with osteoclast-like giant cells. Histopathology 1993;23:187–9.

44. Minervini MI, Demetris AJ, Lee RG, Carr BI, Madariaga J, Nalesnik MA. Utilization of hepatocyte-specific antibody in the immunocytochemical evaluation of liver tumors. Mod Pathol 1997;10:686–92.

45. Moradpour D, Wands JR. Hepatic oncogenesis. In: Zakim D, Boyer TD, eds. Hepatology: a textbook of liver disease, 3rd ed. Philadelphia: WB Saunders, 1996:1490–512.

45a. Murakata LA, Ishak KG, Nzeako UC. Clear cell carcinoma of the liver: a comparative immunohistochemical study with renal clear cell carcinoma. Mod Pathol 2000;13:874–81.

46. Nagasue N, Ito A, Yukaya H, Ogawa Y. Androgen receptors in hepatocellular carcinoma and surrounding parenchyma. Gastroenterology 1985;89:643–7.

47. Nagato Y, Kondo F, Kondo Y, Ebara M, Ohto M. Histological and morphometrical indicators for a biopsy diagnosis of well-differentiated hepatocellular carcinoma. Hepatology 1991;14:473–8.

48. Nakanuma Y, Ohta G. Expression of Mallory bodies in hepatocellular carcinoma in man and its significance. Cancer 1986;57:81–6.

49. Nakashima O, Sugihara S, Kage M, Kojiro M. Pathomorphologic characteristics of small hepatocellular carcinoma: a special reference to small hepatocellular carcinoma with indistinct margins. Hepatology 1995;22:101–5.

50. Nakashima T, Kojiro M. Hepatocellular carcinoma. An atlas of its pathology. Tokyo: Springer-Verlag, 1987.

51. Nakashima T, Okuda K, Kojiro M, et al. Pathology of hepatocellular carcinoma in Japan: 232 consecutive cases autopsied in ten years. Cancer 1983;51:863–77.

52. Ng IO, Lai EC, Ng MM, Fan ST. Tumor encapsulation in hepatocellular carcinoma. A pathologic study of 189 cases. Cancer 1992;70:45–9.

53. Nzeako UC, Goodman ZD, Ishak KG. Hepatocellular carcinoma in cirrhotic and noncirrhotic livers. A clinicohistopathologic study of 804 North American patients. Am J Clin Pathol 1996;105:65–75.

54. Nzeako UC, Goodman ZD, Ishak KG. Comparison of tumor pathology with duration of survival of North American patients with hepatocellular carcinoma. Cancer 1995;76:579–88.

55. Okuda K. Clinical presentation and natural history of hepatocellular carcinoma and other liver cancers. In: Okuda K, Tabor E, eds. Liver cancer. New York: Churchill Livingstone, 1997:1–12.

56. Okuda K. Hepatitis C virus and hepatocellular carcinoma. In: Okuda K, Tabor E, eds. Liver cancer. New York: Churchill Livingstone, 1997:39–50.

57. Okuda K, Arakawa M, Kubo Y, et al. Right-sided pedunculated hepatocellular carcinoma: a form of adrenal metastasis. Hepatology 1998;27:81–5.

58. Okuda K, Nakashima T, Kojiro M, Kondo Y, Wada K. Hepatocellular carcinoma without cirrhosis in Japanese patients. Gastroenterology 1989;97:140–6.

59. Okuda K, Ohtsuki T, Obata H, et al. Natural history of hepatocellular carcinoma in relation to treatment: study of 850 patients. Cancer 1985;56:918–28.

60. Okuda K, Peters RL, Simpson IW. Gross anatomic features of hepatocellular carcinoma from three disparate geographic areas. Proposal of a new classification. Cancer 1984;54:2165–73.

61. Omata M, Peters RL, Tatter D. Sclerosing hepatic carcinoma: relationship to hypercalcemia. Liver 1981;1:33–49.

62. Otsuru A, Nagataki S, Koji T, Tamoki T. Analysis of alpha-fetoprotein gene expression in hepatocellular carcinoma and liver cirrhosis by in situ hybridization. Cancer 1988;62:1105–12.

63. Peters RL. Pathology of hepatocellular carcinoma. In: Okuda K, Peters RL, eds. Hepatocellular carcinoma. New York: John Wiley & Sons, 1976;107–68.

64. Roth JA, Berman E, Befeler D, Johnson FB. A black hepatocellular carcinoma with Dubin-Johnson-like pigment and Mallory bodies: a histochemical and ultrastructural study. Am J Surg Pathol 1982;6:375–82.

65. Sheu JC, Sung JL, Chen DS, et al. Growth rate of asymptomatic hepatocellular carcinoma and its clinical implications. Gastroenterology 1985;89:259–66.

66. Shirabe K, Matsumata T, Adachi E, et al. Prognosis of well differentiated small hepatocellular carcinoma. Is well differentiated hepatocellular carcinoma clinically early cancer? Hepatogastroenterology 1995;42:923–30.

67. Silverman JF, Geisinger KR. Fine needle aspiration of the liver and pancreas. In: Silverberg SG, ed. Principles and practice of surgical pathology and cytopathology, 3rd Ed. New York, Churchill Livingstone, 1997:1941–96.

68. Simonetti, RG, Camma C, Fiorello F, Politi F, D'Amico G, Pagilaro L. Hepatocellular carcinoma: a worldwide problem and the major risk factors. Dig Dis Sci 1991; 36:962–72.

69. Stromeyer FW, Ishak KG, Gerber MA, Mathew T. Ground-glass cells in hepatocellular carcinoma. Am J Clin Pathol 1980;74:254–8.

70. Stuart KE, Anand AJ, Jenkins RL. Hepatocellular carcinoma in the United States. Prognostic features, treatment outcome, and survival. Cancer 1996;77:2217–22.

71. Svenberg T, Hannarstrom S, Hedin A. Purification and properties of biliary glycoprotein I (BGPI). Immunohistochemical relationship to carcinoembryonic antigen. Mol Immunol 1979;16:245–52.

72. Tabor E. The role of tumor suppressor genes in the development of hepatocellular carcinoma. In: Tabor E, DiBisceglie AM, Purcell RH, eds. Etiology, pathology, and treatment of hepatocellular carcinoma in North America. Houston: Gulf Publishing Co, 1991:89–96.

73. Takenaka K, Kawahara N, Yamamoto K, et al. Results of 280 liver resections for hepatocellular carcinoma. Arch Surg 1996;131:71–6.

74. Van Eyken P, Sciot R, Paterson A, Callea F, Kew MC, Desmet VJ. Cytokeratin expression in hepatocellular carcinoma: an immunohistochemical study. Human Pathol 1988;19:562–8.

75. Vauthey JN, Klimstra D, Franceschi D, et al. Factors affecting long-term outcome after resection for hepatocellular carcinoma. Am J Surg 1995;169:28–35.

76. Wogan GN. Aflatoxins as risk factors for hepatocellular carcinoma in humans. Cancer Res (Suppl) 1992;52:2114–8.

77. Wu PC, Lai CL, Lam KC, Lok AS, Lin HJ. Clear cell carcinoma of the liver. Cancer 1983;52:504–7.

78. Wu TC, Tong MJ, Hwang B, Lee SD, Hu MM. Primary hepatocellular carcinoma and hepatitis B infection during childhood. Hepatology 1987;7:46–8.

79. Yokoyama I, Carr B, Saitsu H, Iwatsuki S, Starzl TE. Accelerated growth rates of recurrent hepatocellular carcinoma after liver transplantation. Cancer 1991;68:2095–100.

80. Yuki K, Hirohashi S, Sakamoto M, Kanai T, Shimosato Y. Growth and spread of hepatocellular carcinoma: a review of 240 autopsy cases. Cancer 1990;66:2174–9.

❖❖❖

9
FIBROLAMELLAR HEPATOCELLULAR CARCINOMA

Definition. Fibrolamellar hepatocellular carcinoma (FLC) is a variant of hepatocellular carcinoma (HCC) distinguished by distinctive fibrous lamellae and polygonal tumor cells that have an eosinophilic, coarsely granular ("oncocytic") cytoplasm. It has distinctive clinical features and natural history, which justify its separation from other types of HCC (Table 9-1). It is also known as *fibrolamellar carcinoma* of the liver.

General Features. The clinical and pathologic features of FLC, first described by Edmondson (12), were reported in two series of 23 and 12 cases by Craig et al. (8) and Berman et al. (5), respectively. Berman et al. referred to the tumor as the "polygonal cell type" of HCC with a fibrous stroma. The term fibrolamellar carcinoma proposed by Craig et al. has now been universally adopted. The tumor has distinctive clinical aspects (young patient age of presentation, absence of pre-existing liver disease, a better resectability rate than the usual type of HCC, and a better survival rate following resection or transplantation), as well as distinctive pathologic features (polygonal tumor cells with an eosinophilic cytoplasm packed with mitochondria, and fibrous lamellae). Since these early reports other series larger than three cases (1,4,7,14,17–19,21,23,27,30,33–35,37,39,40), as well as isolated case reports, have been published. The reviews of Rolfes (34a) and Craig (7a) are recommended for further reading.

Clinical Features. Soreide et al. (39) reviewed 80 cases of FLC (including 9 of their own cases) reported from 1980 to 1986. The mean age of patients was 23 years and only 6 percent were older than 50. The male to female ratio was 3 to 4. The disease course is somewhat indolent in comparison to that of the usual type of HCC: in one series symptoms and signs had been present for an average of 11 months compared to 2.8 months for the usual HCC (39). Symptoms include nausea, vomiting, abdominal pain, malaise, and weight loss. Jaundice is rare and is attributable to invasion of the extrahepatic bile ducts by the tumor (2,11). Also rare is presentation with the Budd-Chiari syndrome due to invasion of the inferior vena cava (22).

Liver tests may reveal mild to moderate elevation of the serum aminotransferases, alkaline phosphatase, and bilirubin. In the review of Soreide et al. (39) only 8 percent of patients had a positive test for hepatitis B surface antigen (HBsAg). In a study of 11 cases of HCC in childhood in the Kiehl Pediatric Tumor Registry (25), 3 of the tumors were fibrolamellar carcinomas; all were serologically and immunohistologically negative for hepatitis B virus (HBV) markers. More recently, a patient with FLC, who was seropositive for HBsAg and anti-HBe, was found to have HBV-DNA sequences in both his tumor and nontumor tissue (9). About one tenth of the patients have increased serum alpha-fetoprotein values (39). Other biochemical abnormalities have included increased serum levels of B_{12} (30,39), neurotensin (7,39), and carcinoembryonic antigen (43). Neither the increased serum B_{12} binding capacity (30) nor neurotensin (49) are specific for FLC.

Radiologic Findings. Calcification may be found in plain abdominal films or by computed tomography (CT) in FLC (16,17,42). The tumors are well demarcated and hypodense on unenhanced CT scans (17). The majority are homogeneous, but they may exhibit a central hypodense area that corresponds to a central scar. The central scar may simulate the appearance of focal nodular hyperplasia in imaging studies (44). Angiographically, FLC is hypervascular (17,16,48). Francis et al. (16) found no evidence of arterioportal shunting or venous invasion, but Wong et al. (48) detected early visualization of the inferior vena cava that suggested arteriovenous shunting in their case.

Gross Findings. Two thirds of the cases of FLC are in the left lobe. A single mass is present in 56 percent of cases. The tumor is sharply demarcated but nonencapsulated (figs. 9-1, 9-2). Sections disclose a scalloped margin and a firm to hard consistency. Glistening white fibrous septa, sometimes linked to a central area of scarring and calcification, often give the tumor a lobulated appearance that is somewhat reminiscent of focal nodular hyperplasia (figs. 9-1, 9-2). The tumor tissue itself is light brown, tan, or gray but it may be green

Table 9-1

COMPARISON OF FIBROLAMELLAR HEPATOCELLULAR CARCINOMA WITH ORDINARY HEPATOCELLULAR CARCINOMA

	Fibrolamellar Hepatocellular Carcinoma	Hepatocellular Carcinoma
Clinical Features		
Age range (years)	5–35	50–70
Sex	M=F	M>F
Etiology	Unknown	Viral hepatitis, alcoholic liver disease, aflatoxin, hemochromatosis, other
Surgical resectability	50–75%	10–20%
Mean survival after diagnosis	32–68 months	<6 months
Gross Findings		
Single or multiple	Often single	Single or multiple
Consistency	Firm or hard	Soft or firm
Fibrous septa	Usual	Absent
Bile-stained areas	+/–	+/–
Cirrhosis	–	+
Microscopic Findings		
Fibrous lamellae	+	–
Trabeculae, pseudoglands	+	+
Canaliculi	+	+
Bile production	+	+
Tumor cells	Large, polygonal	Small or large, polygonal, round or irregular
Nuclei	Very large nucleoli ("owl's eye")	Variable size, prominent nucleoli
Mitoses	Rare	Frequent to rare
Cytoplasm	Eosinophilic, coarsely granular	Eosinophilic, fine granularity
Fat, glycogen in cytoplasm	+/–	+/–
Inclusions in cytoplasm	Pale bodies, globules, Mallory bodies (rare)	Globules, Mallory bodies
Ultrastructural Findings		
Mitochondria	Many ("back-to-back")	Scattered
Canaliculi	+	+
Intracellular lumina	+	–
Immunohistochemical Findings		
Polyclonal carcinoembryonic Ag	+	+
Hepatocyte antigen (Hep Par 1)	+	+
Alpha-fetoprotein	–	+/–
Cytokeratins (7,8,18,19)	+/–	+/–
Cytokeratin 20	–	–
Non-Neoplastic Liver		
Cirrhosis	–	+
Dysplastic foci/nodules	–	+/–
Vascular/bile duct invasion	+/–	+/–

if bile production is prominent. The non-neoplastic parenchyma generally appears normal. Cirrhosis had been reported in only 4 percent of cases (39). The distribution of metastases, when present, is similar to that of the usual type of HCC, i.e., to abdominal lymph nodes, peritoneum, and lungs.

Microscopic Findings. The distinctive histopathologic features of FLC are the fibrous stroma and the tumor cells, but there is some overlap with the usual trabecular type of HCC. The fibrous stroma consists of lamellae of varied thickness that contain thick hyalinized bundles

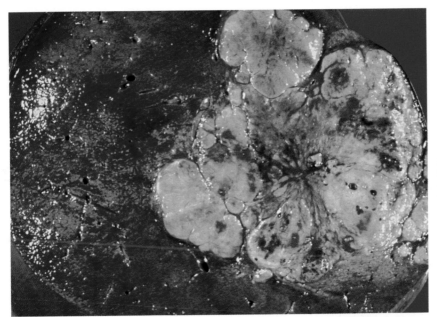

Figure 9-1
FIBROLAMELLAR
HEPATOCELLULAR
CARCINOMA
This section of liver shows a
light tan, nodular mass with an
irregular margin. Note the central
depressed scar and foci of hemorrhage. The non-neoplastic liver is
not cirrhotic.

of collagen as well as thinner collagen and reticulin fibers that support individual and small groups of tumor cells (figs. 9-3–9-5). In needle biopsy specimens the thicker lamellae may not be sampled, but thin fibrous strands are invariably present. In such instances reliance must be placed on the distinctive cytologic features of the tumor cells, as described subsequently. Smooth muscle fibers may be present among the collagen bundles in the septa. A basement membrane may be identified with a periodic acid–Schiff (PAS) stain and by immunostains for laminin and type IV collagen. Many vessels, including peculiar thick-walled arteries, are noted in the stroma (fig. 9-6). Inflammatory cells and rarely, granulomas, may infiltrate the septa and tumor proper (fig. 9-7). Occasional small bile ducts and nerve fibers may be identified in the tumors, as well as focal calcification, often in the center (figs. 9-8–9-10).

The tumor cells have a sheet-like pattern but microtrabeculae may be present (fig. 9-11). Canaliculi in the trabeculae may dilate, resulting in a pseudoglandular pattern (fig. 9-11). Characteristically, the tumor cells are larger than normal liver cells, are polyhedral or rounded, and have a deeply eosinophilic, coarsely granular cytoplasm (fig. 9-12). The granularity is due to the presence of a large number of mitochondria of normal size, that can be well visualized by a phosphotungstic acid hematoxylin stain (fig. 9-13). The cytoplasm

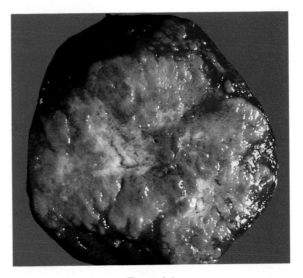

Figure 9-2
FIBROLAMELLAR HEPATOCELLULAR CARCINOMA
The tumor is nodular and tan-brown, with an infiltrative margin and scattered white areas of fibrosis.

and tumor canaliculi may contain bile (fig. 9-14). Glycogen and fat can also be found to a variable extent in the tumor cells. Cytoplasmic inclusions include globular (hyaline), eosinophilic inclusions (that are variably PAS-positive and may be immunoreactive for alpha-1-antitrypsin) (fig. 9-15); ground glass inclusions (41) also referred to "pale bodies" by Craig et al. (8); and rarely, Mallory

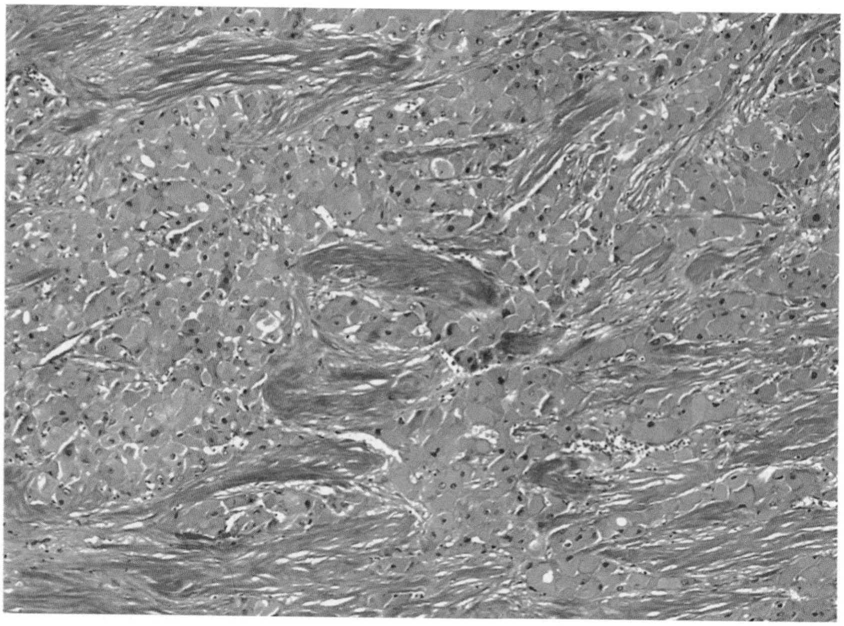

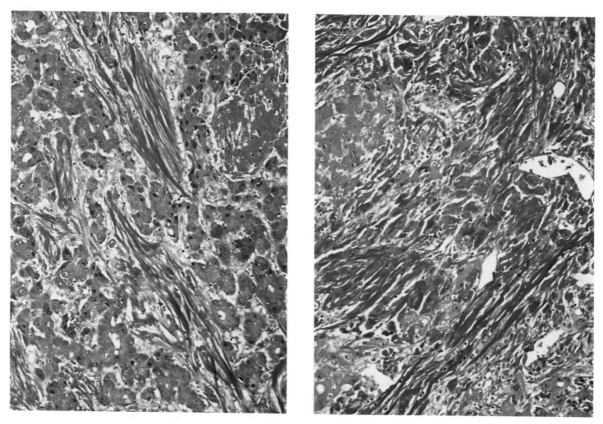

Figure 9-3
FIBROLAMELLAR
HEPATOCELLULAR
CARCINOMA
There is an admixture of fibrous
lamellae and epithelial elements.

Figure 9-4
FIBROLAMELLAR HEPATOCELLULAR CARCINOMA
Left: There are fibrous lamellae of varied thickness (Masson trichrome stain).
Right: Another field shows fibrous lamellae in the matrix (Masson trichrome stain).

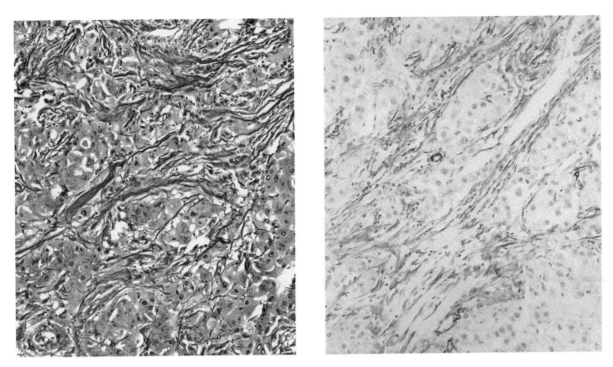

Figure 9-5
FIBROLAMELLAR HEPATOCELLULAR CARCINOMA
A reticulin stain (left) and an immunostain for collagen type IV (right) shows fibrous lamellae.

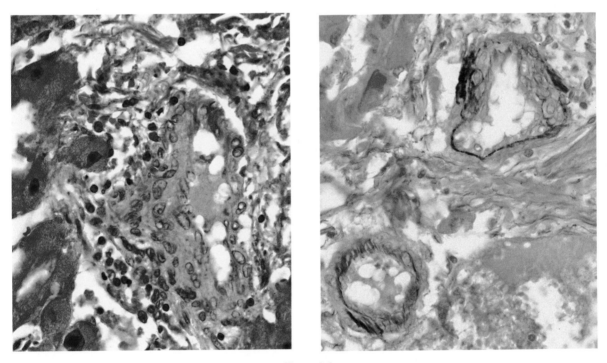

Figure 9-6
FIBROLAMELLAR HEPATOCELLULAR CARCINOMA
A Masson trichrome stain demonstrates the arteries (left) and a Victoria blue stain shows the elastic lamina of the arteries (right).

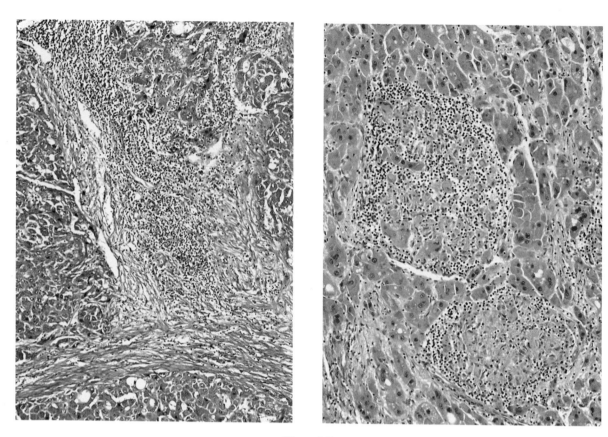

Figure 9-7
FIBROLAMELLAR HEPATOCELLULAR CARCINOMA
Inflammatory cells are shown on the left and epithelioid granulomas on the right.

Figure 9-8
FIBROLAMELLAR
HEPATOCELLULAR
CARCINOMA
Trapped small bile ducts are seen.

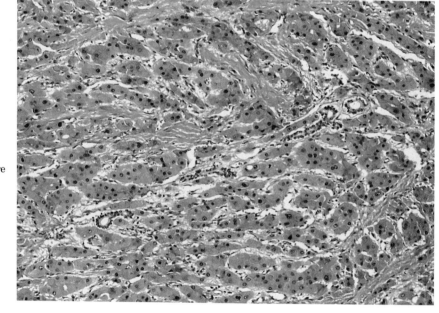

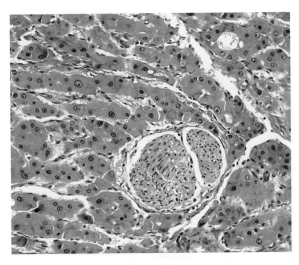

Figure 9-9
FIBROLAMELLAR HEPATOCELLULAR CARCINOMA
A trapped nerve fiber is shown.

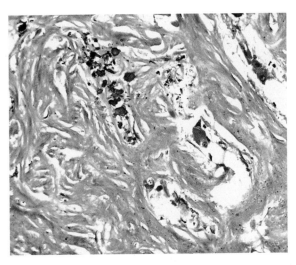

Figure 9-10
FIBROLAMELLAR HEPATOCELLULAR CARCINOMA
Stromal calcification.

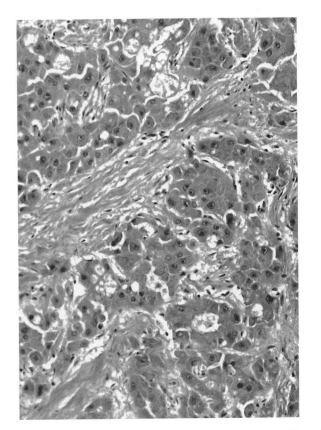

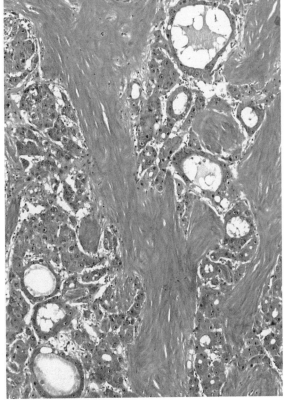

Figure 9-11
FIBROLAMELLAR HEPATOCELLULAR CARCINOMA
An area of tumor showing microtrabeculae is on the left and one with pseudoglands is on the right.

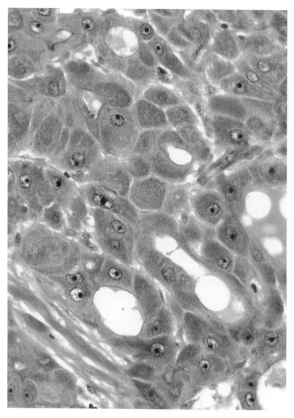

Figure 9-12
FIBROLAMELLAR HEPATOCELLULAR CARCINOMA
The tumor has polygonal, eosinophilic cells with a granular cytoplasm and prominent nucleoli.

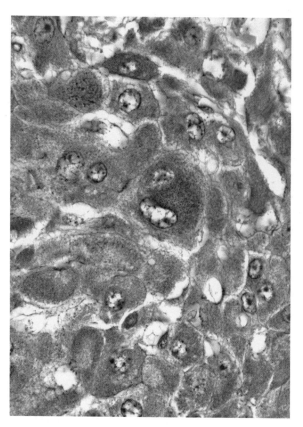

Figure 9-13
FIBROLAMELLAR HEPATOCELLULAR CARCINOMA
Phosphotungstic acid hematoxylin stain demonstrates mitochondria in the cytoplasm of the tumor cells.

Figure 9-14
FIBROLAMELLAR
HEPATOCELLULAR
CARCINOMA
Bile is present in tumor canaliculi.

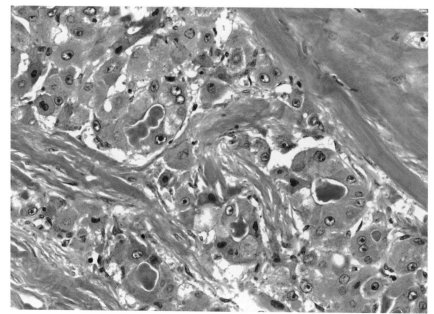

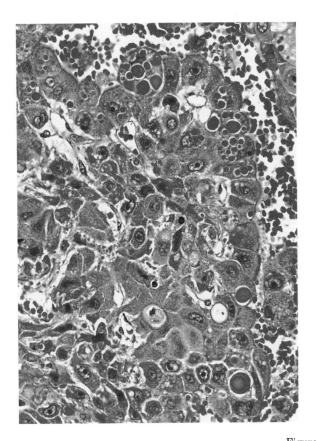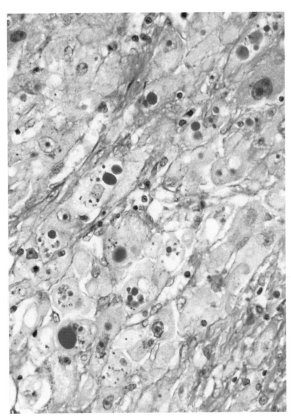

Figure 9-15
FIBROLAMELLAR HEPATOCELLULAR CARCINOMA
Left: Eosinophilic globules are apparent in tumor cells.
Right: The globules are PAS positive after diastase digestion.

bodies (fig. 9-16). The ground glass inclusions are PAS-negative and do not contain HBsAg, but they are immunoreactive for fibrinogen (fig. 9-16, right) (4,41,43). Copper and copper-binding protein can be detected frequently in the cytoplasm of tumor cells (fig. 9-17) (24,43,46,47). Mucin production has been demonstrated in some cases of FLC (18).

The nuclei of the cells of FLC are often large, hyperchromatic, and vesicular, and have prominent, often eosinophilic nucleoli (fig. 9-12). Mitoses and multinucleation are infrequent. Invasion of blood vessels and bile ducts (fig. 9-18) may be observed.

Immunohistochemical Findings. Immunohistopathologic studies have identified alpha-1-antitrypsin (4,6,18,23,24,43,47) as well as ferritin (6) in the cytoplasm of tumor cells. As already noted, fibrinogen is detectable in the ground glass inclusions (fig. 9-16, right). Carcinoembryonic antigen can be identified in a pericanalicular distribution (fig. 9-19) (18,43), as well as C-reactive protein, in a diffuse cytoplasmic distribution (4). The Hep Par 1 (Hepatocyte) immunostain is positive. Alpha-fetoprotein is generally not detected immunohistochemically. Cytokeratin expression was studied in two cases by van Eyken et al. (45): the tumor cells expressed cytokeratin polypeptides 8 and 18 and surprisingly, cytokeratins 7 and even 19 (which are usually expressed by bile ducts cells). Aberrant expression of these cytokeratins has also been found in some HCCs. Expression of cytokeratins 7 and 8 is shown in figure 9-20. An increased amount of fibronectin in FLC (as well as in the clear cell type of HCC and encapsulated HCC) correlates with a better prognosis than that of undifferentiated HCC, which shows a decreased amount of fibronectin (20).

Ultrastructural Findings. The ultrastructure of FLC has been studied extensively (3,6,8,15, 23,26,32,47). The most striking ultrastructural

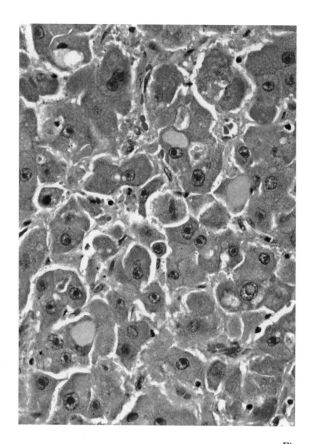
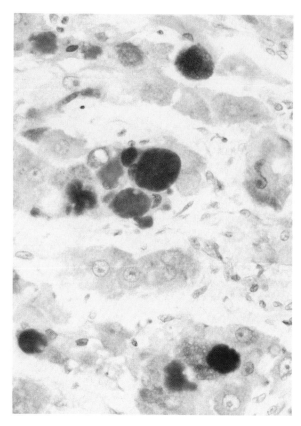

Figure 9-16
FIBROLAMELLAR HEPATOCELLULAR CARCINOMA
Left: Pale bodies are seen in the tumor cell cytoplasm.
Right: Immunostain shows that the pale bodies contain fibrinogen.

Figure 9-17
FIBROLAMELLAR
HEPATOCELLULAR
CARCINOMA
Copper-binding protein in tumor
cells (Victoria blue stain).

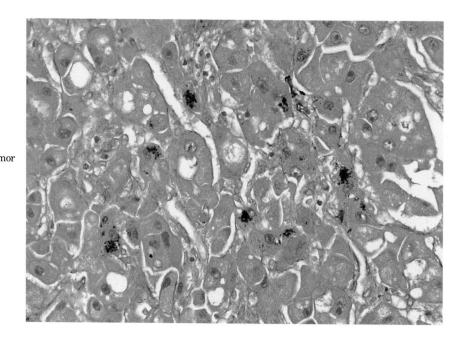

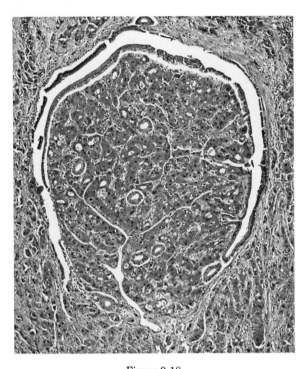

Figure 9-18
FIBROLAMELLAR HEPATOCELLULAR CARCINOMA
The tumor has breached one segment of the duct and herniated into the lumen, but is still covered by the stretched bile duct epithelium.

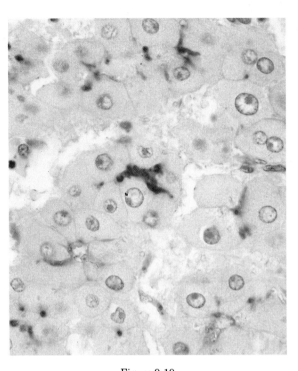

Figure 9-19
FIBROLAMELLAR HEPATOCELLULAR CARCINOMA
Canaliculi are demonstrated immunohistochemically by polyclonal antibodies to carcinoembryonic antigen.

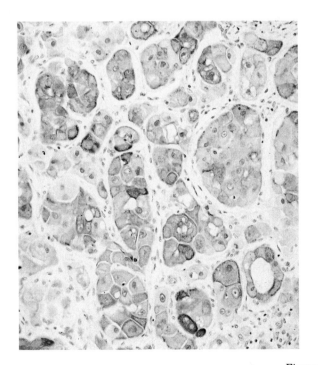

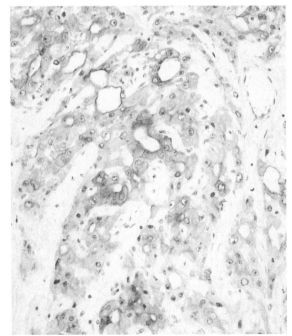

Figure 9-20
FIBROLAMELLAR HEPATOCELLULAR CARCINOMA
Expression of cytokeratins 7 (left) and 8 (right) in tumor cells (immunostain).

feature is the presence of a large number of "back-to-back" mitochondria in the cytoplasm of the tumor cells (fig. 9-21). According to Phillips et al. (32), the mitochondria show changes resembling those of Reye's syndrome. Intercellular spaces lined by microvilli correspond to the canaliculi noted microscopically (44,47). In two studies (26,41) the ground glass inclusions were found to contain an amorphous flocculent material, but in other studies (3,32) they were thought to represent intracellular lumina lined by numerous malformed microvilli. Fibroblasts and myofibroblasts are present in the fibrous lamellae (6).

Differential Diagnosis. This includes one benign lesion, focal nodular hyperplasia (FNH), and several malignant tumors. The septa of FNH lack the dense hyalinization of the lamellae of FLC. They also contain the characteristic thick-walled arteries, and there are numerous ductules interposed between the septa and the hepatic parenchymal component. The cells of FNH resemble normal liver cells, in contrast to the neoplastic cells of FLC.

The typical ("ordinary") HCC usually lacks a fibrous stroma. Rarely, there may be a desmoplastic response (scirrhous variant of HCC). In such tumors the fibrous stroma is loose and lacks the dense hyalinization of the lamellae of FLC. Furthermore, the tumor cells, which may be poorly differentiated, are smaller than normal liver cells, have a high nuclear/cytoplasmic ratio, and lack the coarsely granular, eosinophilic cytoplasm of cells of FLC.

Intrahepatic (peripheral) cholangiocarcinoma often displays a desmoplastic response. Gland formation is usually discernible, canaliculi and bile production are absent, and mucin is often demonstrable by special stains. Additionally, the cells of cholangiocarcinoma are generally small, columnar to cuboidal, and have a lightly stained, clear cytoplasm. The Hep Par 1 immunostain is negative in cholangiocarcinoma but positive in FLC.

Epithelioid hemangioendothelioma is typically characterized by a dense fibrous matrix. Unlike FLC, the tumor cells grow along preformed sinusoids and veins, and also form intracellular vascular lumina. The cells express vascular endothelial cell markers such as factor VIII–related antigen (which is also secreted into the newly formed vascular lumina).

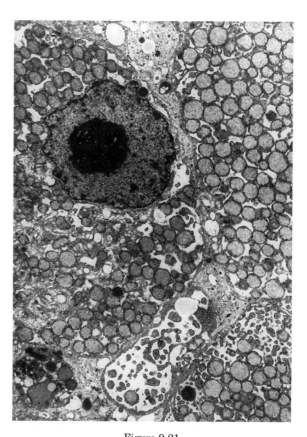

Figure 9-21
FIBROLAMELLAR HEPATOCELLULAR CARCINOMA
Electron micrograph shows numerous mitochondria in the tumor cells. Note the canaliculus-like, cisternal structure (bottom) and the large nucleolus.

The authors have not found metastatic tumors to pose problems in the differential diagnosis of FLC.

Etiology and Pathogenesis. Etiologic and pathogenetic factors in FLC have not been identified. The suggestion that FLC arises in or is the malignant counterpart of focal nodular hyperplasia (3,38,39) remains unsubstantiated. Focal nodular hyperplasia is a relatively frequent benign lesion and has been reported to occur simultaneously with other tumors (such as cavernous hemangioma and hepatocellular adenoma) and, in the case of Saul et al. (36), with FLC. There is a possibility that some fibrolamellar carcinomas may have neuroendocrine features, as demonstrated by the expression of uranaffin by ultrastructural cytochemistry (31), expression of serotonin in several cases (23,31), expression of the neurotensin gene in one case (13), and identification of secretory granules by electron microscopic examination

(23). The lamellar fibrosis of FLC is believed to be due to the action of transforming growth factor–beta produced by the tumor cells (29).

Treatment. The resectability rate of FLC is 58 percent (39). All series have reported long survival periods following excision. The 5-year survival rate , based on the literature survey of Soreide et al. (39), was 56 percent. The longest postresection survival time was 21 years (21). The results of hepatic resection or transplantation from two series of 20 and 41 patients have clearly shown that the most significant determinant of survival is tumor stage (34,37). In one study of 12 cases, DNA ploidy was not found to be related to clinical behavior (28). Various chemotherapeutic regimens have been used in some patients with partial responses (10,19,40,43). A patient of Denis et al. (10) who had bilateral lung metastases was treated with adriamycin and mitomycin; she was in good health 2 years after the initial diagnosis.

REFERENCES

1. Adam A, Soreide O, Hemingway AP, Gibson RN. The radiology of fibrolamellar hepatoma. Clin Radiol 1986;37:355–8.
2. Albaugh JS, Keeffe EB, Krippaehue WW. Recurrent obstructive jaundice of fibrolamellar hepatocellular carcinoma. Dig Dis Sci 1984;29:762–7.
3. An T, Ghatak N, Kastner R, Kay S, Lee HM. Hyaline globules and intracellular lumina in a hepatocellular carcinoma. Am J Clin Pathol 1983;79:392–6.
4. Berman MA, Burnham JA, Sheahan DG. Fibrolamellar carcinoma of the liver: an immunohistochemical study of nineteen cases and a review of the literature. Hum Pathol 1988;19:786–94.
5. Berman MM, Libbey NP, Foster JH. Hepatocellular carcinoma: polygonal cell type with fibrous stroma—an atypical variant with a favorable prognosis. Cancer 1980;46:1448–55.
6. Caballero T, Aneiros J, Lopez-Caballero J, et al. Fibrolamellar hepatocellular carcinoma. An immuno-histochemical and ultrastructural study. Histopathology 1985;9:445–56.
7. Collier NA, Weinbren K, Bloom SR, et al. Neurotension secretion by fibrolamellar carcinoma of the liver. Lancet 1984;i:538–40.
7a. Craig JR. Fibrolamellar carcinoma: clinical and pathologic features. In: Okuda K, Tabor E, eds. Liver cancer. New York: Churchill Livingstone, 1997:255–62.
8. Craig JR, Peters RL, Edmondson HA, Omata M. Fibrolamellar carcinoma of the liver: a tumor of adolescents and young adults with distinctive clinicopathologic features. Cancer 1980;46:372–9.
9. Davison FD, Fagan EA, Portmann B, Williams R. HBV-DNA sequences in tumor and non-tumor tissue in a patient with the fibrolamellar variant of hepatocellular carcinoma. Hepatology 1990;12:676–9.
10. Denis J, Grippon P, Legendre C, Roche J, Goodman BN. Carcinome fibrolamellaire du foie: un carcinome hepatocellulare de pronostic favorable. Gastroenterol Clin Biol 1984;8:920–4.
11. Eckstein RP, Bambach CP, Stiehl D, et al. Fibrolamellar carcinoma as a cause of bile duct obstruction. Pathology 1988;20:326–31.
12. Edmondson HA. Tumors of the liver and intrahepatic bile ducts. Atlas of Tumor Pathology. 1st Series, Fascicle 25. Washington, D.C.: Armed Forces Institute of Pathology, 1958:32.
13. Ehrenfried JA, Zhou Z, Thompson JC, Evers BM. Expression of the neurotensin gene in fetal human liver and fibrolamellar carcinoma. Ann Surg 1994;220:484–91.
14. Farhi DC, Shikes RH, Murari PJ, Silverberg SG. Hepatocellular carcinoma in young people. Cancer 1983;52:1516–25.
15. Farhi DC, Shikes RH, Silverberg SG. Ultrastructure of fibrolamellar oncocytic hepatoma. Cancer 1982;50:702–9.
16. Francis IR, Agha EP, Thompson NW, et al. Fibrolamellar hepatocarcinoma: clinical, radiologic and pathologic features. Gastrointest Radiol 1986;11:67–72.
17. Friedman AC, Lichtenstein JE, Goodman ZD, et al. Fibrolamellar hepatocellular carcinoma. Radiology 1985;157:583–7.
18. Goodman ZD, Ishak KG, Langloss M, Sesterhenn IA, Rabin L. Combined hepatocellular-cholangiocarcinoma: a histologic and immunochemical study. Cancer 1985;55:124–35.
19. Ihde DC, Mathews MJ, Makuch MJ, et al. Prognostic factors in patients with hepatocellular carcinoma receiving systemic chemotherapy: identification of two groups of patients with prospects for prolonged survival. Am J Med 1985;78:399–406.
20. Jagirdar J, Ishak KG, Colombo M, et al. Fibronectin patterns in hepatocellular carcinoma and its clinical significance. Cancer 1985;56:1643–8.
21. Lack EE, Neave C, Vawter GF. Hepatocellular carcinoma. Review of 32 cases in childhood and adolescence. Cancer 1983;52:1510–5.
22. Lamberts R, Nitsche R, de Vivie RE, et al. Budd-Chiari syndrome as the primary manifestation of a fibrolamellar hepatocellular carcinoma. Digestion 1992;23:200–9.
23. Lapis K, Schaff Z, Kopper L, Karacsonyi S, Omos J. Das fibrolamellare Leberkarzinom. Zentralbl Allg Pathol Anat 1990;136:135–49.
24. Lefkowitch JH, Muschel R, Prince JB, et al. Copper and copper binding protein in fibrolamellar carcinoma. Cancer 1983;51:97–100.
25. Leuschner I, Harms D, Schmidt D. The association of hepatocellular carcinoma in childhood with hepatitis B virus infection. Cancer 1988;62:2363–9.

243

26. Mierrau GW, Orisini EN. Case for diagnosis. Ultrastruct Pathol 1983;5:273–9.

27. O'Grady JG, Polson RJ, Rolleska K, et al. Liver transplantation for malignant disease. Results of 93 consecutive patients. Ann Surg 1988;207:373–9.

28. Orsatti G, Greenberg PD, Rolfes DB, Ishak KG, Paronetto F. DNA ploidy of fibrolamellar hepatocellular carcinoma by image analysis. Hum Pathol 1994;25:936–9.

29. Orsatti G, Hytiroglou P, Thung SN, Ishak KG, Paronetto F. Lamellar fibrosis in the fibrolamellar variant of hepatocellular carcinoma: a role for transforming growth factor beta. Liver 1997;17:152–6.

30. Paradinas FJ, Melia WM, Wilkinson ML, et al. High serum vitamin B12 binding capacity as a marker of the fibrolamellar variant of hepatocellular carcinoma. Br Med J 1982;285:840–2.

31. Payne CM, Nagle RB, Paplanus SH, Graham AR. Fibrolamallar carcinoma of the liver: a primary malignant oncocytic carcinoid? Ultrastruct Pathol 1986;10:539–52.

32. Phillips MJ, Poucell S, Patterson J, Valencia P. The liver. An atlas and text of ultrastructural pathology. New York: Raven Press, 1987.

33. Pinna AD, Iwatsuki S, Lee RG, et al. Treatment of fibrolamellar hepatoma with subtotal hepatectomy or transplantation. Hepatology 1997;26:877–83.

34. Ringe B, Wittekind C, Weimann A, Tusch G, Pichlmayr R. Results of hepatic resection and transplantation for fibrolamellar carcinoma. Surg Gynecol Obstet 1992;175:299–305.

34a. Rolfes DB. Fibrolamellar carcinoma of the liver. In: Okuda K, Ishak KG, eds. Neoplasms of the liver. Tokyo, Springer-Verlag, 1987;137:136–42.

35. Ruffin MT. Fibrolamellar hepatoma. Am J Gastroenterol 1990;85:577–81.

36. Saul SH, Titelbaum DS, Gansler TS, et al. The fibrolamellar variant of hepatocellular carcinoma. Its association with focal nodular hyperplasia. Cancer 1987;60:3049–55.

37. Scoazec JY, Flejou JF, D'Errico A, et al. Fibrolamellar carcinoma of the liver: composition of the extracellular matrix and expression of cell-matrix and cell-cell adhesion molecules. Hepatology 1996;24:1120–36.

38. Sheppard KJ, Bradbury DA, Davies J, Ryrie DR. High serum vitamin B12 binding capacity as a marker of the fibrolamellar variant of hepatocellular carcinoma. Br Med J 1983;286:57.

39. Soreide O, Czemiak A, Bradpiece H, Bloom S, Blumgart L. Characteristics of fibrolamellar hepatocellular carcinoma. A study of nine cases and a review of the literature. Am J Surg 1986;151:518–23.

40. Starzl TE, Iwatsuki S, Shaw BW Jr, Nalesnik MA, Farhi DC, Van Thiel DH. Treatment of fibrolamellar hepatoma with partial or total hepatectomy and transplantation of the liver. Surg Gynecol Obst 1986;162:145–8.

41. Stromeyer FW, Ishak KG, Gerber MA, Mathew T. Ground-glass cells in hepatocellular carcinoma. Am J Clin Pathol 1980;74:254–9.

42. Teefey SA, Stephens DH, Weiland LH. Calcification in hepatocellular carcinoma: not always an indication of fibrolamellar histology. Am J Roentgenol 1987;149:1173–4.

43. Teitelbaum DH, Tuttle S, Carey LC, Clausen KP. Fibrolamellar carcinoma of the liver. Review of three cases and the presentation of a characteristic set of tumor markers defining the tumor. Ann Surg 1985;202:36–41.

44. Titelbaum DS, Burke DR, Meranze SG, Saul SH. Fibrolamellar hepatocellular carcinoma: pitfalls in nonoperative diagnosis. Radiology 1988;167:23–30.

45. van Eyken PV, Sciot R, Brock P, et al. Abundant expression of cytokeratin 7 in fibrolamellar carcinoma of the liver. Histopathology 1990;17:101–7.

46. Vecchio FM. Fibrolamellar carcinoma of the liver: a distinct entity within the hepatocellular tumors. A review. Appl Pathol 1988;6:139–48.

47. Vecchio FM, Fabrano A, Ghirlanda G, Manna R, Massi G. Fibrolamellar carcinoma of the liver: the malignant counterpart of focal nodular hyperplasia with oncocytic change. Am J Clin Pathol 1984;81:521–6.

48. Wong LK, Link DP, Frey CF, Ruebner RH, Tesluk H, Pimstone NR. Fibrolamellar hepatocarcinoma: radiology, management and pathology. Am J Roentgenol 1982;139:172–5.

49. Wood JR, Melia WM, Wood SM, et al. Neurotensin and hepatocellular carcinoma. Lancet 1984;1:687.

✧✧✧

10

INTRAHEPATIC CHOLANGIOCARCINOMA AND OTHER MALIGNANT BILIARY TUMORS

INTRAHEPATIC CHOLANGIOCARCINOMA

Definition. Intrahepatic cholangiocarcinoma is an adenocarcinoma arising from the intrahepatic bile ducts that is composed of glands or tubules growing in a moderate or abundant fibrous stroma. Synonyms include *peripheral cholangiocarcinoma, intrahepatic bile duct carcinoma,* and *cholangiocellular carcinoma.*

Epidemiology. It is estimated that there are 46,000 new cases of cholangiocarcinoma worldwide per year (both intrahepatic and extrahepatic) (37). Geographic differences in the frequency of the intrahepatic type (ICC) are well known. For example, ICC is nearly 10 times more common in Japan than in the United States and United Kingdom (93). There are also differences related to the relative frequency of ICC among all primary liver cancers in various countries, e.g., 2.6 percent in Africa and 5.4 percent in Japan (94). Data from the Surveillance, Epidemiology and End Results Program (SEER) of the National Cancer Institute showed that cholangiocarcinoma comprised 19.1 percent of all primary histologically confirmed liver cancers for the years 1973 to 1987 (17).

Etiology. Most cases of ICC are of unknown etiology and arise in a noncirrhotic liver. However, a small number of cases have occurred with nonbiliary cirrhosis (112,127) and in a study by Terada et al. (127) from Japan, 4 to 7 percent of all cholangiocarcinomas arose in a cirrhotic liver. A number of well-known risk factors for ICC have been established over the years and, in part, account for the geographic variability of the tumor; they are listed in Table 10-1 and discussed in the succeeding paragraphs. Of the known associations worldwide, by far the most important are parasitic infections (clonorchiasis and opisthorchiasis) and intrahepatic lithiasis.

Fibrocystic Diseases. Adenocarcinomas can arise in solitary cysts of the liver (6,141), and ICC has been reported in congenital hepatic fibrosis, Caroli's disease, von Meyenburg complexes, and the cysts of autosomal dominant polycystic disease of the liver (46). The overall incidence of carcinomas (mostly cholangiocarcinomas) arising in all cystic dilatations of the bile ducts (including choledochal cyst) is about 3 percent (51).

Inherited Metabolic Diseases. Genetic hemochromatosis is a well-recognized cause of hepatocellular carcinoma, but there are also scattered

Table 10-1

ETIOLOGIC RISK FACTORS IN INTRAHEPATIC CHOLANGIOCARCINOMA

Fibrocystic diseases
    Solitary cyst
    Caroli's disease
    Autosomal dominant polycystic kidney and liver
      disease
    Congenital hepatic fibrosis

Inherited metabolic diseases
    Genetic hemochromatosis
    Alpha-1-antitrypsin deficiency

Extrahepatic biliary atresia

Inflammatory bowel disease

Chronic cholestatic diseases in adults
    Primary sclerosing cholangitis
    Primary biliary cirrhosis

Gallstones

Recurrent pyogenic cholangitis and intrahepatic
    lithiasis

Parasitic diseases
    Clonorchis sinensis
    Opisthorchis viverrini

Infection with hepatitis viruses B and C

Nonbiliary cirrhosis

Thorotrast exposure

External beam radiation

Excessive alcohol consumption

Drugs
    Anabolic/androgenic steroids
    Contraceptive steroids

Occupational exposure

Miscellaneous

reports of ICC in patients with that disease (3, 65). Similarly, alpha-1-antitrypsin deficiency is occasionally associated with ICC (98).

Extrahepatic Biliary Atresia. There are several examples of hepatocellular carcinoma and one of a combined hepatocellular and cholangiocarcinoma complicating biliary atresia, but only one case of an ICC in an 11-year-old girl with biliary cirrhosis (66).

Inflammatory Bowel Disease. Ritchie et al. (104) found the incidence of biliary tract carcinoma in patients with chronic ulcerative colitis to be 1 in 256; one third of the malignancies were intrahepatic. In a series of 32 cases of ICC from the Mayo Clinic (115), 3 patients had chronic ulcerative colitis and 1 each had Crohn's disease and nonspecific colitis. Three other patients with ICC reported by Altaee et al. (3) had chronic ulcerative colitis.

Chronic Cholestatic Diseases in Adults. There are reports of cases of primary sclerosing cholangitis (PSC) (9,36,115,151) and two cases of primary biliary cirrhosis complicated by ICC (1,109). The largest series of patients with PSC and hepatobiliary carcinoma was reported by Bergquist et al. (9). Of their 20 cases, 9 were ICC, 7 were both intrahepatic and extrahepatic cholangiocarcinomas, and only one was extrahepatic cholangiocarcinoma (2 patients had hepatocellular carcinomas and 1 had a carcinoma of the gallbladder). Fifty percent of the patients had cirrhosis, and 60 percent with nontumorous tissue had bile duct dysplasia; 18 had inflammatory bowel disease. The number of cancer patients who smoked or were former smokers was significantly higher than in controls. It should be emphasized that bile duct dysplasia is rare in PSC; in one large series of 60 patients who underwent liver transplantation for end-stage disease only one of the excised livers showed that change (70).

Gallstones. A surprisingly high incidence (17.5 percent) of gallstones (greater than that in the general population) was found in a series of 57 patients with ICC reported from Japan (94). A case-control hospital-based study from the United States showed a significant association between cholelithiasis and biliary tract cancers, but ICC was not mentioned in that study (58).

Recurrent Pyogenic ("Oriental") Cholangitis and Intrahepatic Lithiasis. Recurrent pyogenic cholangitis is an important cause of morbidity and mortality in the Far East, particularly in Hong Kong, Japan, and Korea. It has also been reported in Asian immigrants in Australia, Europe, and the United States. The condition is characterized by recurrent cholangitis and complicated by hepatic abscesses, acute pancreatitis, strictures and dilatations of the larger intrahepatic bile ducts, and in about 10 percent of the cases, stone formation. The strictures and stones tend to have a predilection for the left lobe, which can eventually undergo atrophy (fig. 10-1). Cultures of bile reveal mixed enteric bacteria and sometimes anaerobes. Parasitic infections are not considered to play an etiologic role in this condition, but some cases reported from India were thought to have been initiated by invasion of the biliary tree by *Ascaris lumbricoides* (59). In the majority of cases the intrahepatic stones are composed of calcium bilirubinate (fig. 10-2) (60,134), but cases with cholesterol stones have been reported from Japan (110). About 10 percent of patients with hepatolithiasis in Japan have an associated ICC (63). A series of 12 cases of hepatolithiasis and ICC were reported from that country by Nakanuma et al (87), and another 7 cases were described by Ohta et al. (92). In a series of 19 patients with ICC from Taiwan, 58 percent had associated hepatolithiasis and presented with acute pyogenic abscess (48). Preneoplastic lesions in hepatolithiasis include chronic proliferative cholangitis and atypical epithelial hyperplasia; intestinal metaplasia (goblet and Paneth cell metaplasia) may be an additional precursor lesion (64,68).

Parasitic Diseases. Both *Clonorchis sinensis* and *Opisthorchis viverrini* have been implicated in the causation of ICC in Southeast and East Asia (8,21,35,40,62,67,147). Cases also have been reported in Asian immigrants in the United States (116). Carcinogens in the diet, such as nitrosamine compounds and aflatoxins, may play a synergistic role in the development of ICC, as supported by experimental data (79,138). Adenomatoid hyperplasia with intestinal metaplasia is a characteristic precancerous lesion of the infected bile ducts (figs. 10-3, 10-4).

Hepatitis C Virus. Tomimatsu et al. (142) found hepatitis C virus (HCV) antibody in 13 Japanese patients with cholangiocarcinoma. In another more recent study, Yamamoto et al. (157) studied 50 patients with minute nodular ICC

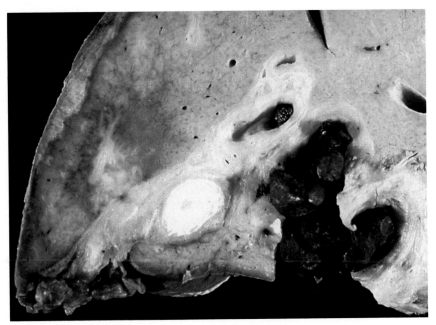

Figure 10-1
RECURRENT
PYOGENIC CHOLANGITIS
This section of liver shows markedly sclerosed bile ducts. One large dilated duct contains dark bilirubin calculi. A small sclerosed duct above it contains a calculus.

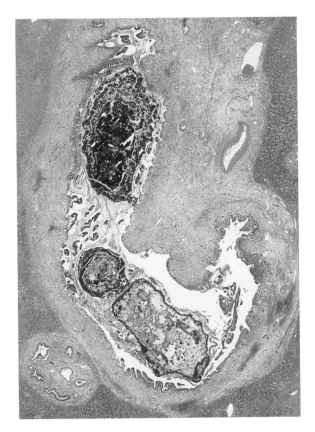

Figure 10-2
RECURRENT PYOGENIC CHOLANGITIS
The dilated duct contains bilirubin calculi. Note the marked chronic inflammation of the wall of the duct and focal epithelial ulceration and hyperplasia.

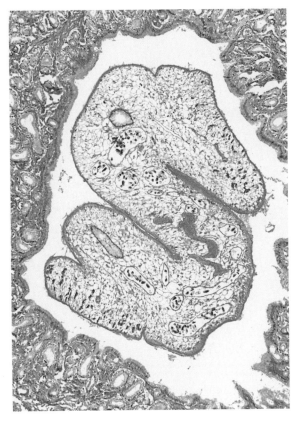

Figure 10-3
CLONORCHIS SINENSIS INFECTION
An adult female worm is present in the lumen of a dilated intrahepatic bile duct. Note the eggs in the uterus of the worm.

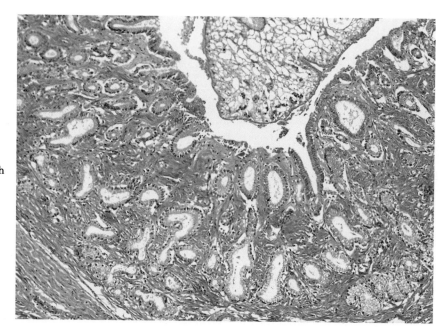

Figure 10-4
ADENOMATOID
HYPERPLASIA
OF A BILE DUCT
This patient was infected with
Clonorchis sinensis.

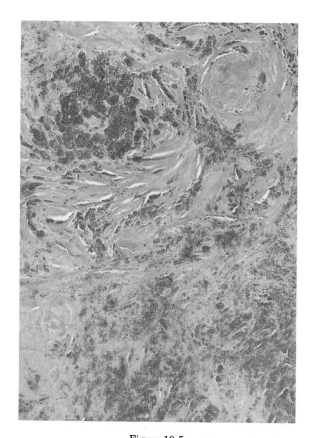

Figure 10-5
THOROTRAST DEPOSITS IN LIVER
The coarse, pink-brown Thorotrast particles are embedded in dense fibrous tissue.

and found that 32 percent were positive for anti-HCV, 10 percent were positive for hepatitis B surface antigen (HBsAg), and 2 percent were positive for both viral markers. Clearly, the relationship of ICC to the hepatotropic viruses requires further investigation.

Thorotrast. This colloidal suspension of thorium dioxide was used as a radiographic contrast medium from 1928 to 1950 in Europe, the United States, and Japan. It accumulates in the reticuloendothelial system in the liver (60 percent) (fig. 10-5), spleen (20 percent), lymph nodes, and bone marrow. The radioactive thorium emits alpha particles and has a very long half-life; in humans its physical half-life is about $1.4 \times 1,010$ years, while its biologic half-life is 400 years. Thorotrast has been implicated as the cause of several types of hepatic malignancy, including ICC, angiosarcoma, and hepatocellular carcinoma (26,47,108,124, 155). Double malignancies (ICC and hepatocellular carcinoma, and ICC and angiosarcoma) have been reported (42,154). In Japan, ICC was the most frequently reported hepatic malignancy (155). The latent period has varied from 12 to over 30 years. Malignancies related to Thorotrast are now only rarely encountered.

Radiotherapy. There is one report of ICC that developed in a young woman whose liver had been included in the field of external beam therapy for Wilms' tumor some 20 years earlier (25).

Excessive Alcohol Consumption. A regular alcohol intake of at least 60 g/day for more than 5 years was documented in 45 percent of patients with ICC reported by Altaee et al. (3). A history of ethanol abuse also was obtained in 45 percent of the Armed Forces Institute of Pathology (AFIP) series of 63 cases of ICC (82).

Drugs. Oral contraceptive use has been reported in eight women who developed ICC (3). An ICC that occurred in a 47-year-old man, who had been treated with anabolic steroids for refractory anemia, was reported by Stromeyer et al. (118); another case was reported by Turani et al. (144).

Occupational Exposure. An excess risk of liver cancer (adenocarcinomas of the liver parenchyma and adenocarcinomas of the biliary passages) was reported in workers in the nonelectrical machinery industry and the primary metal industry by Houten and Sonnesso (41). Malker et al. (75) found an increase in cancer of the biliary tract in asbestos-related workers (such as in shipbuilding), insulation workers, and workers in the wholesale construction materials industry.

Miscellaneous. A number of conditions that have been associated with cancer of the extrahepatic biliary tree have not, to our knowledge, been implicated in ICC. These include an increased incidence of cardiac anomalies with bile duct cancer (13), an association of hereditary nonpolyposis colorectal carcinoma with carcinomas of the biliary tract and papilla of Vater (76), an association between cancers of the bile ducts or papilla of Vater and von Recklinghausen's disease (20), and an association between the typhoid carrier state and hepatobiliary cancer (29,152).

Pathogenesis. Morphologic and cell kinetic studies by Terada et al. (133,135,137) have shown that in hepatolithiasis, carcinogenesis in bile duct epithelial cells progresses in a multistep manner, through hyperplasia, dysplasia, noninvasive adenocarcinoma, and invasive carcinoma. Celli and Que (18) have proposed that all diseases that predispose to cholangiocarcinoma are characterized by chronic inflammation and cholestasis, in particular, exposure to hydrophobic bile acids such as glycoursodeoxycholic acid. This can predispose biliary epithelium to oncogenic mutations and progression to malignancy due, in part, to the failure to activate apoptosis and delete cells with genetic damage, as noted later.

The mutation of oncogenes and tumor suppressor genes is one mechanism for the development and progression of ICC. p53 mutations in ICC have been reported by several groups of investigators (4,22,91,136). In the series of Terada et al. (136), 22 percent of ICCs in Japan had p53 mutations; however, in a study in the United States only one of nine cases of ICC expressed p53 antigen (22). The expression of a variety of oncogenes was studied in a series of 63 cases of ICC by Voravud et al. (148): 95 percent of the tumors expressed p62 c-*myc*, 75 percent expressed p21 c-*ras*, and 73 percent expressed p10 c-*erb* B-2. The expression of c-*myc* and c-*ras*, but not of c-*erb* B-2, correlated directly with tumor differentiation. More recently, Terada et al. (125) found aberrant expression of c-erb B-2 protein in 70 percent of 47 cholangiocarcinomas, and also in noncancerous biliary proliferative lesions such as hepatolithiasis. Conflicting results were, however, reported by Collier et al. (24) who could not detect c-erb B-2 expression in 10 cases of ICC. In addition to the study of Voravud et al. (148), *ras* gene mutations were found in 50 percent of cases of Tada et al. (121) and 88.6 percent of the cases of Nonomura et al. (88).

Alterations of the p53 and *APC* tumor suppressor genes and the K-*ras* proto-oncogene were recently studied in 40 surgically resected ICC cases by Kang et al. (53). An alteration of at least one of the genes was seen in 21 tumors (52.5 percent), and 6 (15 percent) carried an abnormality in more than two genes. Of interest was the correlation between gross tumor type and the genetic alterations: the p53 mutation was prominent in the ICC of "mass-forming type" while the K-*ras* mutation occurred more frequently in the "periductal extension type" of ICC (p<0.05). It was concluded that each of the examined genes is involved in the development of ICC, and that the p53 and K-*ras* mutations may play a role in the type of tumor growth pattern.

Overexpression of c-*neu* (the rat proto-oncogene homologue of c-*erb* B-2) was found to be a prominent feature of the furan rat model of cholangiocarcinoma and its precursor lesions by Sirica et al. (117). In a more recent study both c-*neu* and c-*met* were found to be expressed relatively early in furan-induced cholangiocarcinoma in rat liver, and thus may play a potentially important role in its pathogenesis (103).

An alternative mechanism of carcinogenesis involving dysregulation or inhibition of apoptosis has been suggested by Harnois et al. (34). These investigators compared *bcl*-2 expression in two human cell lines: nonmalignant cholangiocytes and cells of a human cholangiocarcinoma cell line. *Bcl*-2 expression was 15-fold greater in malignant than nonmalignant cholangiocytes. The authors concluded that resistance to apoptosis is a characteristic of cholangiocarcinoma cells; it appears to be mediated, in part, by overexpression of *bcl*-2. Celli and Que (18) have further suggested that dysregulation of *bcl*-2 expression may also lead to the loss of the tumor suppressor gene p53.

Clinical Features. In an AFIP series of 63 cases, 46 (73 percent) were males and 17 (27 percent) were females (82). In another series of 57 cases reported from Japan by Okuda et al. (94), 63 percent of the patients were males. The age range of the patients in the AFIP series was 30 to 81 years, with an average age of 62 years, a figure almost identical to that (62.2 years) of the cases of Okuda et al. The majority (90.5 percent) of the AFIP patients were Caucasian. The diagnosis of ICC is established by biopsy and/or imaging studies.

Symptoms in the AFIP patients included upper abdominal pain (33 percent), ascites and/or edema (35 percent), weight loss (24 percent), weakness or fatigue (15 percent), anorexia (18 percent), and nausea and/or vomiting (7 percent). Jaundice was noted in 20 percent of the AFIP patients, and in 25 percent of the patients of Okuda et al. (94). Unusual presentations have included rupture (150), pyogenic liver abscess (48), portal hypertension (120), and Cushing's syndrome (97). A mass was palpated in 31 percent of patients in the Mayo Clinic series (3) but only in 5.3 percent of those in the series of Okuda et al.

Laboratory Findings. Liver tests in the AFIP series (82) included increased alkaline phosphatase activity in 74 percent of patients (average, 702 IU/L), an elevated total serum bilirubin in 70 percent (average, 13.5 mg/dl), and an elevated aspartate aminotransferase value (average, 157 IU/L) in 85 percent. The combination of elevated serum levels of carcinoembryonic antigen (CEA) and CA19-9 are thought to be helpful in distinguishing ICC from hepatocellular carcinoma (86,94). The serum alpha-fetoprotein value is usually normal or slightly increased, but values greater than 1,000 ng/dl have been reported in a few patients (94,158). Hypercalcemia was present in one of the AFIP patients and has been reported in others (95,159).

Radiologic Findings. Plain abdominal films may show tumoral calcification, and dense Thorotrast deposits in the liver in Thorotrast-related cases (106). The ultrasound findings in 101 cases of ICC reported from Thailand showed the tumor masses to be hyperechoic in 55.4 percent, hypoechoic in 14.8 percent, isoechoic in 9.9 percent, and mixed echoic in 19.8 percent; calcification was noted in 3 percent of the cases (153). Angiographically, ICC has a variable appearance with avascular, hypovascular, and hypervascular patterns possible (106).

The most common appearance of ICC on computed tomography (CT) is that of a single, homogeneous, low-attenuation mass, but multiple low-attenuation lesions may be seen (106). Two-phase spiral CT scans have shown thin, incomplete, rim-like contrast enhancement at the tumor periphery, and markedly low intratumoral attenuation with amorphous areas of slightly high attenuation during both scanning phases (21,61). Magnetic resonance imaging (MRI) studies of eight patients with ICC were described by Fan et al. (30): the characteristic appearance was that of a large mass with an irregular margin, satellite nodules, and a central scar. Tumors were hypointense relative to liver parenchyma on T1-weighted spin-echo images and hyperintense on T2-weighted spin-echo images. On dynamic MRI studies, tumors characteristically had minimal or moderate rim enhancement with progressive and concentric filling with contrast material.

The presence of somatostatin receptors was demonstrated recently in seven cholangiocarcinomas by Tan et al. (123). Using gamma camera imaging with an ^{111}In-SS analogue, a histologically proven cholangiocarcinoma was localized in one patient. These investigators have suggested that these analogues could be useful for diagnosis, localization, and treatment of biliary tract malignancies.

Gross Findings. Cholangiocarcinomas may be massive and nodular or diffuse (figs. 10-6–10-8). Sasaki et al. (111) classified their tumors into "mass forming" and "periductal infiltrating" types. The liver is typically noncirrhotic, and may be moderately to markedly enlarged. The tumors are usually firm or hard, and vary from white to

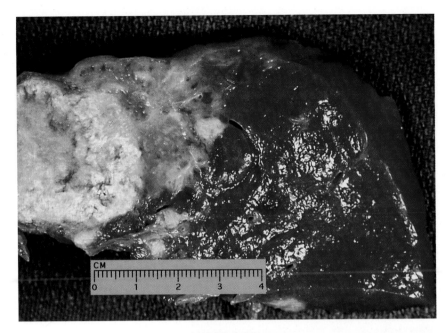

Figure 10-6
INTRAHEPATIC
CHOLANGIOCARCINOMA
The large tumor has an irregular, infiltrative margin. The central white area is calcified. There is no cirrhosis in the non-neoplastic liver.

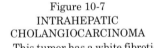

Figure 10-7
INTRAHEPATIC
CHOLANGIOCARCINOMA
This tumor has a white fibrotic center and a pink-tan infiltrative margin.

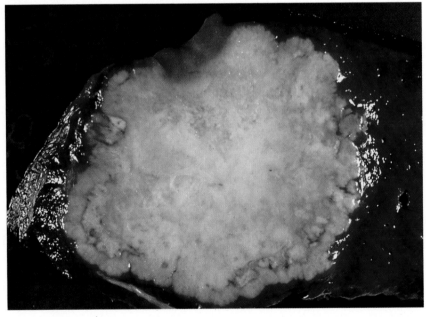

tan-white. Nodules beneath Glisson's capsule tend to be umbilicated. Primary growth is somewhat more frequent in the right lobe, but the tumor may arise in any lobe and can spread widely within the liver via the portal vein. Of 60 cases in the AFIP series (82), 35 percent were in the right lobe, 22 percent in the left, and 12 percent were "central," e.g., involved both lobes; the entire liver was riddled by multiple tumors in 31 percent of the cases. The tumor formed a single mass in 22 percent of cases, and a single mass with satellite nodules in another 33 percent of cases; the remainder had multiple tumors. None of the AFIP cases were of the periductal infiltrating type of Sasaki et al. (111). Necrosis, hemorrhage, and other degenerative changes are not as marked in ICC as in hepatocellular carcinoma. Some tumors undergo focal calcification.

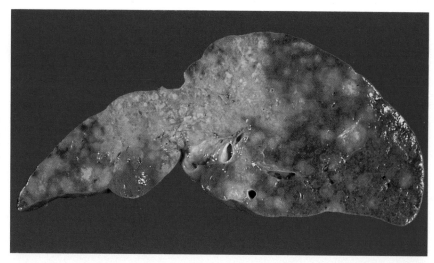

Figure 10-8
INTRAHEPATIC
CHOLANGIOCARCINOMA
The section of the liver discloses one large, tan tumor mass, as well as multiple smaller lesions. Note the yellow foci of necrosis in the large mass.

Microscopic Findings. Cholangiocarcinoma resembles many glandular carcinomas of extrahepatic origin (45,81). The diagnosis often depends upon exclusion of other primary sites. The tumor cells are arranged in tubules (fig. 10-9), acini (fig. 10-10), nests (fig. 10-11), or trabeculae (fig. 10-12). Micropapillary areas may be seen in some tumors (fig. 10-13). The trabeculae of ICC are surrounded by fibrous tissue rather than sinusoids, as is the case in hepatocellular carcinoma. Most cholangiocarcinomas tend to be well differentiated, and are composed of columnar to cuboidal epithelial cells with a moderate amount of clear or slightly granular, lightly eosinophilic cytoplasm. Mucin production is minimal to moderate. Nuclei are relatively small and lack the prominent, eosinophilic nucleoli of cells of hepatocellular carcinoma.

Histologic parameters that are helpful in distinguishing well-differentiated ICC from benign lesions are variation and irregularity of nuclear size, mitoses, and secondary gland formation (focal cribriform pattern) (83,84). The tumors show varying degrees of differentiation (figs. 10-14, 10-15). In a recent study of 43 cases of surgically resected ICC, Sugawara et al. (117) found that interleukin-6 expression is inversely related to cell proliferation but positively related to the degree of differentiation. Conversely, Ki-67 was expressed infrequently in well differentiated areas of ICC, but was expressed frequently in moderately and poorly differentiated areas. Multinucleation is rare in ICC (fig. 10-15). Papillary tumors usually arise from the larger ducts (fig. 10-16). A desmoplastic response, sometimes with hyalinization, may be marked (fig.

10-17). Patients with ICC with a fibrous stroma more than or equal to the tumor cells (scirrhous type) have a significantly lower survival rate than those with ICC with a scanty stroma (nonscirrhous type), according to Kajiyama et al. (52).

The well-known hypovascularity of ICC, in comparison to hepatocellular carcinoma, may be related to the relative increase of thrombospondin-1 and the relative decrease of vascular endothelial growth factor (55). The enhanced expression of thrombospondin-1 was observed in the fibroblasts of the stroma as well as in cancer cells, suggesting that it may negatively regulate angiogenesis in ICC. Alpha-smooth muscle actin–positive cells have been identified in the stroma of ICC (128). It is believed that these actin-positive cells become activated into myofibroblasts, which in turn produce the extracellular matrix proteins that lead to tumoral fibrosis. Tenascin expression in the peritumoral stroma of ICC may stimulate cell growth and proliferation (129). Thorotrast-related tumors show the characteristic pink-brown granular deposits, which are refractile and non-birefringent, in macrophages and Kupffer cells or embedded in dense connective tissue (fig. 10-5).

Variants of ICC include *mucinous, adenosquamous* and *mucoepidermoid carcinomas, clear cell carcinomas,* and *spindle cell carcinomas,* which are discussed later. The existence of a *cholangiolocellular carcinoma,* i.e., one presumed to arise from cholangioles or canals of Hering (37), is disputed. Such a tumor is said to have cells arranged in small cores with a central lumen, with the individual cuboidal cells resembling

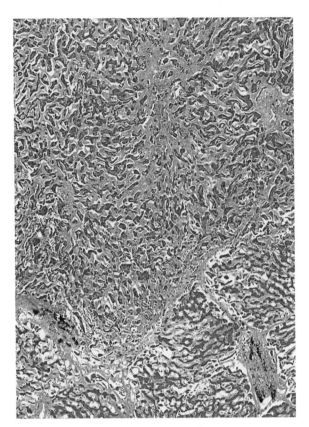

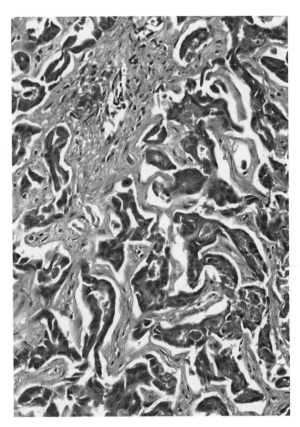

Figure 10-9
INTRAHEPATIC CHOLANGIOCARCINOMA, TUBULAR PATTERN
Left: The tubules are surrounded by a fibrous stroma.
Right: Higher magnification shows a low columnar lining of the tubules.

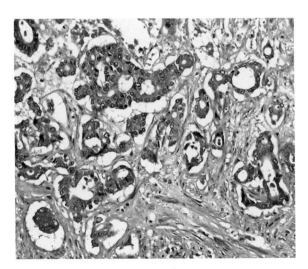

Figure 10-10
INTRAHEPATIC CHOLANGIOCARCINOMA,
ACINAR PATTERN
A moderately differentiated adenocarcinoma.

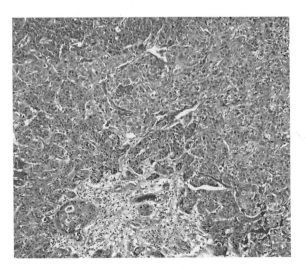

Figure 10-11
INTRAHEPATIC CHOLANGIOCARCINOMA,
GLANDULAR PATTERN WITH SOLID NESTS

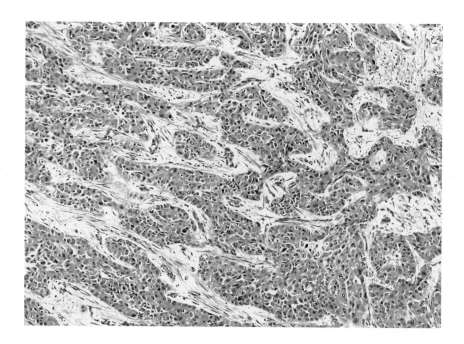

Figure 10-12
INTRAHEPATIC
CHOLANGIOCARCINOMA
WITH TRABECULAR
PATTERN

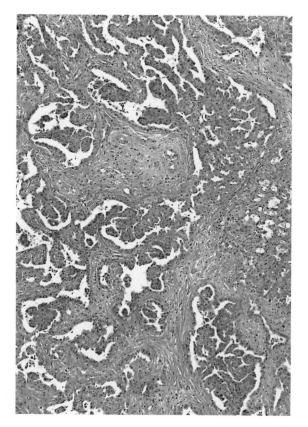

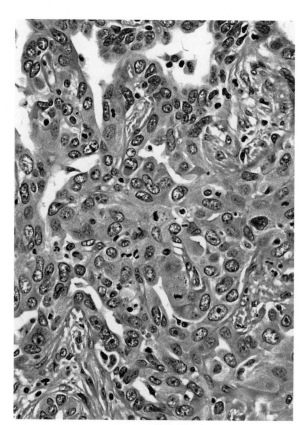

Figure 10-13
INTRAHEPATIC CHOLANGIOCARCINOMA, MICROPAPILLARY PATTERN
The high-power (right) view shows marked pleomorphism and mitotic figures.

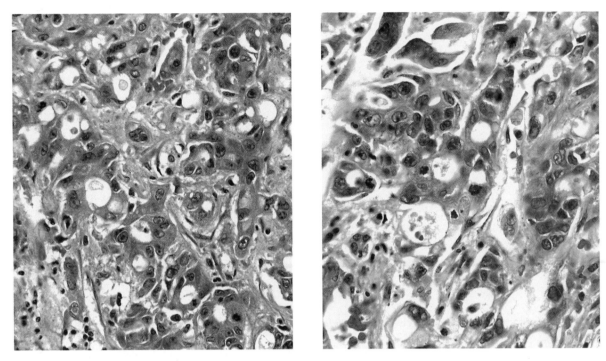

Figure 10-14
INTRAHEPATIC CHOLANGIOCARCINOMA, MODERATELY DIFFERENTIATED
Glandular lumina are present (left), but not well-formed; on the right there are glandular lumina as well as solid areas.

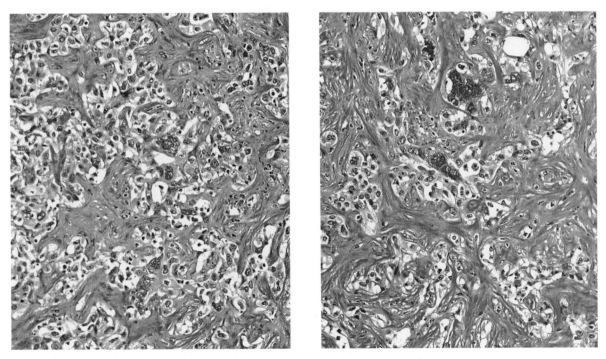

Figure 10-15
INTRAHEPATIC CHOLANGIOCARCINOMA, POORLY DIFFERENTIATED
There are poorly formed glands in a desmoplastic stroma (left); many of the tumor cells (right) have anaplastic nuclei.

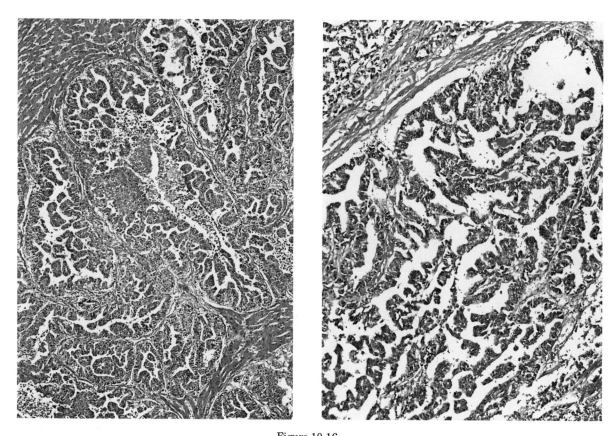

Figure 10-16
INTRAHEPATIC CHOLANGIOCARCINOMA, PAPILLARY TYPE
Left: This papillary tumor arose in the large intrahepatic ducts (not shown) of a patient with *Clonorchis sinensis* infection.
Right: Higher magnification of the left view.

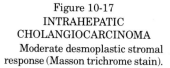

Figure 10-17
INTRAHEPATIC
CHOLANGIOCARCINOMA
Moderate desmoplastic stromal
response (Masson trichrome stain).

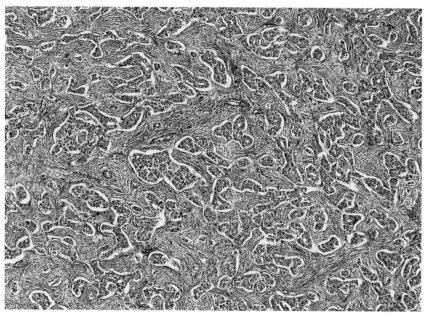

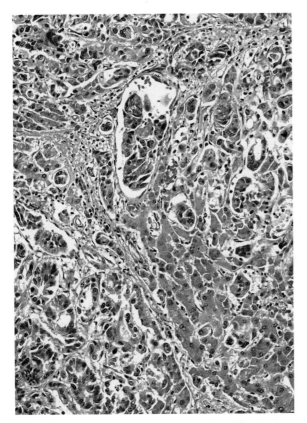 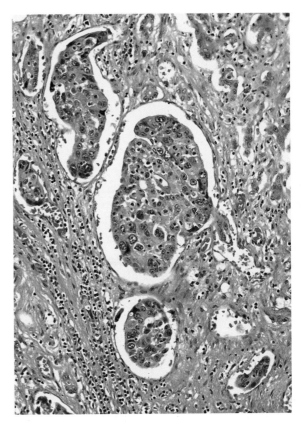

Figure 10-18
INTRAHEPATIC CHOLANGIOCARCINOMA
Vascular spread is shown in sinusoids and veins (left) and in portal vein branches (right).

those of cholangioles. We are highly skeptical that such a tumor exists.

The tumor cells can grow along sinusoids and spread extensively throughout the liver via the portal venous system (fig. 10-18). The endothelial lining of blood vessels may serve as a basement membrane for intravascular extension (27). Perineural invasion also occurs, but can only be appreciated in large portal areas close to the liver hilum.

Preneoplastic lesions of the intrahepatic bile ducts include intestinal metaplasia (both goblet and Paneth cell), hyperplasia (sometimes papillary), atypical hyperplasia, and carcinoma in situ. Papillary and atypical hyperplasia of the peribiliary glands has been noted in some cases, raising the possibility of cholangiocarcinomas arising from those glands (87).

Immunohistochemical Findings. Cells of cholangiocarcinoma can express a large number of proteins detectable by immunohistochemical methods (Table 10-2). These "markers" include polyclonal cytokeratin, cytokeratins 7 and 19, carcinoembryonic antigen, CA19-9, epithelial membrane antigen, BER-EP4, and blood group antigens (fig. 10-19A–C). Cytokeratin 20 was positive in 10 percent of the cases studied by Maeda et al. (73). The Hepatocyte (Hep Par 1) antigen is usually not expressed by cells of cholangiocarcinoma (fig. 10-19D). In the AFIP series of 63 cases of ICC, 2 (3 percent) showed neuroendocrine differentiation (82). The expression of HLA-DR in ICC was considered to have prognostic significance by Torri et al. (143): these authors found that the 5-year survival rate for patients with tumors that were positive was better than that of those with tumors with negative staining. The use of immunohistochemistry in the differential diagnosis is discussed in the next section.

Ultrastructural Findings. In this era of immunohistochemistry the use of electron microscopy to identify ICC or differentiate it from other tumors is of no practical value. Readers interested in the

257

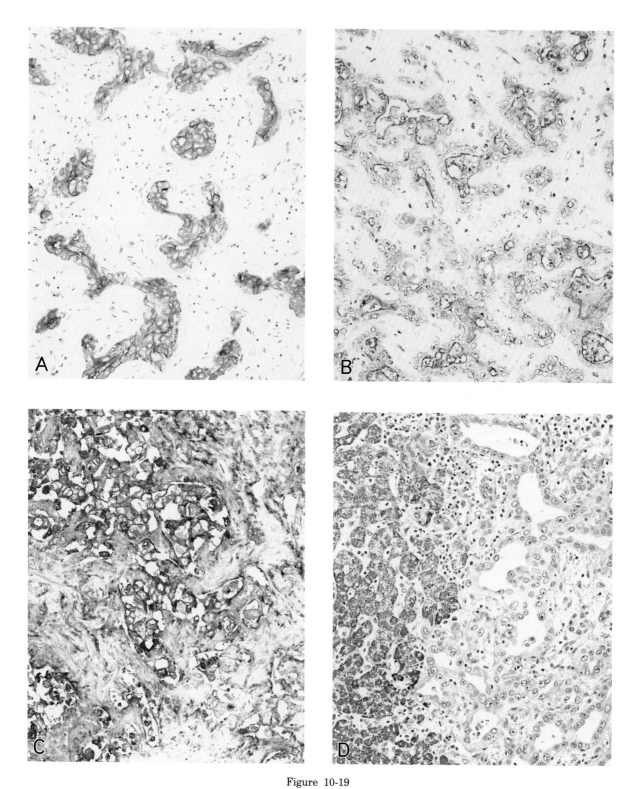

Figure 10-19

INTRAHEPATIC CHOLANGIOCARCINOMA: IMMUNOHISTOCHEMICAL EXPRESSION OF ANTIGENS

A: Cytokeratin 7, cytoplasmic staining.

B: Epithelial membrane antigen, luminal staining.

C: Carcinoembryonic antigen, polyclonal antiserum, cytoplasmic staining.

D: Hepatocyte antigen, liver cells on the left show positive granular staining, while the cholangiocarcinoma on the right is negative.

ultrastructure of cholangiocarcinoma and hepatocellular carcinoma are referred to the reports of Ordonez and Mackay (96) and others (2).

Variants of Intrahepatic Cholangiocarcinoma. Rare types of cholangiocarcinoma include:

Mucinous Intrahepatic Cholangiocarcinoma. Two cases have been described, one of which complicated hepatolithiasis and recurrent pyogenic cholangitis (23,84). As the name implies these tumors are characterized by an abundance of cytoplasmic and extracellular mucin (fig. 10-20).

Adenosquamous Carcinoma. A small number of these cases have been published (7,9,33,44,74, 84,122,145). They resemble similar but more common tumors in the gallbladder or pancreas. The largest series of eight cases arising in the liver was reported by Maeda et al. (74). Six of the tumors were surgically resected but all the patients died within 1 year of diagnosis, leading to the conclusion that patients with adenosquamous carcinoma have a poorer prognosis than do those with the usual type of ICC. This grim prognosis was also found in other surgically resected cases (44,122). Microscopically, these tumors are composed of malignant squamous and glandular components in varied proportions (fig. 10-21). Expression of involucrin, a specific marker for squamous epithelium, was demonstrated in one adenosquamous

Table 10-2

ANTIGENS THAT HAVE BEEN DESCRIBED IN INTRAHEPATIC CHOLANGIOCARCINOMA

Antigen	References
A, B, H, and Lewis blood group antigens	50,77
Alpha-fetoprotein	15,88,94
Amylase	130
Apomucins (MUC1, MUC5AC, MUC6)	112,113
Carcinoembryonic antigen	72,89
Carbohydrate antigen 19-9	77,83
Cell adhesion molecules (E-cadherin, α-catenin, β-catenin, and CD44)	5
Epithelial membrane antigen	12
Gastrin	16
Hepatocyte (Hep Par 1)	78
Human chorionic gonadotropin	88
Interleukin 6	119
Keratins (7,8,18,19,20)	49,72
Ki-67	119
Lipase	131
Parathyroid hormone-related peptide	107
Secretory component	83
Thrombospondin-1	55
Tissue polypeptide antigen	99
Trypsinogen/trypsin	136

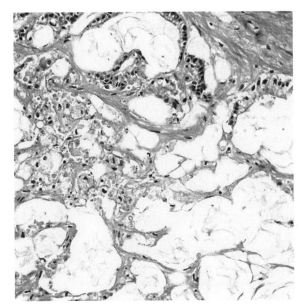 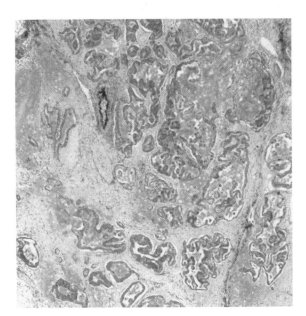

Figure 10-20
INTRAHEPATIC CHOLANGIOCARCINOMA, MUCINOUS VARIANT
Pools of mucin are evident (left) and are demonstrated by Alcian blue stain (right).

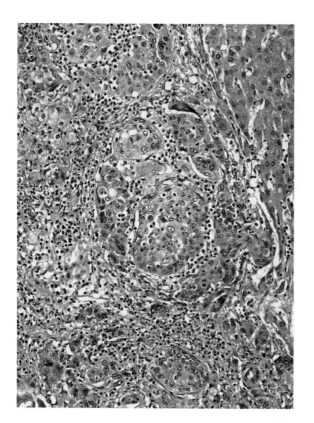 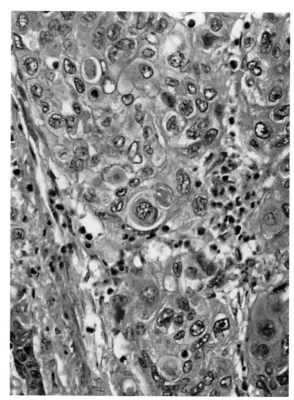

Figure 10-21
INTRAHEPATIC CHOLANGIOCARCINOMA, ADENOSQUAMOUS VARIANT
Left: Squamous component shows nests of tumor cells surrounded by inflammatory cells.
Right: Higher magnification reveals keratinized cells (center).

carcinoma (44). A spindle cell ("sarcomatous") variant of this tumor has been reported (114). There is general agreement that they arise from malignant transformation of squamous metaplastic foci in an ICC. However, one unique case arose in a biliary cystadenocarcinoma (80).

Squamous Cell Carcinoma. This is not, strictly speaking, a variant of ICC, but it is discussed here because we believe it is closely related to ICC. Most but not all reported cases of squamous cell carcinoma of the liver have arisen in solitary cysts (see chapter 3, fig. 3-3) (11,31,32,71,84,102), but one tumor was associated with multiple biliary cysts (14). It is assumed that squamous carcinomas arise in metaplastic squamous epithelium in a bile duct cyst, or in a chronically inflamed bile duct, e.g., in intrahepatic lithiasis.

Mucoepidermoid Carcinoma. Only one example of this tumor has been reported (100), and there is one case on file at AFIP that was associated with prior exposure to Thorotrast. The tumors resemble

those arising in salivary glands (28). The AFIP case is illustrated in figures 10-22 and 10-23.

Clear Cell Carcinoma. This type of carcinoma is very rare; two examples have been reported (69,139). The tumor cells in one case were negative for mucicarmine and periodic acid–Schiff (PAS) stains (69), but the other case (140) showed diastase-sensitive PAS-positive material and focal mucicarmine positivity in tumor cells. Ten examples of clear cell carcinoma of the gallbladder and extrahepatic bile ducts have been described (146). The case of Tihan et al. (139), accessioned at the AFIP, is illustrated in figure 10-24.

Spindle Cell Variant. This type, ICC with "sarcomatous" or "sarcomatoid" change, is rare. Nakajima et al. (85a) reported seven cases and alluded to several previously reported cases; another case was subsequently described (43). The spindle cell change may be focal or involve most of the tumor. The spindle cells express cytokeratin and epithelial membrane antigen.

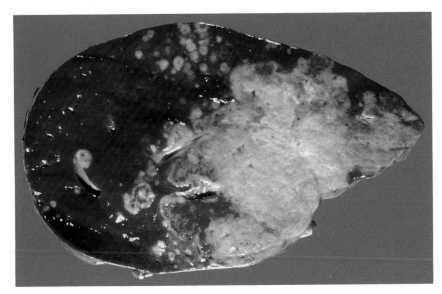

Figure 10-22
INTRAHEPATIC
CHOLANGIOCARCINOMA,
MUCOEPIDERMOID VARIANT
Section of liver shows a large, tan to white tumor with a congested periphery. There are multiple, small satellite tumors.

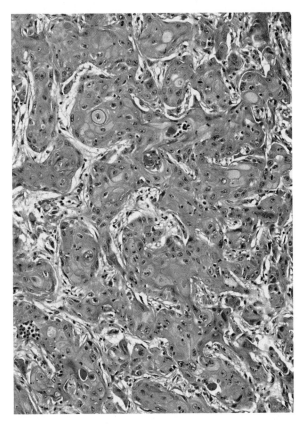
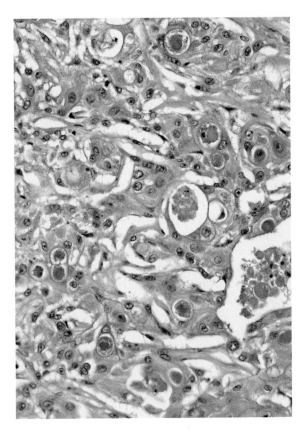

Figure 10-23
INTRAHEPATIC CHOLANGIOCARCINOMA, MUCOEPIDERMOID VARIANT
Left: The tumor cells form nests of moderately differentiated squamous carcinoma.
Right: Mucicarmine stain demonstrates mucin production.

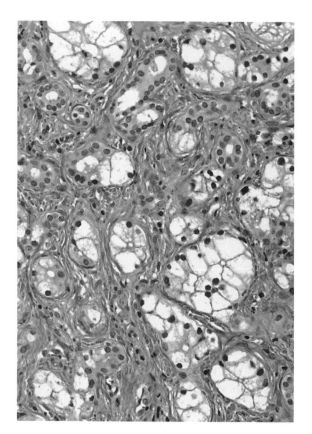 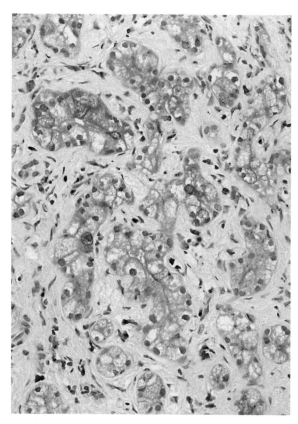

Figure 10-24
INTRAHEPATIC CHOLANGIOCARCINOMA, CLEAR CELL VARIANT
Left: The tumor cells are large and have an empty cytoplasm due to glycogen accumulation (not shown); small eccentric nuclei are seen. Some glands are partly composed of columnar cells.
Right: The tumor cells are decorated by polyclonal antibodies to carcinoembryonic antigen.

Differential Diagnosis. There are several tumors that may be confused with ICC. Peribiliary gland hamartoma (bile duct adenoma) is discussed in chapter 3. It is usually an incidental finding, but the discovery of a small white lesion on the surface of the liver at laparotomy, particularly in a patient with a known extrahepatic primary malignancy, can be of concern to the surgeon. It is often a problem for the pathologist as well, particularly if the extrahepatic primary is an adenocarcinoma. Helpful features distinguishing peribiliary gland hamartoma from ICC are the lack of secondary gland formation with a focal cribriform pattern, and the absence of nuclear pleomorphism or hyperchromasia, mitotic figures, or lymphatic or vascular invasion. Typically, portal areas in their normal spatial arrangement are scattered in the lesion. Peribiliary gland hamartomas express antigens that are shared with peribiliary glands, and are therefore believed to

arise from those glands (10). Cholangiocarcinoma has only rarely developed in a preexisting peribiliary gland hamartoma (see chapter 3).

There are no reliable morphologic or immunohistochemical findings that can differentiate ICC from metastatic adenocarcinoma, with the exception of organ-specific carcinoma antigens, e.g., those of the prostate, breast, etc. Thus, the diagnosis of ICC is largely one of exclusion of an extrahepatic primary, with the possible exception of one marker, parathyroid hormone–related peptide. Roskams et al. (107) found expression of the peptide in ICC, but not in metastatic adenocarcinoma from the gastrointestinal tract or hepatocellular carcinoma; however, two of five metastatic breast adenocarcinomas were positive. These interesting findings will require confirmation by other investigators.

One of the recognized patterns of hepatocellular carcinoma (HCC), the pseudoglandular (pseudoacinar) one, should be differentiated from ICC.

Unlike the true glands of ICC there is no mucin production by the cells lining the pseudoglands. Instead, bile plugs may be present in the lumen. Furthermore, the pseudoglands of HCC are lined by a canalicular membrane that can be demonstrated immunohistochemically by a polyclonal immunostain for carcinoembryonic antigen. Cells of HCC but not ICC express hepatocyte antigen (Hep Par 1) (78). Additionally, cells of ICC, but not HCC, express cytoplasmic polyclonal carcinoembryonic antigen, CA19, epithelial membrane antigen, Ber EP4, amylase, and lipase (Table 10-2). Cytokeratins 7 and 19 (bile duct markers) and 8 and 18 (liver cell markers) may also be helpful, but there may be some overlap of cytokeratin phenotypes. In a recent study, Yamaguchi et al. (156) found albumin mRNA (by in situ hybridization) in 50 of 53 (94 percent) HCCs but in none of 8 ICCs or 14 metastatic adenocarcinomas. These investigators are of the opinion that this technique could be helpful in differentiating malignant liver tumors.

Epithelioid hemangioendothelioma can deceptively mimic ICC, since intracellular and intercellular vascular lumina may suggest gland formation. It is reliably differentiated by lack of mucin production and by the expression of endothelial cell markers such as factor VIII–related antigen, CD34, and CD31 (see chapter 12).

Spread and Metastases. In the AFIP series metastasis occurred in 46 (73 percent) of the 63 cases (82). The most frequently involved organs and tissues were lymph nodes and lungs (74 percent), peritoneum and adrenal gland (20 percent), kidney (15 percent), and bone (13 percent).

Treatment and Prognosis. The median survival period in two relatively large series was 5.7 months (82) and 6.5 months (94). Chemotherapy and radiation therapy are of no value in treatment, and transplantation has been abandoned in the majority of liver transplant centers. Resection offers the only hope of cure, but many of the patients present with unresectable tumors; in the series of Schlinkert et al. (115) 81 percent of patients had unresectable tumors. Nevertheless, in recent years a significantly improved survival rate has been reported after resection. Some studies have found that survival rate depends on the TNM tumor stage (101,149). In the series of Washburn et al. (149), of 88 patients, those undergoing resection survived significantly longer (median, 23.2 months) than palliated patients (median 7.7 months). The median survival time in a series of 50 patients reported by Pichlmayr et al. (101) after resection was 12.8 months. In another recent study, patients with lymph node metastases had a lower survival rate than those without metastases, but patients with only regional metastases (in the hepatoduodenal ligament) did not differ in survival from those with distant metastases (nodes around the cardiac portion of the stomach or along the common hepatic artery) (90). Kajiyama et al. (52) correlated several histologic parameters with prognosis in a series of 58 surgically resected ICCs. They found that the scirrhous type of ICC, lymphatic permeation, perineural invasion, and higher proliferation activity of the tumor cells were associated with a poor prognosis. The spindle cell (sarcomatous) variant of ICC also has a poorer prognosis than the ordinary type (85). Other predictors of outcome in surgically resected cases in one study were tumor size, positive margins, presence of satellite nodules, and degree of tumor necrosis (105). Survival of more than 5 years has now been reported in several series (19,57,56,101, 115,158); the longest period was 12 years (39).

HEPATOBILIARY CYSTADENOCARCINOMA

Definition. This adenocarcinoma, usually papillary, arises in a multilocular hepatobiliary cystadenoma or, infrequently, in a unilocular bile duct cyst.

Clinical Features. Hepatobiliary cystadenocarcinomas can occur in both females and males (164,166), unlike their benign counterparts, the cystadenomas, which occur predominantly in women. Ten of 18 AFIP cases reported by Devaney et al. (164) occurred in women (56 percent). The mean age at presentation was 59 years and the median age, 61 years (age range, 24 to 90 years).

Of the 18 AFIP patients with cystadenocarcinoma, half presented with upper abdominal pain of variable duration. Four patients had an asymptomatic mass in the upper abdomen, while the tumors of the remaining five were incidental findings (four at laparotomy and one at autopsy).

Radiologic Findings. These have been reported in several series (161,163,168). The largest series of 34 cases was studied at the AFIP (161).

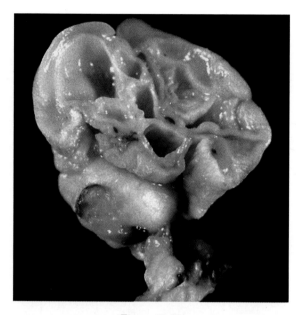

Figure 10-25
HEPATOBILIARY CYSTADENOCARCINOMA
Resected specimen shows some locules filled in with solid tumor.

Imaging features suggestive of cystadenocarcinoma include internal septation and nodularity.

Gross Findings. Of the 18 AFIP cases, 10 arose in the right lobe, 6 in the left lobe, and 2 involved both lobes (161). Seven were less than 10 cm, 10 were between 10 and 18 cm, and 1 was 25 cm in diameter. All 18 tumors were multilocular. The wall can be thick and the mucinous contents bile stained, "muddy," or blood stained. Polypoid masses may project into the cyst cavities, or some of the cysts may be replaced by solid tumor growth (fig. 10-25).

Microscopic Findings. Adenocarcinomas can arise in both solitary (162,165,167) and multilocular biliary cysts (160,164,166). By definition, these are both cystadenocarcinomas. Additionally, cholangiocarcinomas can coexist with bile duct cysts, as already mentioned in the section on etiology, and as noted by Azizah et al. (160a) and others (169,171). However, the majority of cystadenocarcinomas have arisen in an underlying multilocular hepatobiliary cystadenoma. Fifteen of the 18 cases of Devaney et al. (164) were

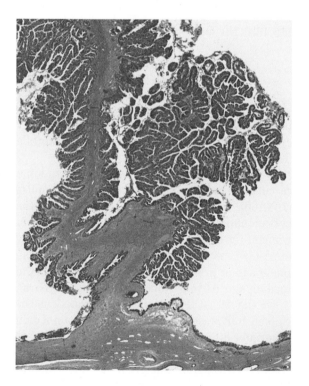 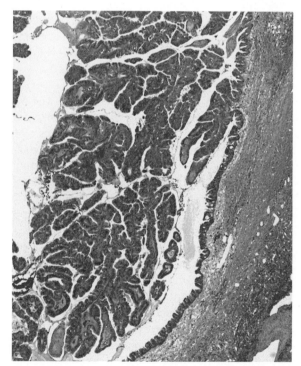

Figure 10-26
HEPATOBILIARY CYSTADENOCARCINOMA
Left: Low-power view shows a papillary growth with a fibrovascular stalk projecting into one of the cyst cavities.
Right: A higher magnification reveals fronds of a papillary adenocarcinoma.

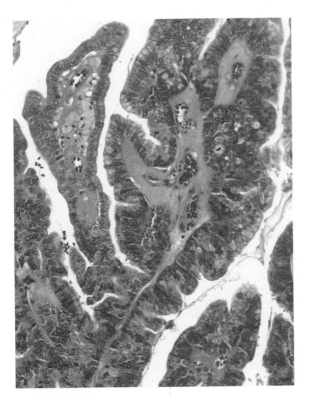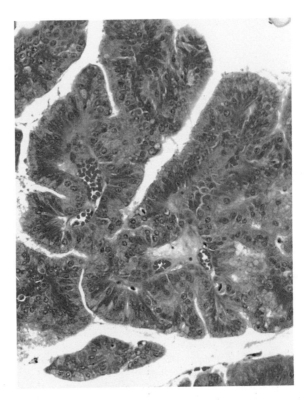

Figure 10-27
HEPATOBILIARY CYSTADENOCARCINOMA
Left: Medium-power view of papillary intracystic adenocarcinoma with multilayering, loss of polarity, and mitoses.
Right: Higher power view of papillary fronds.

tubulopapillary carcinomas (figs. 10-26, 10-27); one cystadenocarcinoma had a solid or tubular composition resembling cholangiocarcinoma, while another was an adenosquamous carcinoma. Another example of an adenosquamous carcinoma that arose in a cystadenocarcinoma was reported by Moore et al. (170a). Other variants have included a papillary cystadenocarcinoma with spindle cell (pseudosarcomatous) metaplasia (173), and a cystadenocarcinoma with oncocytic differentiation (174). In females the stroma is densely cellular (ovarian-like) with a small amount of collagen and smooth muscle fibers, but is collagenous in males. There may be invasion through the cyst wall into the adjacent liver. Vascular invasion was prominent in one of the AFIP cases (164).

Putative preneoplastic lesions in hepatobiliary cystadenoma and cystadenocarcinoma include epithelial dysplasia and intestinal metaplasia. Epithelial dysplasia is defined as enlargement of the lining cells, multilayering, hyperchromasia, loss of polarity, and scattered

mitoses. Ten of the 18 AFIP cystadenocarcinomas displayed foci of epithelial dysplasia in addition to the malignant areas (164). Focal intestinal metaplasia may also be present; it is not clear that this change represents a marker of significantly enhanced risk of progression of cystadenoma to cystadenocarcinoma.

Immunohistochemical Findings. Both hepatobiliary cystadenoma and cystadenocarcinoma express cytokeratins, epithelial membrane antigen, carcinoembryonic antigen, and CA19-9. A minority show neuroendocrine differentiation. The immunohistochemical profile is not helpful in distinguishing the benign from the malignant lesions.

Treatment and Prognosis. There is general agreement that the prognosis of patients with hepatobiliary cystadenocarcinoma after surgical excision is much better than for those with ICC (160,164,166,170,172). A number of patients have survived from 3 to 8 years after surgical excision of their tumor (164,166).

REFERENCES

Intrahepatic Cholangiocarcinoma

1. Akisawa N, Maeda T, Tsuda K, et al. Primary biliary cirrhosis associated with cholangiocarcinoma. Dig Dis Sci 1998;43:2138–42.

2. Alpert LI, Zak FG, Werthamer S, Bochetto JE. Cholangiocarcinoma: a clinicopathologic study of five cases with ultrastructural observations. Hum Pathol 1974;5:709–28.

3. Altaee MY, Johnson PJ, Farrant JM, Williams R. Etiologic and clinical characteristics of peripheral and hilar cholangiocarcinoma. Cancer 1991;68:2051–5.

4. Arora DS, Ramsdale J, Lodge JP, Wyatt JI. P53 but not bcl-2 is expressed by most cholangiocarcinomas: a study of 28 cases. Histopathology 1999;34:497–501.

5. Ashida K, Terada T, Kitamura Y, Kaibara N. Expression of E-catenin, alpha-catenin, beta-catenin, and CD44 (standard and variant isoforms) in human cholangiocarcinoma: an immunohistochemical study. Hepatology 1998;27:974–82.

6. Azizah N, Paradinas FJ. Cholangiocarcinoma coexisting with developmental liver cysts: a distinct entity different from the cystadenocarcinoma. Histopathology 1980;4:391–400.

7. Barr RJ, Hancock DE. Adenosquamous carcinoma of the liver. Gastroenterology 1975;69:1326–30.

8. Belamaric J. Intrahepatic bile duct carcinoma and C sinensis infection in Hong Kong. Cancer 1973;31:488–93.

9. Bergquist A, Glaumann H, Persson B, Boomé U. Risk factors and clinical presentation of hepatobiliary carcinoma in patients with primary sclerosing cholangitis: a case-control study. Hepatology 1998;27:311–6.

10. Bhathal PS, Hughes NR, Goodman ZD. The so-called bile duct adenoma is a peribiliary gland hamartoma. Am J Surg Pathol 1996;20:858–64.

11. Bloustein PA, Silverberg SG. Squamous cell carcinoma originating in an hepatic cyst. Case report with a review of the hepatic cyst-carcinoma association. Cancer 1976;38:2002–5.

12. Bonetti F, Chilosi M, Pisa R, Novelli P, Zamboni G, Menestrina F. Epithelial membrane antigen expression in cholangiocarcinoma. An useful immunohistochemical tool for differential diagnosis with hepatocarcinoma. Virchows Arch [A] 1983;401:307–13.

13. Brandt-Rauf PW, Pincus MR, Adelson S. Bile duct cancer and cardiac anomalies. NY State J Med 1986;86:7–9.

14. Burroughs AK, Barter SJ, Jenkins WJ. Malignant epithelioma of the liver. Postgrad Med J 1981;57:304–5.

15. Brumm C, Schultze C, Charels K, Morohashi T, Kloppel G. The significance of alpha-fetoprotein and other tumour markers in differential immunocytochemistry of primary liver tumours. Histopathology 1989;14:503–13.

16. Caplin M, Khan K, Savage K, et al. Expression and processing of gastrin in hepatocellular carcinoma, fibrolamellar carcinoma and cholangiocarcinoma. J Hepatol 1999;30:519–26.

17. Carriaga MT, Henson DE. Liver, gallbladder, extrahepatic bile ducts, and pancreas. Cancer 1995;75:171–90.

18. Celli A, Que FG. Dysregulation of apoptosis in the cholangiopathies and cholangiocarcinoma. Semin Liver Dis 1998;18:177–85.

19. Chen MF, Jan YY, Wang CS, Jeng LB, Huang TL. Clinical experience in 20 hepatic resections for peripheral cholangiocarcinoma. Cancer 1989;64:2226–32.

20. Ching CK, Greer AJ. Metachronous biliary tract cancers in a patient with von Recklinghausen's disease. Am J Gastroenterol 1993;88:1124–5.

21. Choi BI, Park JH, Kim YI, et al. Peripheral cholangiocarcinoma and clonorchiasis: CT findings. Radiology 1988;169:149–53.

22. Choi SW, Hytiroglou P, Geller SA, et al. The expression of p53 malignant epithelial tumors of the liver: an immunohistochemical study. Liver 1993;13:172–6.

23. Chow LT, Ahuja AT, Kwong KH, Fung KS, Lai CK, Lau JW. Mucinous cholangiocarcinoma: an unusual complication of hepatolithiasis and recurrent pyogenic cholangitis. Histopathology 1997;30:491–4.

24. Collier JD, Guo K, Mathew J, et al. C-erbB-2 oncogene expression in hepatocellular carcinoma and cholangiocarcinoma. J Hepatol 1992;14:377–80.

25. Cunningham JJ. Cholangiocarcinoma occurring after childhood radiotherapy for Wilm's tumor. Hepatogastroenterology 1990;37:395–7.

26. da Silva Horta J. Late effects of Thorotrast on the liver and spleen and their efferent lymph nodes. Ann NY Acad Sci 1976;145:676–99.

27. Edmondson HA. Tumors of the liver and intrahepatic bile ducts. Atlas of Tumor Pathology, 1st Series, Fascicle 25. Washington, D.C.: Armed Forces Institute of Pathology, 1958.

28. Ellis GL, Auclair PL. Tumors of the salivary glands. Atlas of the Tumor Pathology, 3rd Series, Fascicle 17. Washington D.C.: Armed Forces Institute of Pathology, 1995.

29. El-Zayadi A, Ghoneim M, Kabil SM, el Tawil A, Sherif A, Selim O. Bile duct carcinoma in Egypt: possible etiological factors. Hepatogastroenterology 1991;38:337–40.

30. Fan ZM, Yamashita Y, Harada M, et al. Intrahepatic cholangiocarcinoma: spin-echo and contrast-enhanced dynamic MR imaging. AJR Am J Roentgenol 1993;161:313–7.

31. Greenwood N, Orr WM. Primary squamous-cell carcinoma arising in a solitary non-parasitic cyst of the liver. J Pathol 1972;107:145–8.

32. Gresham GA, Rue LW. Squamous cell carcinoma of the liver. Hum Pathol 1985;16:413–6.

33. Hamaya K, Nose S, Mimura T, Sasaki K. Solid adenosquamous carcinoma of the liver. A case report and review of the literature. Acta Pathol Jpn 1991;41:834–40.

34. Harnois DM, Que FG, Celli A, LaRusso NF, Gores GJ. Bcl-2 is overexpressed and alters the threshold for apoptosis in a cholangiocarcinoma cell line. Hepatology 1997;26:884–90.

35. Haswell-Elkins MR, Satarug S, Elkins DB. Opisthorchis viverrini infection in northeast Thailand and its relationship to cholangiocarcinoma. J Gastroenterol Hepatol 1992;7:538–48.

36. Haworth AC, Manely PN, Groll A, et al. Bile duct carcinoma and biliary tract dysplasia in chronic ulcerative colitis. Arch Pathol Lab Med 1989;113:434–6.

37. Higginson J, Steiner PE. Definition and classification of malignant epithelial neoplasms of the liver. Acta Un Int Cancer 1961;17:593–603.

38. Holzinger F, Baer HU, Büchler MW. Mechanism of biliary carcinogenesis and preneoplastic lesions. Dig Surg 1995;12:208–14.

39. Horie Y, Akamizu H, Nishimura Y, et al. Intrahepatic cholangiocarcinoma with a long-term survival of 12 years after surgical resection: report of a case and review of the literature. Hepatogastroenterology 1995;42:506–9.

40. Hou PC. The relationship between primary carcinoma of the liver and infestation with Clonorchis sinensis. J Pathol Bacteriol 1956;73:239–46.

41. Houten L, Sonnesso G. Occupational exposure and cancer of the liver. Arch Environ Hlth 1980;35:51–3.

42. Imanishi T, Hamasato S, Soda M, et al. An autopsy case of Thorotrast induced liver cancer (hepatocellular carcinoma-cholangiocarcinoma). Acta Hepatol Jpn 1986;27:1616–21.

43. Imazu H, Ochiai M, Funabiki T. Intrahepatic sarcomatous cholangiocarcinoma. J Gastroenterol 1995;30:677–82.

44. Isa T, Kusano T, Muto Y, et al. Clinicopathologic features of resected adenosquamous carcinomas of the liver. J Clin Gastroenterol 1997;25:623–7.

45. Ishak KG, Anthony PP, Sobin LH. Histopathological typing of tumours of the liver. Berlin, Springer-Verlag, 1994.

46. Ishak KG, Sharp HL. Developmental abnormalities and liver disease in childhood. In: MacSween RN, Anthony PP, Scheuer PJ, Burt AD, Portmann BC, eds. Pathology of the liver, 3rd ed. Edinburgh: Churchill Livingstone, 1994:83–122.

47. Ito Y, Kojiro M, Nakashima T, Mori T. Pathomorphologic characteristics of 102 cases of thorotrast-related hepatocellular carcinoma, cholangiocarcinoma, and hepatic angiosarcoma. Cancer 1988;62:1153–62.

48. Jan YY, Yeh TS, Chen MF. Cholangiocarcinoma presenting as pyogenic liver abscess: is its outcome influenced by hepatolithiasis? Am J Gastroenterol 1998;93:253–5.

49. Johnson DE, Herndier BG, Medeiros LJ, Warnke RA, Rouse RV. The diagnostic utility of the keratin profile of hepatocellular carcinoma and cholangiocarcinoma. Am J Surg Pathol 1988;12:187–97.

50. Jovanovic R, Jagirdar J, Thung SN, Paronetto F. Blood-group-related antigen Lewis X and Lewis Y in the differential diagnosis of cholangiocarcinoma and hepatocellular carcinoma. Arch Pathol Lab Med 1989;113:139–42.

51. Kagawa Y, Kashihara S, Kuramoto S, Maetani S. Carcinoma arising in a congenitally dilated biliary tract. Report of a case and review of the literature. Gastroenterology 1978;74:1286–94.

52. Kajiyama K, Maeda T, Takenaka K, Sugimachi K, Tsuneyoshi M. The significance of stromal desmoplasia in intrahepatic cholangiocarcinoma. A special reference of "scirrhous-type" and "nonscirrhous-type" growth. Am J Surg Pathol 1999;23:892–902.

53. Kang YK, Kim WH, Lee HW, Lee HK, Kim YI. Mutation of p53 and K-ras, and loss of heterozygosity of APC in intrahepatic cholangiocarcinoma. Lab Invest 1999;79:477–8.

54. Karashina M, Kozuka S, Nakashima N, et al. Relationship of intrahepatic bile duct hyperplasia to cholangiocellular carcinoma. Cancer 1988;61:2469–74.

55. Kawahara N, Ono M, Taguchi KI, et al. Enhanced expression of thrombospondin-1 and hypovascularity in human cholangiocarcinoma. Hepatology 1998;28:1512–7.

56. Kawarada Y, Mitzumoto R. Cholangiocellular carcinoma of the liver. Am J Surg 1984;147:354–9.

57. Kawarada Y, Mitzumoto R. Diagnosis and treatment of cholangiocellular carcinoma of the liver. Hepatogastroenterology 1990;37:176–81.

58. Khan ZR, Neugut AI, Ahsan H, Chabot JA. Risk factors for biliary tract cancers. Am J Gastroenterol 1999;94:149–52.

59. Khuroo MS, Dar MY, Yattoo GN, et al. Serial cholangiographic appearances in recurrent pyogenic cholangitis. Gastrointest Endosc 1993;39:674–9.

60. Kim MH, Sekijima J, Lee SP. Primary intrahepatic stones. Am J Gastroenterol 1995;90:540–8.

61. Kim TK, Choi BI, Han JK, Jeng HJ, Cho SG, Han MC. Peripheral cholangiocarcinoma of the liver: two-phase spiral CT findings. Radiology 1997;204:539–43.

62. Kim YI. Liver carcinoma and liver fluke infection. Drug Res 1984;34:1121–4.

63. Kinami Y, Noto K, Miyazaki I, Matsubara F. A study of hepatolithiasis related to cholangiocarcinoma (in Japanese). Acta Hepatol Jpn 1978;19:578–83.

64. Koga A, Ichimiya H, Yamaguchi K, Miyazaki K, Nakayama F. Hepatolithiasis associated with cholangiocarcinoma. Possible etiologic significance. Cancer 1985;55:2826–9.

65. Kowdley KV, Hassanein T, Kaur S, et al. Primary liver cancer and survival in patients undergoing liver transplantation for hemochromatosis. Liver Transpl Surg 1995;1:237–41.

66. Kulkarni PB, Beatty EC Jr. Cholangiocarcinoma associated with biliary cirrhosis due to congenital biliary atresia. Am J Dis Child 1977;131:442–4.

67. Kurathong S, Lerdverasirikul P, Wongpaitoon V, et al. Opisthorchis viverrini infection and cholangiocarcinoma. A prospective, case-controlled study. Gastroenterology 1985;89:151–6.

68. Kurumaya H, Terada T, Nakanuma Y. "Metaplastic lesions" in intrahepatic bile ducts in hepatolithiasis: a histochemical and immunohistochemical study. J Gastroenterol Hepatol 1990;5:530–6.

69. Logani S, Adsay V. Clear cell cholangiocarcinoma of the liver is a morphologically distinctive entity [Letter]. Hum Pathol 1998;29:1548–9.

70. Ludwig J, Wahlstrom HE, Batts KP, Wiesner RH. Papillary bile duct dysplasia in primary sclerosing cholangitis. Gastroenterology 1992;102:2134–8.

71. Lynch MJ, McLeod MK, Weatherbee L, Gilsdorf JR, Guice KS, Eckhauser FE. Squamous cell cancer of the liver arising from a solitary benign nonparasitic cyst. Am J Gastroenterol 1988;83:426–31.

72. Ma CK, Zarbo RJ, Frierson HF, Lee MW. Comparative immunohistochemical study of primary and metastatic carcinoma of the liver. Am J Clin Pathol 1993;99:551–7.

73. Maeda T, Kajiyama K, Adachi E, Takenaka K, Sugimachi K, Tsuneyoshi M. The expression of cytokeratins 7, 19, and 20 in primary and metastatic carcinomas of the liver. Mod Pathol 1996;9:901–9.

74. Maeda T, Takenaka K, Taguchi K, et al. Adenosquamous carcinoma of the liver: clinicopathologic characteristics and cytokeratin profile. Cancer 1997;80:364–71.

75. Malker HS, McLaughlin JK, Malker BK, et al. Biliary tract cancer and occupation in Sweden. Br J Ind Med 1986;43:257–62.

76. Mecklin JP, Järvinen HJ, Virolainen M. The association between cholangiocarcinoma and hereditary nonpolyposis colorectal carcinoma. Cancer 1992;69:1112–4.

77. Minato H, Nakanuma Y, Terada T. Expression of blood group-related antigens in cholangiocarcinoma in relation to non-neoplastic bile ducts. Histopathology 1996;28:411–9.

78. Minervini MI, Demetris AJ, Lee RG, Carr BI, Madariaga J, Nalesnik MA. Utilization of hepatocyte-specific antibody in the immunohistochemical evaluation of liver tumors. Mod Pathol 1997;10:686–92.

79. Moore M, Fukushima, Ichihara A, Sato K, Ito N. Intestinal metaplasia and altered enzyme expression in propylnitrosamine-induced Syrian hamster cholangiocellular and gallbladder lesions. Virchows Arch [Cell Pathol] 1986;51:29–38.

80. Moore S, Gold RP, Lebwohl O, et al. Adenosquamous carcinoma of the liver arising in biliary cystadenocarcinoma: clinical, radiologic, and pathologic features with review of the literature. J Clin Gastroenterol 1984;6:267–75.

81. Mori W, Nagasako K. Cholangiocarcinoma and related lesions. In: Okuda K, Peters RL, eds. Hepatocellular carcinoma. New York: John Wiley & Sons, 1976:227–46.

82. Murakata LA, Ishak KG, Goodman ZG. Intrahepatic cholangiocarcinoma. A clinicopathologic study of 63 cases. [Unpublished observation, 2000.]

83. Nakajima T, Kondo Y. Well differentiated cholangiocarcinoma. Diagnostic significance of morphologic and immunohistochemical parameters. Am J Surg Pathol 1989;13:569–73.

84. Nakajima T, Kondo Y, Miyazaki M, Okui K. A histopathologic study of 102 cases of intrahepatic cholangiocarcinoma: histologic classification and modes of spreading. Hum Pathol 1988;19:1228–34.

85. Nakajima T, Tajima Y, Sugano I, Nagao K, Kondo Y, Wada K. Intrahepatic cholangiocarcinoma with sarcomatous change. Clinicopathologic and immunohistochemical evaluation of seven cases. Cancer 1993;72:1872–7.

86. Nakanuma Y, Hoso M, Terada T. Clinical and pathologic features of cholangiocarcinoma. In: Okuda K, Tabor E, eds. Liver cancer. New York: Churchill Livingstone, 1997:279–90.

87. Nakanuma Y, Terada T, Tanaka Y, Ohta G. Are hepatolithiasis and cholangiocarcinoma etiologically related? A morphological study of 12 cases of hepatolithiasis associated with cholangiocarcinoma. Virchows Arch [A] 1985;406:45–58.

88. Nonomura A, Mizukami Y, Matsubara F, et al. Human chorionic gonadotropin and alpha-fetoprotein in cholangiocarcinoma in relation to the expression of ras p21: an immunohistochemical study. Liver 1989;9:205–15.

89. Nonomura A, Ohta G, Hayashi M, et al. Immunohistochemical localization of ras p21 and carcinoembryonic antigens (CEA) in cholangiocarcinoma. Liver 1987;7:142–8.

90. Nozaki Y, Yamamoto M, Ikai I, et al. Reconsideration of the lymph node metastasis pattern (N factor) from intrahepatic cholangiocarcinoma using the International Union Against Cancer TNM Staging System for primary liver carcinoma. Cancer 1998;83:1923–9.

91. Ohashi K, Nakajima Y, Kanchiro H, et al. Ki-ras mutations and p53 protein expressions in intrahepatic cholangiocarcinomas: relation to gross tumor morphology. Gastroenterology 1995;109:1612–7.

92. Ohta T, Nagakawa T, Koniski I, et al. Clinical experience of intrahepatic cholangiocarcinoma associated with hepatolithiasis. Jap J Surg 1988;18:47–53.

93. Okuda K, Kojiro M, Okuda H. Neoplasms of the liver. In: Schiff L, Schiff ER, eds. Diseases of the liver, 7th ed. Philadelphia: JB Lippincott, 1993:1236–96.

94. Okuda K, Kubo Y, Okazaki N, Arishima T, Hashimoto M. Clinical aspects of intrahepatic bile duct carcinoma including hilar carcinoma: a study of 57 autopsy-proven cases. Cancer 1977;39:232–46.

95. Omata M, Peters RL, Tatter D. Sclerosing hepatic carcinoma: relationship to hypercalcemia. Liver 1981;1:33–49.

96. Ordonez NG, Mackay B. Ultrastructure of liver cell and bile duct carcinoma. Ultrastr Pathol 1983;5:201–41.

97. Ouazzani HC, Fadli F, Dafiri N, et al. Hépatocholangiome et Cushing paranéoplastique. Sem Hôp (Paris) 1985;61:3021–23.

98. Parham DM, Paterson RJ, Gunn A, Guthrie W. Cholangiocarcinoma in two siblings with emphysema and alpha-1-antitrypsin deficiency. Q J Med 1989;71:359–67.

99. Pastolero GC, Wakabayashi T, Oka T, Moris S. Tissue polypeptide antigen—a marker antigen differentiating cholangiolar tumors from other hepatic tumors. Am J Clin Pathol 1987;87:168–73.

100. Pianzola LE, Drut R. Mucoepidermoid carcinoma of the liver. Am J Clin Pathol 1971;56:758–61.

101. Pichlmayr R. Lameshc P, Weimann A, Tusch G, Ringe B. Surgical treatment of cholangiocellular carcinoma. World J Surg 1995;19:83–8.

102. Pliskin A, Cualing H, Stenger RJ. Primary squamous cell carcinoma originating in congenital cysts of the liver. Report of a case and review of the literature. Arch Pathol Lab Med 1992;166:105–7.

103. Radaeva S, Ferreira-Gonzalez A, Sirica AE. Overexpression of c-neu and c-met during rat liver cholangiocarcinogenesis: a link between biliary intestinal metaplasia and mucin-producing cholangiocarcinoma. Hepatology 1999;29:1453–62.

104. Ritchie JK, Allan RN, Macartney J, Thompson H, Hawley PR, Cooke WT. Biliary tract carcinoma associated with ulcerative colitis. Q J Med 1974;170:263–79.

105. Roayaie S, Guarrera JV, Thung SN, et al. Aggressive surgical treatment of intrahepatic cholangiocarcinoma: predictors of outcome. J Am Coll Surg 1998;187:365–72.

106. Ros PR, Buck JL, Goodman ZD, Ros AM, Olmsted WW. Intrahepatic cholangiocarcinoma: radiologic-pathologic correlation. Radiology 1988;167:689–93.

107. Roskams T, Willems M, Campos RV, Drucker DJ, Yap SH, Desmet VJ. Parathyroid hormone-related peptide expression in primary and metastatic liver tumours. Histopathology 1993;23:519–25.

108. Rubel LR, Ishak KG. Thorotrast-associated cholangiocarcinoma: an epidemiologic and clinicopathologic study. Cancer 1982;50:1408–15.

109. Ryorin H, Ohta H, Terada T, et al. Cholangiocarcinoma with primary biliary cirrhosis (in Japanese). Acta Hepatol Jpn 1995;36:175.

110. Saito K, Nakanuma Y, Ohta T, et al. Morphological study of cholesterol hepatolithiasis. Report of three cases. J Clin Gastroenterol 1990;12:585–90.

111. Sasaki A, Aramaki M, Kawano K, et al. Intrahepatic peripheral cholangiocarcinoma: mode of spread and choice of surgical treatment. Br J Surg 1998;85:1206–9.

112. Sasaki M, Nakanuma Y, Ho SB, Kim YS. Cholangiocarcinomas arising in cirrhosis and combined hepatocellular-cholangiocellular carcinomas share apomucin profiles. Am J Clin Pathol 1998;109:302–8.

113. Sasaki M, Nakanuma Y, Kim YS. Characterization of apomucin expression in intrahepatic cholangiocarcinomas and their precursor lesions: an immunohistochemical study. Hepatology 1996;24:1074–8.

114. Sasaki M, Nakanuma Y, Nagai Y, Nonomura A. Intrahepatic cholangiocarcinoma with sarcomatous transformation: an autopsy case. J Clin Gastroenterol 1991;13:220–5.

115. Schlinkert RT, Nagorney DM, Van Heerden JA, Adson MA. Intrahepatic cholangiocarcinoma: clinical aspects, pathology and treatment. HPB Surgery 1992;5:95–102.

116. Schwartz DA. Cholangiocarcinoma associated with liver fluke infection: a preventable source of morbidity in Asian immigrants. Am J Gastroenterol 1986;81:76–9.

117. Sirica A, Radaeva S, Caran N. NEU overexpression in the furan rat model of cholangiocarcinogenesis compared with biliary ductal cell hyperplasia. Am J Pathol 1997;151:1685–94.

118. Stromeyer FW, Smith DH, Ishak KG. Anabolic steroid therapy and intrahepatic cholangiocarcinoma. Cancer 1979;443:440–3.

119. Sugawara H, Yasoshima M, Katayanagi K, et al. Relationship between interleukin-6 and proliferation and differentiation in cholangiocarcinoma. Histopathology 1998;33:145–53.

120. Sugihara S, Kojiro M. Pathology of cholangiocarcinoma. In: Okuda K, Ishak KG, eds. Neoplasms of the liver. Tokyo, Springer-Verlag, 1987:143–58.

121. Tada M, Omata M, Ohto M. High incidence of ras gene mutation in intrahepatic cholangiocarcinoma. Cancer 1992;69:1115–8.

122. Takahashi H, Hayakawa H, Tanaka M, et al. Primary adenosquamous carcinoma of liver resected by right trisegmentectomy: report of a case and review of the literature. J Gastroenterology 1997;32:843–7.

123. Tan CK, Podila PV, Taylor JE, et al. Human cholangiocarcinomas express somatostatin receptors and respond to somatostatin with growth inhibition. Gastroenterology 1995;108:1908–16.

124. Telles NC, Thomas LB, Popper H, Ishak K, Falk H. Evolution of Thorotrast-induced hepatic angiosarcomas. Environ Res 1979;18:74–87.

125. Terada T, Ashida K, Endo K, et al. C-erb B-2 protein is expressed in hepatolithiasis and cholangiocarcinoma. Histopathology 1998;33:325–31.

126. Terada T, Kida T, Kananuma Y, Noguchi T. Extensive portal tumor thrombi in an autopsy case of intrahepatic cholangiocarcinoma. Am J Gastroenterol 1992;87:1513–8.

127. Terada T, Kida T, Nakanuma Y, Kurumaya H, Doishita K, Takayangi N. Intrahepatic cholangiocarcinomas associated with nonbiliary cirrhosis. A clinicopathologic study. J Clin Gastroenterol 1994;18:335–42.

128. Terada T, Makimoto K, Terayama N, et al. Alpha-smooth muscle actin-positive stromal cells in cholangiocarcinoma, hepatocellular carcinoma and metastatic liver carcinoma. J Hepatol 1996;24:706–12.

129. Terada T, Nakanuma Y. Expression of tenascin, type IV collagen and laminin during human intrahepatic bile duct development and intrahepatic cholangiocarcinoma. Histopathology 1994;25:143–50.

130. Terada T, Nakanuma Y. An immunohistochemical survey of amylase isoenzymes in cholangiocarcinoma and hepatocellular carcinoma. Arch Pathol Lab Med 1993;117:160–2.

131. Terada T, Nakanuma Y. Pancreatic lipase is a useful phenotypic marker of intrahepatic large and septal bile ducts, peribiliary glands, and their malignant counterparts. Mod Pathol 1993;6:419–26.

132. Terada T, Nakanuma Y. Pathological observations of intrahepatic peribiliary glands in 1000 consecutive autopsy livers. II. A possible source of cholangiocarcinoma. Hepatology 1990;12:92–7.

133. Terada T, Nakanuma Y, Ohta T, Nagakawa T. Histological features and interphase nucleolar organizer regions in hyperplastic, dysplastic and neoplastic epithelium of intrahepatic bile ducts in hepatolithiasis. Histopathology 1992;21:233–40.

134. Terada T, Nakanuma Y, Saito K, Kono N. Biliary sludge and microcalculi in intrahepatic bile ducts. Morphologic and X-ray microanalytical observations in 18 among 1,179 consecutively autopsied livers. Acta Pathol Jpn 1990;40:894–901.

135. Terada T, Nakanuma Y, Sirica AE. Immunohistochemical demonstration of MET overexpression in human intrahepatic cholangiocarcinoma and hepatolithiasis. Hum Pathol 1998;29:175–80.

136. Terada T, Ohta T, Minato H, Nakanuma Y. Expression of pancreatic trypsinogen/trypsin and cathepsin B in human cholangiocarcinoma and hepatocellular carcinomas. Hum Pathol 1995;26:746–52.

137. Terada T, Shimizu K, Izumi R, Nakanuma Y. Methods in pathology. p53 expression in formalin-fixed, paraffin-embedded archival specimens of intrahepatic cholangiocarcinoma: retrieval of p53 antigenicity by microwave oven heating of tissue sections. Mod Pathol 1994;7:249–52.

138. Thamavit W, Kongkanuntn R, Tiwawech D, Moore A. Level of opithorchis infestation and carcinogen dose-dependence of cholangiocarcinoma induction in Syrian golden hamsters. Virchows Arch [Cell Pathol] 1987;54:52–8.

139. Tihan T, Blumgart L, Klimstra DS. Clear cell papillary carcinoma of the liver: an unusual variant of peripheral cholangiocarcinoma. Hum Pathol 1998;29:196–200.

140. Toda M, Omata M, Ohto M. High incidence of ras gene mutation in intrahepatic cholangiocarcinoma. Cancer 1992;69:1115–8.

141. Todani T, Tabuchi K, Watanabe Y, Kobayashi T. Carcinoma arising in the wall of congenital bile duct cysts. Cancer 1979;44:1134–41.

142. Tominatsu M, Ishiguro N, Taniai M, et al. Hepatitis C virus antibody in patients with primary liver cancer (hepatocellular carcinoma, cholangiocarcinoma, and combined hepatocellular-cholangiocarcinoma) in Japan. Cancer 1993;72:683–88.

143. Torrii A, Harada A, Nakao A, et al. Expression of HLA-DR in intrahepatic cholangiocarcinoma. Cancer 1992;70:1057–61.

144. Turani H, Levi J, Zevin D, Kessler E. Hepatic lesions in patients on anabolic androgenic therapy. Israel J Med Sci 1983;19:332–7.

145. Urushizaki I, Kitago M, Natori H, et al. A rare case of adenoacanthoma originally developed from intrahepatic bile duct (in Japanese). Jap J Cancer Clin 1973;19:152–5.

146. Vardaman C, Albores-Saavedra J. Clear cell carcinomas of the gallbladder and extrahepatic bile ducts. Am J Surg Pathol 1995;19:91–9.

147. Vatananasapt V, Uttaravichien T, Mairiang EO, Pairojkul C, Chartbanchachai W. Cholangiocarcinoma in north-east Thailand. Lancet 1990;1:116–7.

148. Voravud N, Foster CS, Gilbertson JA, Sikora K, Waxman J. Oncogene expression in cholangiocarcinoma and in normal hepatic development. Hum Pathol 1989;20:1163–8.

149. Washburn WK, Lewis WD, Jenkins RL. Aggressive surgical resection for cholangiocarcinoma. Arch Surg 1995;130:270–6.

150. Watanabe M, Akagi S, Hamamoto S. Intraperitoneal rupture of cholangiocarcinoma in a patient with liver cirrhosis, type C, with hepatocellular carcinoma [Letter]. Am J Gastroenterol 1999;94:2320–1.

151. Wee A, Ludwig J, Coffey RJ, LaRusso NF, Wiesner RH. Hepatobiliary carcinoma associated with primary sclerosing cholangitis and chronic ulcerative colitis. Hum Pathol 1985;16:719–26.

152. Welton JC, Marr JS, Friedman SM. Association between hepatobiliary cancer and typhoid carrier state. Lancet 1979;1:791–4.

153. Wibulpolprasert B, Dhiensiri T. Peripheral cholangiocarcinoma: sonographic evaluation. J Clin Ultrasound 1992;20:303–14.

154. Winberg CD, Ranchod M. Thorotrast induced hepatic cholangiocarcinoma and angiosarcoma. Hum Pathol 1979;10:108–12.

155. Yamada S, Hosoda S, Tateno H, Kido C, Takahashi S. Survey of Thorotrast-associated liver cancer in Japan. JNCI 1983;70:31–5.

156. Yamaguchi K, Nalesnik MA, Carr BI. In situ hybridization of albumin mRNA in normal liver and liver tumors: identification of hepatocellular origin. Virchows Arch [Cell Pathol] 1993;64:361–5.

157. Yamamoto M, Takasaki K, Nakano M, Saito A. Minute nodular intrahepatic cholangiocarcinoma. Cancer 1998;82:2145–9.

158. Yamanaka N, Okamoto E, Ando T, et al. Clinicopathologic spectrum of resected extraductal mass-forming intrahepatic cholangiocarcinoma. Cancer 1995;76:2249–56.

159. Zelissen PM, Van Hattum EJ. Een jonge vrouw met een lever tumor en hypercalciëmie. Neder Tijdsch Genees 1986;38:1705–7.

Hepatobiliary Cystadenocarcinoma

160. Akwari OE, Tucker A, Seigler HF, Itani KM. Hepatobiliary cystadenocarcinoma with mesenchymal stroma. Ann Surg 1990;211:18–27.

160a. Azizah N, Paradinas FJ. Cholangiocarcinoma coexisting with developmental liver cysts: a distinct entity different from the cystadenocarcinoma. Histopathology 1980;4:391–400.

161. Buetow PC, Buck JL, Patongrag-Brown L, et al. Biliary cystadenoma and cystadenocarcinoma: clinical-imaging-pathologic correlation with emphasis on the importance of ovarian stroma. Radiology 1995;196:803–10.

162. Choi BI, Lim JH, Han MC, et al. Biliary cystadenoma and cystadenocarcinoma: CT and sonographic findings. Radiology 1989:171:57–61.

163. Dean DL, Bauer HM. Primary cystic carcinoma of the liver. Am J Surg 1969;117:416–20.

164. Devaney K, Goodman ZD, Ishak KG. Hepatobiliary cystadenoma and cystadenocarcinoma. A light microscopic and immunohistochemical study of 70 patients. Am J Surg Pathol 1994;18:1078–91.

165. Huguier M, Cherqui D, Houry S, et al. Kystes biliares du foie. Presse Med (Paris) 1986;15:827–9.

166. Imamura M, Miyashita T, Tani T, Naito A, Tobe T, Takahashi K. Cholangiocellular carcinoma associated with multiple liver cysts. Am J Gastroenterol 1984;79:790–5.

167. Ishak KG, Willis GW, Cummins SD, Bullock AA. Biliary cystadenoma and cystadenocarcinoma: report of 14 cases and review of the literature. Cancer 1976;38:322–38.

168. Kashima S, Asanuma Y, Niwa M, Koyama K. A case of true hepatic cyst with malignant change. Acta Hepatol Jpn 1988;29:1265–8.

169. Korobkin M, Stephens D, Lee J, et al. Biliary cystadenocarcinoma: CT and sonographic findings. AJR Am J Roentgeneol 1989;153:507–11.

170. Madariaga JR, Iwatsuki S, Starzl TE, Todo S, Selby R, Zetti G. Hepatic resection for cystic lesions of the liver. Ann Surg 1993;218:610–4.

170a. Moore S, Gold RP, Lebwohl O, et al. Adenosquamous carcinoma of the liver arising in biliary cystadenocarcinoma: clinical, radiologic, and pathologic features with review of the literature. J Clin Gastroenterol 1984;6:267–75.

171. Rossi RL, Silverman ML, Braasch JW, Munson JL, ReMine SG. Carcinoma arising in cystic conditions of the bile ducts. A clinical and pathologic study. Ann Surg 1987;205:377–84.

172. Shimada M, Kajiyama K, Saitoh A, Kano T. Cystic neoplasms of the liver: a report of two cases with special reference to cystadenocarcinoma. Hepatogastroenterology 1996;43:249–54.

173. Unger PD, Thung SN, Kaneko M. Pseudosarcomatous cystadenocarcinoma of the liver. Hum Pathol 1987;18:521–3.

174. Wolf HK, Garcia JA, Bossen EH. Oncocytic differentiation in intrahepatic biliary cystadenocarcinoma. Mod Pathol 1992;5:665–8.

◇◇◇

11

MISCELLANEOUS MALIGNANT TUMORS

NONHEPATOCYTIC MALIGNANT MIXED TUMOR

A number of neoplasms that do not fit into other categories have been reported as "mixed tumors" of the liver. Among these are sometimes included spindle cell variants of hepatocellular carcinoma (chapter 8) and cholangiocarcinoma (chapter 10), as well as true carcinosarcomas that contain elements of hepatocellular carcinoma and rare cases of malignancy arising in an hepatic teratoma (chapter 5). Kawarada et al. (1) reported two cases that they classified as nonhepatocytic malignant mixed tumor, and they reviewed 22 other cases of mixed tumors gathered from the literature, but most of these were felt to be variants of hepatocellular carcinoma or epithelioid hemangioendothelioma. There are two cases in the Armed Forces Institute of Pathology (AFIP) files that appear similar to those of Kawarada et al. (1).

Definition. These tumors are true *carcinosarcomas* in which the epithelial elements are glandular rather than hepatocellular. As such, they could be regarded as a variant of cholangiocarcinoma, but they are so rare and distinctive that they are considered here separately.

Clinical Features. The cases of Kawarada et al. (1) were both men, aged 43 and 49. The similar AFIP cases included a 79-year-old man with alcoholic cirrhosis and a 33-year-old woman with no preexisting liver disease. All presented with abdominal pain and a large hepatic mass. The 43-year-old man was alive with no evidence of disease at 2 years 8 months after resection. The other patients died of their disease.

Gross Findings. The tumors were described as firm, large, and bulky, replacing much of the liver. Areas of hemorrhage were noted in one case.

Microscopic Findings. The tumors all had an element of adenocarcinoma that was mixed with a poorly differentiated spindle cell tumor. In addition, there were heterologous elements with variable amounts of osteoid, areas that resembled chondrosarcoma, and sometimes foci of rhabdomyoblasts (fig. 11-1).

Differential Diagnosis. As noted, if the spindled component is fibrosarcoma-like and does not have features of a specific sarcoma, then the tumor should be considered a spindle cell or sarcomatoid variant of cholangiocarcinoma (chapter 10). If the epithelial component shows hepatocellular differentiation, then the tumor is considered a carcinosarcoma or sarcomatoid variant of hepatocellular carcinoma. If there are both malignant hepatocellular and glandular elements to the epithelial component, then the tumor is a combined hepatocellular-cholangiocarcinoma with spindle cell metaplasia.

YOLK SAC TUMOR

Yolk sac tumor or endodermal sinus tumor, a well-recognized neoplasm of the ovary and testis, sometimes arises in extragonadal sites. There are, to our knowledge, 11 reported cases of primary yolk sac tumor of the liver (3,5–7) as well as one case each of hepatoblastoma (2) and hepatocellular carcinoma (4) that had yolk sac elements. There are two primary hepatic yolk sac tumors in the files of the AFIP.

Clinical Features. Patients have ranged in age from 8 months to 62 years. The typical presentation is with abdominal distention and pain due to a rapidly growing hepatic mass. One patient was successfully treated and cured with combination chemotherapy followed by surgical resection (6).

Gross Findings. The tumors are usually described as variegated and may have areas of hemorrhage.

Microscopic Findings. As in the gonads, the tumors may have reticular, pseudopapillary, or sheet-like growth patterns. With sufficient sections there are invariably Schiller-Duval bodies (fig. 11-2), consisting of a papillary structure that contains a central, thin-walled blood vessel surrounded by primitive columnar cells, which in turn are surrounded by a space lined by hobnail-shaped cells. Periodic acid–Schiff (PAS)-positive hyaline globules are usually present in some of the epithelial cells, and the epithelial cells stain for alpha-fetoprotein and alpha-1-antitrypsin.

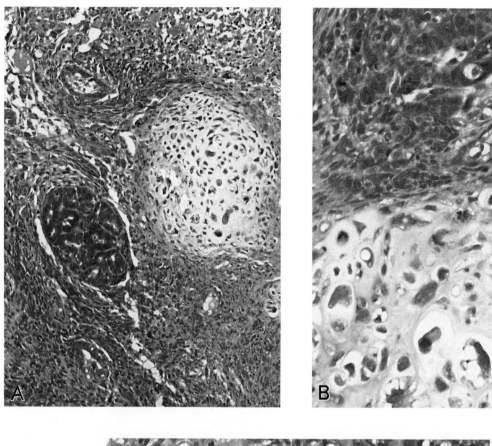

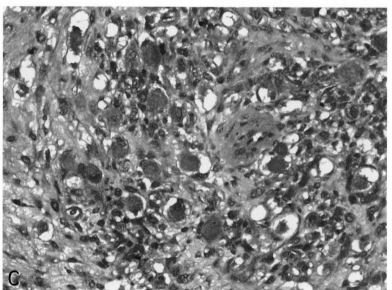

Figure 11-1
NONHEPATOCYTIC MALIGNANT MIXED TUMOR

A: The tumor has areas of adenocarcinoma that merge into a poorly differentiated spindle cell tumor with heterologous elements.

B: Adenocarcinoma with spindle cell metaplasia is present at the top of the field, while cartilage with malignant nuclear features is present at the bottom.

C: Rhabdomyoblasts are among the spindle cells.

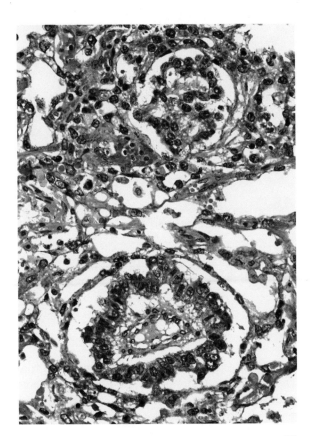 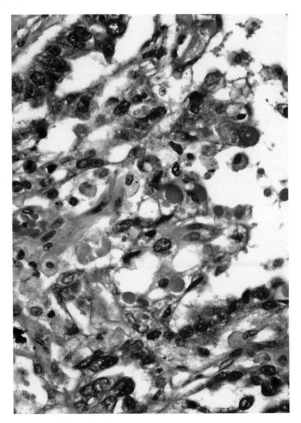

Figure 11-2
YOLK SAC TUMOR OF THE LIVER
Left: Schiller-Duval bodies consisting of a central thin-walled blood vessel are surrounded by primitive columnar cells.
Right: Many of the tumor cells contain hyaline globules.

Differential Diagnosis. In a young child, embryonal hepatoblastoma (chapter 6) is far more common and is the principal diagnosis that should be considered. If there is no evidence of hepatocellular differentiation, and if typical Schiller-Duval bodies are present, the diagnosis of yolk sac tumor is not in doubt. Metastasis from a gonadal primary must be excluded, but there is little else that would be seriously considered.

MALIGNANT RHABDOID TUMOR

Rhabdoid tumors are distinctive childhood neoplasms of uncertain histogenesis that arise most frequently in the kidney, where they have been distinguished from Wilms' tumor. Identical tumors may arise in extrarenal sites, and there are 18 cases reported in the liver (9,10). There are five primary hepatic rhabdoid tumors in the files of the AFIP, one of which has been reported (8).

Clinical Features. Nearly all cases have occurred in the first 2 years of life, usually presenting as a rapidly growing abdominal mass. As in other sites, the patients have a very poor prognosis and uniformly fatal outcome.

Gross Findings. Reported patients have had large bulky tumors with a fleshy, variegated appearance on sectioning. The tumors replace large portions of the liver, and have infiltrative margins and often satellite nodules.

Microscopic Findings. The tumors characteristically have sheets of large, polygonal or round cells with large, vesicular nuclei, prominent nucleoli, and abundant eosinophilic cytoplasm, imparting the "rhabdoid" appearance to the tumor (fig. 11-3). PAS-positive globular cytoplasmic hyaline inclusions may be present. Ultrastructurally, the eosinophilic cytoplasm contains whorls of intermediate filaments, and immunostains are frequently positive for both

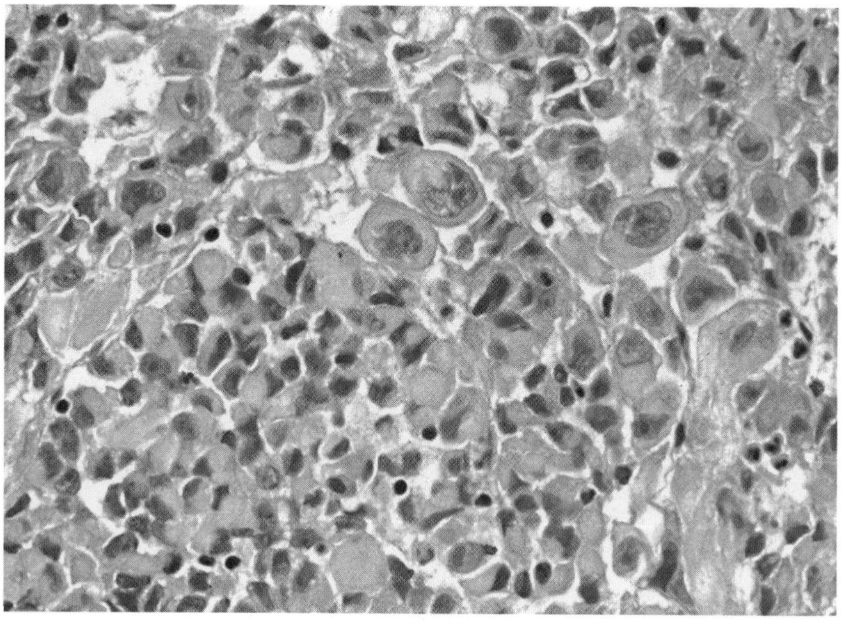

Figure 11-3
MALIGNANT RHABDOID
TUMOR OF THE LIVER
The tumor cells have abundant eosinophilic cytoplasm and large vesicular nuclei with prominent nucleoli.

vimentin and cytokeratin; neural markers such as S-100 protein, neuron-specific enolase, and MIC-2 may also be present (10).

Differential Diagnosis. The "rhabdoid" appearance of the tumor cells always raises the differential diagnosis of embryonal rhabdomyosarcoma (chapter 12), but the presence of cytokeratin and absence of myoglobin and other muscle markers distinguishes the rhabdoid tumor. Hepatoblastoma (chapter 6) should always be the first consideration in the diagnosis of a malignant hepatic tumor in a young child, but the high-grade nature of the tumor and lack of hepatocellular differentiation should help rule this out.

CARCINOID TUMOR

Primary carcinoid tumors of the liver have been reported (11,13,14), with over 20 purported cases in the literature, but many of these may in fact have been metastatic or may have represented focal neuroendocrine differentiation in other tumors. Carcinoids are notorious for producing large hepatic metastases from small primaries in the ileum or rectum (12), and so a complete and thorough autopsy with careful attention to the entire intestinal tract is mandatory before one can be certain that the tumor was primary in the liver. Carcinoid tumors are also frequently indolent and slow growing (12), so that prolonged survival fol-

lowing resection cannot be considered proof that the tumor was primary in the liver. A carcinoid tumor that is seen in a surgical specimen or biopsy should be considered metastatic, even if no primary is found with the usual clinical evaluation. There are cases in which the primary tumor may only be detected with a special diagnostic test using single photon emission computed tomography and ^{111}In-DTPA octreotide, which binds to somatostatin receptors that are present in the majority of carcinoids (fig. 11-4) (12). Cells with neuroendocrine differentiation can be found in the liver in some pathologic conditions (15), so it seems likely that a carcinoid tumor might arise from the same pleuripotential cells that give rise to these. However, in the files of the AFIP, of 410 cases of carcinoid tumor in the liver diagnosed between 1970 and 1998 there is only one that was definitely primary.

Clinical Features. In view of the difficulty in establishing the diagnosis of primary carcinoid, it is hard to generalize the clinical features from the literature. The cases reported as primary hepatic carcinoid tumors have all been in adults, with about equal numbers in men and women. Carcinoid syndrome is rare (13).

Gross Findings. Some of the reported tumors have been multiple (raising the question of whether they are actually metastases) while others have been solitary. Some have been described as "large"; one measured 17 cm (13). The case in the AFIP files was a 1 cm subcapsular nodule that was an incidental autopsy finding in a 93-year-old man who died of a cerebral hemorrhage.

Microscopic Findings. Carcinoid tumors in any location have a typical appearance consisting of nests of uniform cells, and sometimes trabecular or ribbon-like growth within the nests (fig. 11-5). Immunostains for endocrine markers, such as chromogranin and synaptophysin, are usually positive and confirm the diagnosis. Serotonin and other hormones are variably positive. Ultrastructural examination reveals typical dense core neuroendocrine granules.

Differential Diagnosis. It can be difficult at times to distinguish hepatocellular carcinoma from a carcinoid tumor, as both may have eosinophilic cells growing in a trabecular pattern. A positive stain for a neuroendocrine marker indicates that the tumor is a carcinoid, while an immunostain for carcinoembryonic antigen that shows intercellular canaliculi or a positive stain for Hep Par 1 antigen (Hepatocyte) (see chapter 8), indicates that the tumor is actually hepatocellular carcinoma. Cholangiocarcinomas occasionally have areas that mimic carcinoid tumors, but in those tumors immunostains for cytokeratin 7 are usually strongly positive while stains for endocrine markers are negative.

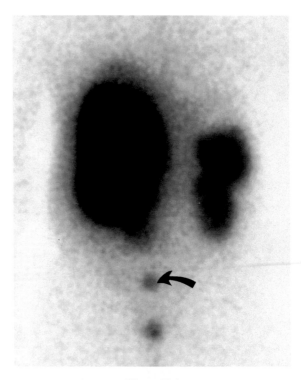

Figure 11-4
"PSEUDO-PRIMARY" HEPATIC CARCINOID TUMOR
This ^{111}In-DPTA octreotide scan shows a massive carcinoid tumor replacing the right lobe of the liver, as well as tracer in the spleen, kidneys, and bladder. The primary tumor, a small carcinoid in the rectum (arrow), would not have been detected without this special study, and the tumor might have been called a "primary hepatic carcinoid," even though it is actually a metastasis.

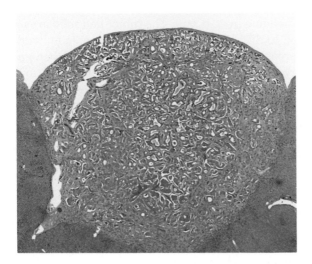 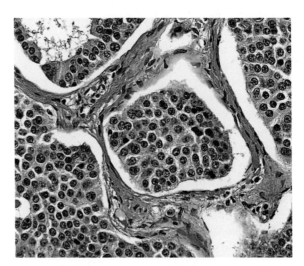

Figure 11-5
PRIMARY HEPATIC CARCINOID TUMOR
This 1 cm nodule (left) was an incidental autopsy finding in a 93-year-old man. It is the only case in the AFIP files that we are sure was a primary hepatic carcinoid. The tumor is a typical carcinoid with a fibrous stroma and nests and ribbons of monomorphic cells with prominent nucleoli. High magnification (right) shows the typical cytologic features of a carcinoid.

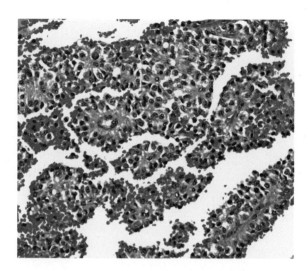
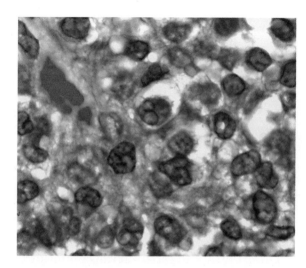

Figure 11-6
SOLID-PSEUDOPAPILLARY TUMOR, PRIMARY IN THE LIVER
This tumor, although identical to the solid-pseudopapillary tumor of the pancreas, was primary in the liver. There has been degeneration of many of the tumor cells, leaving a pseudopapillary configuration of cells that cling to fibrovascular stalks. At high magnification (right), the tumor cells have a moderate amount of cytoplasm and lobulated or grooved nuclei.

SOLID-PSEUDOPAPILLARY TUMOR

The low-grade malignant tumor of the pancreas (17) that is called *solid-pseudopapillary tumor, solid-cystic tumor, papillary-cystic tumor,* or *solid and papillary epithelial neoplasm* may rarely occur as a primary tumor of the liver. There is one reported case (16) and one other case on file at the AFIP.

Clinical Features. In the pancreas, these are tumors of young and middle-aged women. The two primary liver tumors were in women, aged 41 and 56 years. One had an asymptomatic left lobe liver mass detected on routine examination, while the other presented with abdominal pain and distension. Both underwent resection. Long-term follow-up is not available in these two cases, but in the pancreas most tumors are cured by resection.

Gross Findings. The reported case had two large masses, one each in the right and left lobes. Both tumors were multicystic with necrotic and hemorrhagic contents.

Microscopic Findings. The tumor cells grow in solid sheets; the pseudopapillary appearance is produced by cystic degeneration of poorly vascularized parts of the tumor and preservation of cells surrounding fibrovascular stalks (fig. 11-6). The tumor cells are small and cuboidal, and often have lobulated or grooved nuclei. In pancreatic tumors, electron microscopy may occasionally demonstrate zymogen granules, but usually the tumor cells show no evidence of specific differentiation, and the histogenesis of the tumor is unknown.

MALIGNANT CYSTIC MESOTHELIOMA

There is one reported case (18), which was reviewed at the AFIP, of a malignant cystic mesothelioma in an infant. The tumor had solid areas of undifferentiated malignant neoplasm and areas that resembled the more typical benign cystic mesothelioma of the abdomen, with transitional forms that appeared to merge into these (fig. 11-7). Electron microscopy confirmed mesothelial differentiation. The tumor grew into and replaced large parts of the liver, and the patient died within a few months. We know of no other similar cases.

OSSIFYING STROMAL-EPITHELIAL TUMOR

There are three cases in the files of the AFIP which we believe represent a hitherto unreported tumor with unique clinical and histopathologic features.

Clinical Features. Two of the cases were in women, aged 28 and 32 at the time of diagnosis,

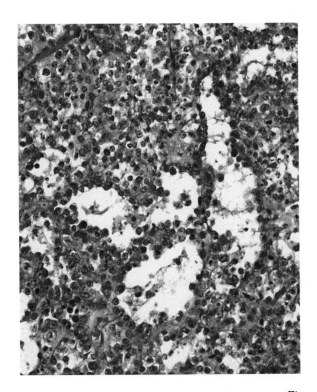
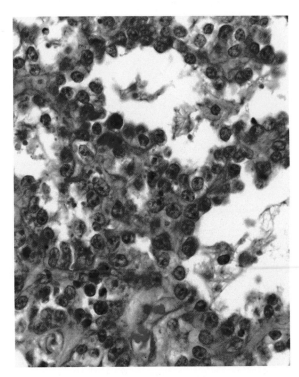

Figure 11-7
MALIGNANT CYSTIC MESOTHELIOMA
Left: The tumor consists of sheets of cells that in places form cyst-like clefts.
Right: The clefts are lined with cells that have a hobnail appearance.

and the third was in a 19-year-old man. All had been known to have a calcified liver mass since childhood. Both women underwent hepatic resection because of recent enlargement of the mass, while the man only had a needle biopsy for diagnosis. One of the women was alive with a recurrence 6 years later. No follow-up was available on the other two patients. However, based on the histologic appearance and the fact that one tumor recurred, we believe that this is a low-grade malignancy.

Gross Findings. The tumors were 10 to 12 cm in diameter. One resected tumor was described as firm and gray-white on section with a 3-cm area of calcification.

Microscopic Findings. All three tumors had mixtures of primitive spindled stromal cells and myofibroblasts (actin positive) surrounding nests and islands of epithelial cells. The epithelial cells had a moderate amount of basophilic to clear cytoplasm and single, round nuclei (fig. 11-8A,B). Scattered mitoses were present in the epithelial elements (fig. 11-8B). The epithelial cells formed occasional glands, and displayed spindling in

some areas. There were also areas of osteoid production that appeared to merge with epithelial elements (fig. 11-8C), and some of these were calcified (fig. 11-8A). Immunostains showed the epithelial cells to be strongly positive for cytokeratin. S-100 protein was also strongly positive in one case (fig. 11-8D) and focally positive in the other two. Stains for hepatocyte antigen, carcinoembryonic antigen (for canaliculi), endocrine markers, and melanoma antigens (to rule out angiomyolipoma and related tumors) were negative. Stains for smooth muscle actin and vimentin decorated the stromal cells. The histogenesis of this unusual tumor remains unknown.

SQUAMOUS CELL CARCINOMA

Since nearly all of the rare, primary squamous cell carcinomas of the liver arise in congenital cysts, and since cholangiocarcinomas occasionally have squamous components (adenosquamous), squamous cell carcinoma is included in chapter 10, along with these other related entities.

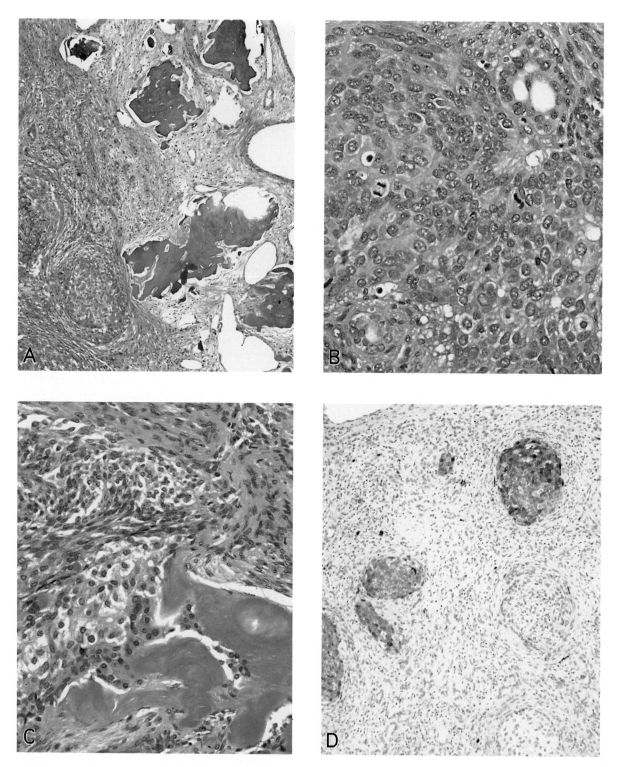

Figure 11-8
OSSIFYING STROMAL-EPITHELIAL TUMOR
A: The tumor consists of islands of epithelial cells in a spindle cell stroma (left) and areas of ossification (right).
B: At higher magnification, the epithelial cells form occasional glandular lumina and have scattered mitoses.
C: There is osteoid production adjacent to epithelial cells and spindled stroma.
D: Some of the epithelial islands are strongly positive for S-100 protein (immunostain).

OTHER RARE TUMORS

There are a few other rarely reported malignant hepatic neoplasms of which we have no examples at the AFIP. Four cases of *osteoblastoma-like giant cell tumor* of the liver have been reported (20,22). There is one reported case of a primary *extramedullary plasmacytoma* of the liver (24). Two cases of *primary pheochromocytoma* of the liver (not necessarily malignant, but included here for completeness) have been reported (19,21). And finally there is a report of a *lymphoepithelioma-like carcinoma* of the liver that was associated with Epstein-Barr virus infection (23).

REFERENCES

Malignant Mixed Tumor

1. Kawarada Y, Uehara S, Noda M, Yatani R, Mizumoto R. Nonhepatocytic malignant mixed tumor primary in the liver. Cancer 1985;55:1790–8.

Yolk Sac Tumor

2. Cross SS, Variend S. Combined hepatoblastoma and yolk sac tumor of the liver. Cancer 1992;69:1323–6.
3. Higuchi T, Kikuchi M. Yolk sac tumor of the liver treated with transcatheter arterial embolization. Am J Gastroenterol 1993;88:1125–6.
4. Morinaga S, Nishiya H, Inafuku T. Yolk sac tumor of the liver combined with hepatocellular carcinoma. Arch Pathol Lab Med 1996;120:687–90.
5. Wakely PJ Jr, Krummel TM, Johnson DE. Yolk sac tumor of the liver. Mod Pathol 1991;4:121–5.
6. Whelan JS, Stebbiings W, Owen RA, Calne R, Clark PI. Successful treatment of a primary endodermal sinus tumor of the liver. Cancer 1992;70:2260–2.
7. Wong NA, D'Costa H, Barry RE, Alderson D, Moorghen M. Primary yolk sac tumor of the liver in adulthood. J Clin Pathol 1998;51:939–40.

Malignant Rhabdoid Tumor

8. Parham DM, Peiper SC, Robicheaux G, Ribeiro RC, Douglass EC. Malignant rhabdoid tumor of the liver. Arch Pathol Lab Med 1988;112:61–4.
9. Parham DM, Weeks DA, Beckwith JB. The clinicopathologic spectrum of putative extrarenal rhabdoid tumors: an analysis of 42 cases studied with immunohistochemistry or electron microscopy. Am J Surg Pathol 1994;18:1010–29.
10. Scheimberg I, Cullinane C, Kelsey A, Malone M. Primary hepatic malignant tumor with rhabdoid features: a histological, immunocytochemical, and electron microscopic study of four cases and a review of the literature. Am J Surg Pathol 1996;20:1394–400.

Carcinoid Tumor

11. Andreola S, Lombardi L, Audisio RA, et al. A clinicopathologic study of primary hepatic carcinoid tumors. Cancer 1990;65:1211–8.
12. Kvols LK. Gastrointestinal carcinoid tumors and the malignant carcinoid syndrome. In: Feldman M, Scharschmidt BF, Sleisenger MH, eds. Sleisenger & Fordtran's gastrointestinal and liver disease, 6th ed. Philadelphia: WB Saunders, 1998:1831–43.
13. Mehta DC, Warner RR, Rarnes I, Weiss M. An 18-year follow-up of primary hepatic carcinoid with carcinoid syndrome. J Clin Gastroenterol 1996;23:60–2.
14. Miura K, Shirasawa H. Primary carcinoid tumor of the liver. Am J Clin Pathol 1988;89:561–4.
15. Roskams T, De Vos R, Van den Oord J, Desmet V. Cells with neuroendocrine features in regenerating human liver. APMIS Suppl 1991;23:32–39.

Solid-Pseudopapillary Tumor

16. Kim YI, Kim ST, Lee GK, Choi BI. Papillary cystic tumor of the liver. A case report with the ultrastructural observation. Cancer 1990;65:2740–6.
17. Solcia E, Capella C, Kloppel G. Tumors of the pancreas. Atlas of Tumor Pathology, 3rd series, Fascicle 20. Washington, D.C.: Armed Forces Institute of Pathology, 1995.

Malignant Cystic Mesothelioma

18. DeStephano DB, Wesley JR, Heidelberger KP, Hutchinson RJ, Blane CE, Coran AG. Primitive cystic hepatic neoplasm of infancy with mesothelial differentiation: report of a case. Pediatr Pathol 1985;4:291–302.

Other Tumors

19. Craig JR, Peters RL, Edmondson HA. Tumors of the liver and intrahepatic bile ducts. Atlas of Tumor Pathology, 2nd Series, Fascicle 26. Washington, D.C., Armed Forces Institute of Pathology, 1989:105–6.
20. Hood DL, Bauer TW, Leibel SA, McMahon JT. Hepatic giant cell carcinoma. An ultrastructural and immunohistochemical study. Am J Clin Pathol 1990;93:111–6.
21. Jaeck D, Paris F, Welsch M, et al. Primary hepatic pheochromocytoma: a second case. Surgery 1995;117:586–90.
22. Munoz PA, Rao MS, Reddy JK. Osteoclastoma-like giant cell tumor of the liver. Cancer 1980;46:771–9.
23. Vortmeyer AO, Kingma DW, Fenton RG, Curti BD, Jaffe ES, Duray PH. Hepatobiliary lymphoepithelioma-like carcinoma associated with Epstein-Barr virus. Am J Clin Pathol 1998;109:90–5.
24. Weichhold W, Labouyrie E, Merlio JP, Basson B, de Mascarel A. Primary extramedullary plasmacytoma of the liver. A case report. Am J Surg Pathol 1995;19:1197–202.

12

MALIGNANT MESENCHYMAL TUMORS

Primary malignant mesenchymal tumors of the liver are much rarer than epithelial neoplasms, but figures regarding their incidence are quite limited. Of the 405 primary malignant tumors collected by Edmondson and Peters (2), 1.2 percent were sarcomas. Data from the Surveillance, Epidemiology and End Results Program (SEER) of the National Cancer Institute for the years 1973 to 1987 revealed a total of 6,391 primary liver cancers (all histologically confirmed), of which 127 (2 percent) were sarcomas (1 percent angiosarcomas and 1 percent other sarcomas) (1). Metastatic sarcomas must be rigorously excluded clinically and radiographically before inferring that a sarcoma is primary in the liver. In one small series of hepatic sarcomas (2a) only 60 percent of tumors believed to be primary in the liver were confirmed as such after extensive evaluation. The most common site for an occult primary was the retroperitoneum. At the Armed Forces Institute of Pathology (AFIP), 232 primary hepatic sarcomas were on file from 1981 to 1990 (3). The number of cases of each of the sarcomas, together with the age and sex of

the patients, are listed in Table 12-1. The malignant vascular tumors, angiosarcoma and epithelioid hemangioendothelioma, are by far the most frequent sarcomas of the liver.

Primary sarcomas usually develop in a noncirrhotic liver, although various degrees of fibrosis may be present in angiosarcoma related to prior exposure to Thorotrast or vinyl chloride. Sarcoma and carcinoma occurring simultaneously in a cirrhotic liver are exceptionally rare (4). The diagnosis should be made with caution since hepatocellular carcinoma can show a spindle cell (pseudosarcomatous) pattern. Carcinosarcomas (admixtures of carcinoma, either hepatocellular or cholangiocellular, and various differentiated sarcomatous elements) also are rare.

The clinical course of some sarcomas, such as epithelioid hemangioendothelioma, is unpredictable, but in general, hepatic sarcomas are rapidly growing and uniformly fatal. Therapy remains unsatisfactory, although some progress has been made in the treatment of the childhood sarcomas such as embryonal (undifferentiated) sarcoma and embryonal rhabdomyosarcoma. Etiologic factors

Table 12-1

PRIMARY HEPATIC SARCOMAS ON FILE AT THE
ARMED FORCES INSTITUTE OF PATHOLOGY (1981–1990)*

Tumor	No. of Cases (%)	Mean Age (Years)	Age Range (Years)	Sex (M/F)
Angiosarcoma	65 (28.01)	56.3	3–96	44/21
Epithelioid hemangioendothelioma	61 (26.29)	44.3	12–80	19/42
Embryonal sarcoma	38 (16.37)	16.5	8 mo–73 yr	15/23
Leiomyosarcoma	30 (12.93)	57.5	9–89	15/15
Malignant fibrous histiocytoma	11 (4.74)	56.0	23–77	6/5
Fibrosarcoma	6 (2.58)	57.3	38–69	3/3
Rhabdomyosarcoma	3 (1.29)	39.6	6–74	2/1
Schwannoma	1 (0.43)	22.0	22	0/1
Unclassified tumors	17 (7.37)	57.1	21–91	15/2

*Total number of cases 232.

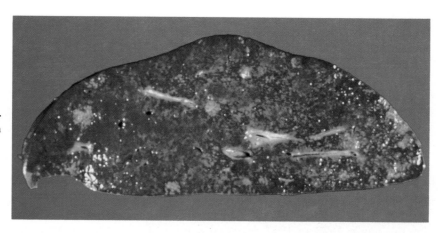

Figure 12-1
EPITHELIOID
HEMANGIOENDOTHELIOMA
Section of liver with tan tumor nodules of varied size scattered in both lobes.

for sarcomas are largely unknown, except for angiosarcoma, which has been linked to exposure to Thorotrast, vinyl chloride, and arsenic.

EPITHELIOID HEMANGIOENDOTHELIOMA

Definition. Epithelioid hemangioendothelioma is a low-grade malignant neoplasm of endothelial cells, invariably associated with a stroma that varies from loose and myxoid to dense and fibrous. The tumor cells often have an abundant cytoplasm and thus mimic epithelial tumors, but they often form intracellular vascular lumina. Epithelioid hemangioendothelioma can involve other organs, such as lung (sometimes simultaneously with the liver), soft tissue, and bone (12,30).

Clinical Features. Since the publication of a series of 32 cases involving the liver by Ishak et al. (17), a considerable number of other cases have been reported (6–9,13–16,19,23–28,31). The largest series consists of 137 cases studied by Makhlouf et al. (20) at the AFIP. The age at presentation of the AFIP patients ranged from 12 to 86 years; 62 percent were women. Symptoms and signs included weakness, anorexia, nausea, episodic vomiting, upper abdominal aching and pain, jaundice, and hepatosplenomegaly (17,20). An acute abdomen from rupture of the tumor with hemoperitoneum (17), a Budd-Chiari-like syndrome (13, 29), and portal hypertension or liver failure (11, 24) were less common presentations. However, in a significant number (42 percent) of the AFIP cases the tumor was an incidental finding.

Liver tests do not offer clues to the diagnosis, although increased serum alkaline phosphatase activity is demonstrable in about two thirds of the patients (12). An elevated serum factor VIII level was found in one of the cases reviewed at the AFIP and another reported one (18). Hepatic scintigraphy generally reveals "filling defects" throughout the liver. Calcification may be evident in plain films of the abdomen. On computed tomography (CT) tumor nodules have low attenuation, are peripherally based, and are associated with capsular retraction or flattening (14). Contrast-enhanced CT scans show a peripheral enhancement pattern of alternating attenuation values that correlate with the hyperemic rim noted on pathologic examination (23). In one CT study, lesions that were initially nodular later became diffuse (23). Ultrasound examination reveals predominantly hypoechoic lesions (14,23). On magnetic resonance imaging (MRI), the tumor signal is low on T1-weighted and high on T2-weighted images, with a low signal halo present around the nodules (23). It should be emphasized that although epithelioid hemangioendothelioma is a vascular tumor, angiographic examination typically reveals avascular lesions (20). At the present time, a definitive diagnosis of epithelioid hemangioendothelioma can only be established by liver biopsy.

Gross Findings. Epithelioid hemangioendothelioma usually consists of multiple lesions involving the entire liver (17,20); these were described as mostly peripheral in one study (21). The lesions vary from a few millimeters to several centimeters in diameter (figs. 12-1, 12-2). The neoplastic tissue is tan to white, firm, and sometimes gritty when sectioned. The margins of the lesions may be hyperemic. The tumor generally does not arise on a background of

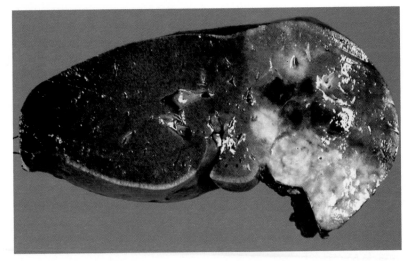

Figure 12-3
EPITHELIOID
HEMANGIOENDOTHELIOMA
The lightly stained tumor has infiltrated and destroyed several adjacent acini.

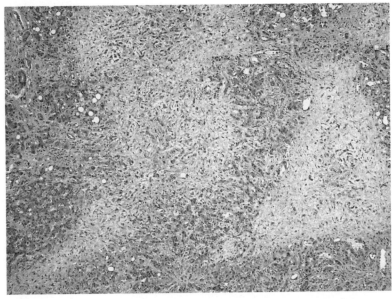

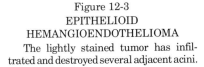

chronic liver disease, with the exception of two reported cases that occurred in cirrhotic livers (17,26). Some cases are associated with nodular regenerative hyperplasia (17).

Microscopic Findings. The tumor nodules are ill-defined, and often involve multiple contiguous acini (fig. 12-3). In actively proliferating lesions the acinar landmarks, such as terminal hepatic venules and portal areas, can be recognized despite extensive infiltration by the tumor (figs. 12-3, 12-4). The tumor cells grow along preexisting sinusoids, terminal hepatic venules and portal vein branches, and often invade Glisson's capsule (figs. 12-5–12-8). Growth within the acini

is associated with gradual atrophy and eventual disappearance of liver cell plates (fig. 12-9). Intravenous growth may be in the form of a solid plug, or a polypoid or tuft-like projection. Invasion of arteries in portal areas is rare. Neoplastic cells are either "epithelioid," with a rounded shape and abundant cytoplasm (fig. 12-10); intermediate (fig. 12-11); or "dendritic," with spindle or irregular shapes and multiple interdigitating processes (fig. 12-12). Nuclear atypia and mitoses are mainly observed in the epithelioid cells. Cytoplasmic vacuoles, representing intracellular vascular lumina, are often identified and may contain erythrocytes (figs. 12-9, 12-11, 12-13).

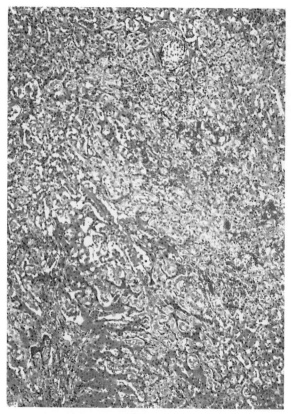

Figure 12-4
EPITHELIOID HEMANGIOENDOTHELIOMA
Cords and nests of tumor cells have infiltrated hepatic sinusoids and destroyed the liver plates.

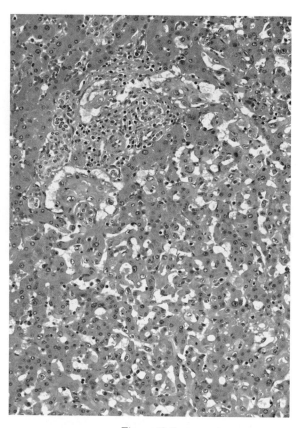

Figure 12-5
EPITHELIOID HEMANGIOENDOTHELIOMA
Epithelioid tumor cells have diffusely infiltrated the sinusoids, particularly those surrounding a portal area (top).

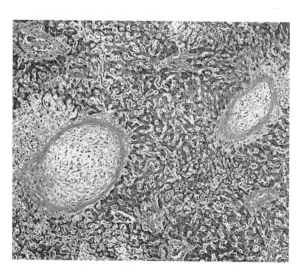

Figure 12-6
EPITHELIOID HEMANGIOENDOTHELIOMA
Neoplastic occlusion of two terminal hepatic venules.

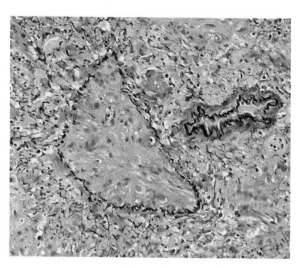

Figure 12-7
EPITHELIOID HEMANGIOENDOTHELIOMA
The portal vein branch is infiltrated by tumor cells surrounded by a myxoid (pale green) matrix. Note the uninvolved artery to right of the vein (Musto pentachrome stain).

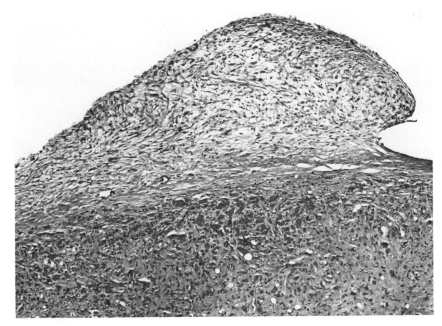

Figure 12-8
EPITHELIOID
HEMANGIOENDOTHELIOMA
A capsular nodule of dendritic tumor cells (brick red) is set in a loose fibrous stroma (Masson trichrome stain).

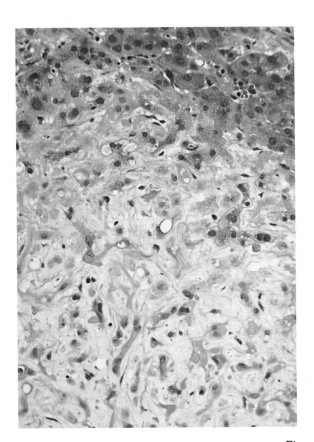
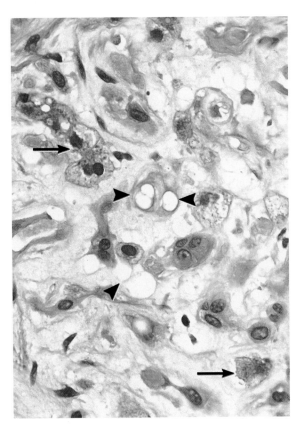

Figure 12-9
EPITHELIOID HEMANGIOENDOTHELIOMA

Left: Interconnected epithelioid tumor cells have destroyed the hepatic parenchyma.

Right: Higher magnification shows some tumor cells with intracytoplasmic vascular lumina (arrow heads). Several disrupted liver cells (arrows) are also present.

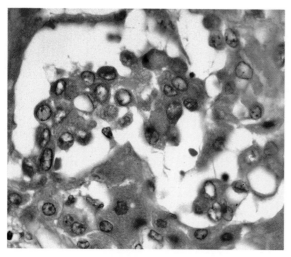

Figure 12-10
EPITHELIOID HEMANGIOENDOTHELIOMA
There are polypoid clusters of epithelioid tumor cells in dilated sinusoidal lumina. Note the vesicular nuclei and inconspicuous nucleoli.

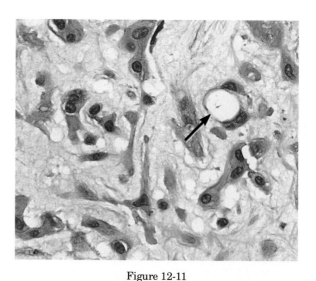

Figure 12-11
EPITHELIOID HEMANGIOENDOTHELIOMA
Tumor cells ("intermediate") are separated by a loose myxoid stroma. Note the cytoplasmic vascular lumina, one of which is indicated by an arrow.

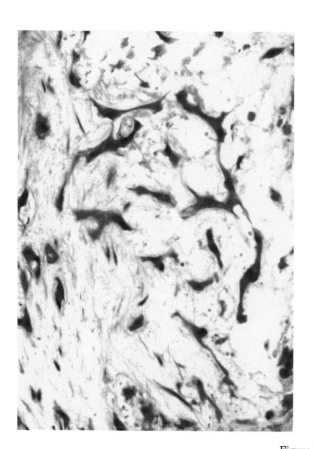

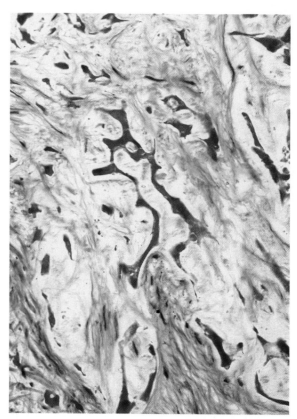

Figure 12-12
EPITHELIOID HEMANGIOENDOTHELIOMA
Left: The tumor cells are dendritic and interconnected by cytoplasmic processes.
Right: Dendritic tumor cells (red) are embedded in a collagenous matrix (Masson trichrome stain).

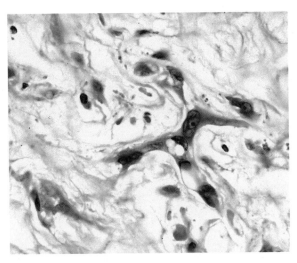

Figure 12-13
EPITHELIOID HEMANGIOENDOTHELIOMA
High magnification of a dendritic tumor cell with a triple-barreled vascular lumen.

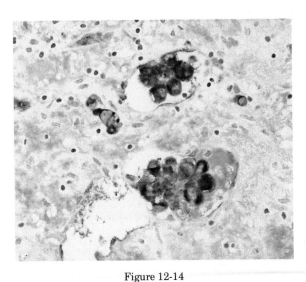

Figure 12-14
EPITHELIOID HEMANGIOENDOTHELIOMA
Tumor cells show strong cytoplasmic expression of von Willebrand factor (immunostain).

Immunohistochemical Findings. The tumor cells synthesize von Willebrand factor (factor VIII–related antigen), which can be demonstrated in the cytoplasm or in the neoplastic vascular lumina (fig. 12-14). Other endothelial cell markers, such as CD31 and CD34 (QBEND/10), are also positive (5,20,22,29,30) but the most useful is expression of von Willebrand factor. Tumor cells also express vimentin (fig. 12-15) and laminin. The stroma of actively proliferating lesions has a myxoid appearance due to an abundance of sulfated mucopolysaccharide (fig. 12-16). Reticulin fibers surround nests of tumor cells (fig. 12-17). Basement membrane can be demonstrated around the cells by the periodic acid–Schiff (PAS) stain (fig. 12-18), as well as ultrastructurally and immunohistochemically (fig. 12-19). Variable numbers of smooth muscle cells surround the basement membrane (fig. 12-20). In our experience the tumor cells infrequently express cytokeratins (fig. 12-21). As the lesions evolve they are associated with progressive fibrosis and calcification (figs. 12-22, 12-23). Eventually, tumor cells (and indeed, the vascular nature of the lesion) may be difficult if not impossible to recognize in the densely sclerosed areas (figs. 12-24, 12-25). Needle biopsy specimens taken from such areas often pose problems for inexperienced pathologists.

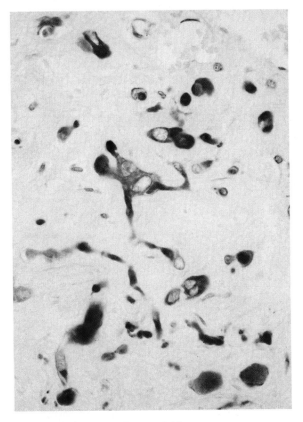

Figure 12-15
EPITHELIOID HEMANGIOENDOTHELIOMA
The tumor cells and their processes express vimentin (immunostain).

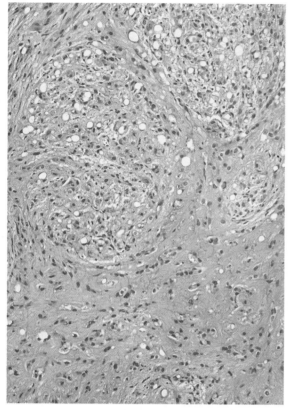

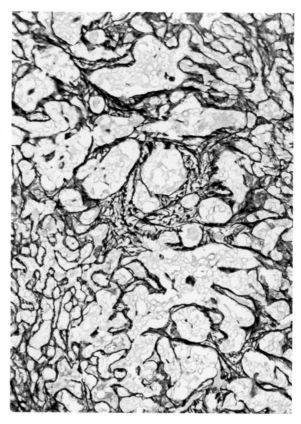

Figure 12-16
EPITHELIOID HEMANGIOENDOTHELIOMA
Tumor cells (pink) are surrounded by a sulfated muco-polysaccharide matrix (blue) (Alcian blue stain). Vacuoles represent intracellular vascular lumina.

Figure 12-17
EPITHELIOID HEMANGIOENDOTHELIOMA
Nests of tumor cells are surrounded by reticulin fibers (Manuel reticulin stain).

Figure 12-18
EPITHELIOID
HEMANGIOENDOTHELIOMA
A basement membrane surrounds many of the cords and nests of tumor cells (PAS after diastase digestion).

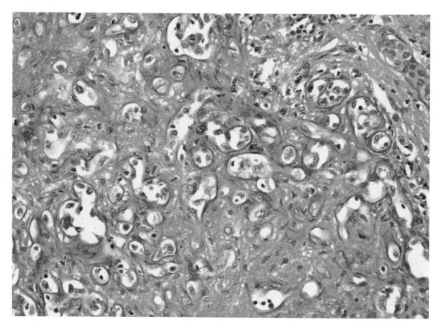

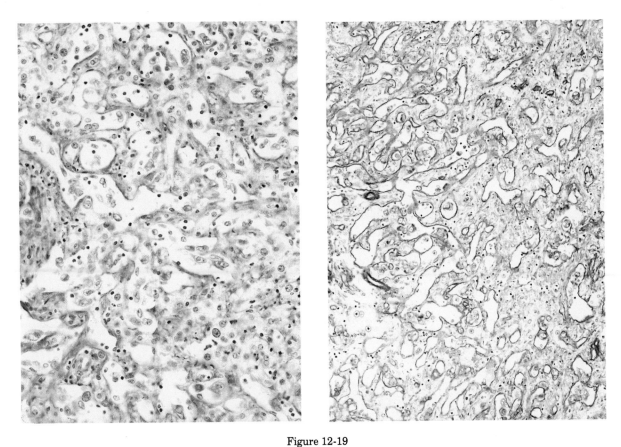

Figure 12-19
EPITHELIOID HEMANGIOENDOTHELIOMA
The basement membrane is decorated by collagen IV antibody (immunostain) (left) and laminin antibody (immunostain) (right).

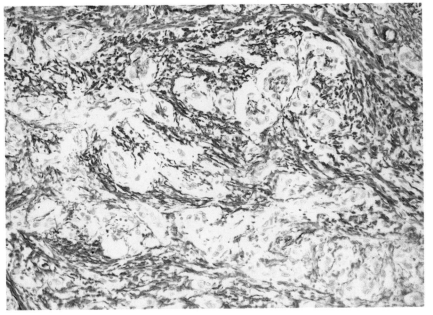

Figure 12-20
EPITHELIOID
HEMANGIOENDOTHELIOMA
Smooth muscle fibers are present in the tumor matrix (alpha-smooth muscle immunostain).

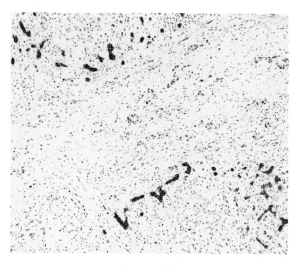

Figure 12-21
EPITHELIOID HEMANGIOENDOTHELIOMA
Tumor cells are not expressing cytokeratin. Stained bile ductules surround the tumor (pancytokeratin immunostain).

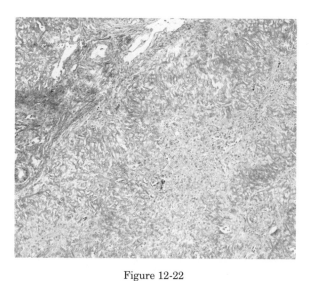

Figure 12-22
EPITHELIOID HEMANGIOENDOTHELIOMA
Large areas of the tumor are densely sclerosed. Note the preserved portal area in upper left corner (Masson trichrome stain).

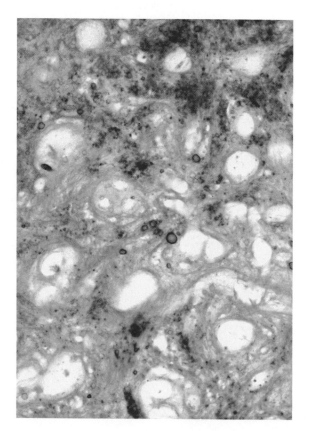

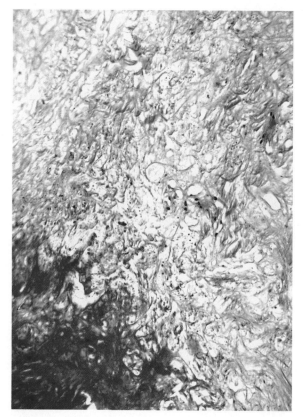

Figure 12-23
EPITHELIOID HEMANGIOENDOTHELIOMA
Left: Basophilic granules and spherules of calcification in a densely sclerosed area of a tumor. There are no viable tumor cells.
Right: Another part of the same sclerosed area. A calcific plaque is present in the lower left corner.

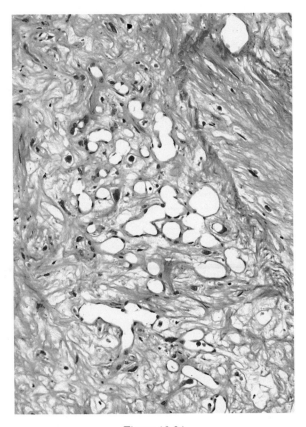

Figure 12-24
EPITHELIOID HEMANGIOENDOTHELIOMA
A sclerosed area of tumor with capillaries; only a few tumor cells are viable. The lumen of a segment of a terminal hepatic venule (top right) is replaced by fibrous tissue.

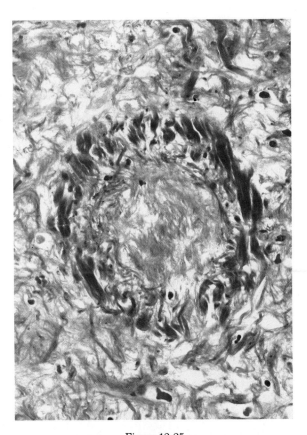

Figure 12-25
EPITHELIOID HEMANGIOENDOTHELIOMA
A terminal hepatic venule in a sclerosed area of tumor is occluded by fibrous tissue (Masson trichrome stain).

Ultrastructural Findings. The cells of epithelioid hemangioendothelioma have many of the characteristics of endothelial cells, including a basal lamina, pinocytotic vesicles, and Weibel-Palade bodies. Intracellular lumina are frequently seen. Unlike normal endothelial cells, the tumor cells contain a large number of intermediate filaments which account for their "epithelioid" appearance by light microscopy; dense bodies may also be present.

Differential Diagnosis. The histopathologic differential diagnosis (Table 12-2) includes other benign and malignant vascular tumors and epithelial tumors (e.g., cholangiocarcinoma) as well as non-neoplastic conditions (17,20). Angiosarcoma is much more destructive than epithelioid hemangioendothelioma, obliterates acinar landmarks, and results in cavity formation. The cells are not epithelioid but are spindled or show considerable pleomorphism, and intracellular lumina are not seen. Both tumors invade veins (terminal hepatic venules and portal vein branches) and the cells of both tumors express the vascular endothelial cell markers. Acinar landmarks, such as portal areas, are more likely to be preserved in epithelioid hemangioendothelioma than in angiosarcoma. Cholangiocarcinomas display tubular, glandular, or papillary patterns, and often produce mucin. Their cells are cuboidal or columnar but can be pleomorphic, are cytokeratin positive, and do not express endothelial cell markers. Many cases of epithelioid hemangioendothelioma seen in consultation at the AFIP are misdiagnosed as non-neoplastic diseases, such as cirrhosis, precirrhotic fibrosis, or veno-occlusive disease. Awareness of epithelioid hemangioendothelioma and recognition of the characteristic epithelioid or dendritic cells and intravascular growth should prevent misdiagnoses.

Table 12-2

MORPHOLOGIC DIFFERENTIAL DIAGNOSIS OF VASCULAR NEOPLASMS OF THE LIVER

Morphologic Features	Cavernous Hemangioma	Infantile Hemangioendothelioma	Kaposiform Angiosarcoma	Kaposi's Sarcoma	Epithelioid Hemangioendothelioma	Angiosarcoma
Gross involvement	Usually single	Single or multiple	Usually single	Multiple	Usually multiple	Usually multiple
Microscopic involvement	Replaces acini	Replaces acini	Infiltrates and destroys acini	Grows in portal areas	Infiltrates and partly destroys acini (spares portal areas)	Infiltrates and destroys acini
Remnants of hepatic acini	No	No	Yes	No	Yes	Yes
Infiltration of preexisting sinusoids	No	No	Yes	Yes, periportal (rare)	Yes	Yes
Invasion of veins (terminal hepatic venules, portal vein branches)	No	No	Yes	No	Yes	Yes
Invasion of capsule	No	No	No	No	Yes	Yes
Cells lining neoplastic vessels						
Pleomorphism	No	No	No	No	Yes	Yes
Mitoses	No	No	Yes	Yes	Yes	Yes
Epithelioid change	No	No	No	No	Yes	No
Multinucleation/giant cells	No	No	No	No	Yes (rare)	Yes
"Dendritic" cells	No	No	No	No	Yes	No
"Glomeruloid" foci	No	No	Yes	No	No	No
Von Willebrand factor in tumor cells	Yes	Yes	No	Yes (rare)	Yes	Yes
CD31, CD34 in tumor cells	Yes	Yes	Yes	Yes	Yes	Yes
Eosinophilic, PAS-positive globules in tumor cells	No	No	Yes	Yes	No	No
Bile ducts in tumor*	No	Yes	No	No	No	No
Collagenous matrix	Yes	Yes (central)	Yes	Yes (rare)	Yes (diffuse)	No
Inflammation (other than in necrotic foci)	No	No	Yes	Yes	Yes	No
Hemosiderin (other than in old hemorrhages or infarcts)	No	No	Yes	Yes	Yes	No
Hematopoietic cells in neoplastic vessels	No	Yes	No	No	No	Yes
Nodular regenerative hyperplasia in non-neoplastic liver	No	No	No	No	Yes (some cases)	Yes (some cases)
Extrahepatic metastases	No	No	Yes (lung, pleura, lymph nodes, spleen)	Yes (Simultaneous foci in skin, GI tract, etc.)	Yes (lung, peritoneum, lymph nodes, spleen)	Yes (lung, spleen, lymph nodes, bone marrow)

*Excluding ducts trapped in portal areas.

Etiology and Pathogenesis. Etiologic factors in hepatic hemangioendothelioma are unknown. Some of the female patients had used oral contraceptives (9,23), and one patient had had prior exposure to vinyl chloride (15). A number of other associated or antecedent conditions are mentioned by Makhlouf et al. (20).

The pathogenesis of epithelioid hemangioendothelioma remains undetermined. On the basis of recurrence in an hepatic allograft and tumor immunophenotype, Demetris et al. (10) have speculated that these tumors may derive from primitive "reticuloendothelial" cells that can differentiate along endothelial and dendritic cell pathways, and may represent a neoplastic analogue of wound healing.

Treatment and Prognosis. The prognosis of patients with epithelioid hemangioendothelioma is unpredictable. About 28 percent of the tumors metastasize (17,20), but the development of metastases does not preclude a long survival. Follow-up information on 60 of the 137 patients reported by Maklouf et al. (20) is available. Of these, 43 percent died of the disease at intervals that ranged from 4 months to 28 years. Overall, 43 percent of patients survived 5 years or longer irrespective of the type of treatment received (surgery, chemotherapy, radiation, liver transplantation, or no therapy at all). Some 40 other patients have been treated by hepatic transplantation (19–21,24,25,31). Metastatic spread was not considered a contraindication to surgery in two series, and in some of the cases did not correlate with length of survival (19,21). In the series of Kelleher et al. (19), 9 of 10 patients who underwent transplantation were alive 5 to 134 months postoperatively (5 disease free and 4 with tumor). In the series of Marino et al. (21), the projected 5-year actuarial survival rate was 76 percent. One patient with unresectable tumor survived 4 years after therapy with hepatic intra-arterial 5-fluorouracil (16).

Makhlouf et al. (20) studied several histologic parameters of epithelioid hemangioendothelioma using univariate analysis in an attempt to predict behavior. No significant correlation was found with mitoses, capsule invasion, or nuclear atypia. High cellularity correlated significantly with a poor clinical outcome (p=0.00012), while the association with tumor necrosis approached significance (p=0.057).

ANGIOSARCOMA

Definition. Angiosarcoma is a high-grade malignant neoplasm of endothelial cells. In contrast to epithelioid hemangioendothelioma there is little stromal response. The tumor cells may appear epithelioid, but more typically they are spindled.

Etiology. This is unknown in the majority of cases. A survey of angiosarcomas in the United States from 1964 through 1974 by Falk et al. (50) disclosed 168 cases; 75 percent of these were of uncertain etiology while the remainder were related to exposure to vinyl chloride, Thorotrast, inorganic arsenic, and androgenic/anabolic steroids. Etiologic factors implicated in angiosarcoma in humans are discussed by Falk et al. and are listed in Table 12-3. The most important are vinyl chloride, arsenic, and Thorotrast, but cases attributed to these agents have declined dramatically in the past decade. In reference to vinyl chloride, a gas used to make polyvinyl chloride, the exposure was occupational. The angiosarcomas related to arsenic were reported in German vineyard workers exposed to arsenical insecticides, in persons who had taken Fowler's solution (potassium arsenite) medicinally for prolonged periods for asthma or psoriasis, in a patient who had been treated for syphilis with dioxidiaminoarsenobenzol, and in a few persons exposed to high levels of arsenic in drinking water. Colloidal thorium dioxide (Thorotrast) was used as a radiographic contrast medium from the 1930s through the 1950s. After injection, nearly all the material remains permanently in the body, accumulating in the liver and to lesser degrees in the spleen, lymph nodes, and bone marrow. Thorium is weakly radioactive and emits predominantly alpha and beta particles. The first hepatic angiosarcoma in a person who had received Thorotrast was reported in 1947. Subsequently, numerous other Thorotrast-associated angiosarcomas, as well as hepatocellular carcinomas and cholangiocarcinomas, have been reported. The interval between receiving the Thorotrast and development of angiosarcoma may has varied from 12 to 60 years.

Clinical Features. Although rare, this malignant vascular tumor is the most common sarcoma arising in the liver. Worldwide, over 200 cases are diagnosed annually (32,34,50). The peak age incidence is in the sixth and seventh decades, with a male to female ratio of 3:1 (74). The modes of

Table 12-3

ETIOLOGY OF ANGIOSARCOMA*

Physical/ Chemical Agent	Circumstances of Exposure	Latent Period (years)	References
Thorotrast	Used as contrast medium for radiographic studies	15–60	36,40,41,43,45a,52,64, 68,69,73,76,77,86,92,101, 105,106,108,111,112
Radium	Radium needle implanted for treatment of breast carcinoma (1 case)	3	90
External radiation	Atomic bomb explosion, Hiroshima (1 case)	36	79
Vinyl chloride	Industrial exposure during manufacture of poly-vinyl chloride; exposure to sprays containing vinyl chloride as propellant	9–35	37,45,49,54,55,60, 72,83,85,86,102
Arsenical compounds	Insecticide for spraying of vineyards; medicinal use of Fowler's solution; dioxidiaminoarsenobenzol for treatment of syphilis; high levels of arsenic in drinking water (India, Bangladesh)	6–46	48,51,65,71,87–89, 91,92a
Copper sulfate	Used for spraying vineyards (1 case)	35	84
Pesticides	Farmers exposed to organophosphorous and organochlorine containing pesticides in Egypt	14	47
Iron	Idiopathic hemochromatosis in cirrhotic stage	?	35,70,99
Androgenic/anabolic steroids	Treatment of Fanconi's anemia and other disorders	2–35	53,80
Contraceptive steroids	Birth control (1 case)	10	95
Diethylstilbestrol	Treatment of prostatic cancer (1 case)	13	59
Phenelzine	Treatment of depression (1 case)	6	42

*Cases arising in preexisting benign vascular tumors, such as infantile hemangioendothelioma, are excluded.

presentation include: 1) symptoms and signs indicative of liver disease (62 percent), such as hepatomegaly, ascites, abdominal pain, anorexia, nausea and occasional vomiting, weight loss, and fever; 2) signs and symptoms of an acute abdomen from hemoperitoneum due to rupture of the tumor (15 percent); 3) splenomegaly, with or without pancytopenia (5 percent); and 4) symptoms or signs referable to metastases to distant organs such as the skeleton or lungs (9 percent) (63). Portal hypertension, a recognized complication of vinyl chloride exposure (38,96), may antedate the development of angiosarcoma (63). The diagnosis is best established by open liver biopsy following suggestive radiographic studies.

Laboratory data include anemia, sometimes a microangiopathic hemolytic anemia, leukocytosis (65 percent) or leukopenia (22 percent), and thrombocytopenia (62 percent) (63). Disseminated intravascular coagulopathy is a rare complication (103). Liver tests are abnormal in about two thirds of patients (63,74). The most consistent abnormalities are bromosulfophthalein (BSP) retention (100 percent), increased serum alkaline phosphatase activity (83 percent), and a prolonged prothrombin time (72 percent). Hyperbilirubinemia develops in about 60 percent of patients, while mild to modest aminotransferase elevations are found in less than half.

Radiographic Findings. Chest roentgenograms reveal elevation of the diaphragm (32 percent of cases) or much less frequently, pleural effusions, atelectasis, or pleural masses (63). Plain films of the abdomen in Thorotrast-related angiosarcomas invariably disclose opacification of the liver, spleen, and abdominal lymph nodes

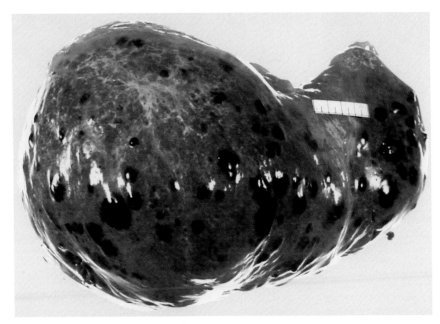

Figure 12-26
ANGIOSARCOMA
The external surface of the liver is riddled with raised, black tumor nodules of varied size. Note the yellow-white reticular fibrosis.

(72). Hepatic scans are abnormal in the majority of cases, but definite filling defects are recorded in only 70 percent of cases (63). CT has been utilized in diagnosis (73,75,106,110), as well as in detecting rupture of the tumor (75). The smallest tumor detected by CT in the large series of Van Kaick et al. (106) was 3 cm in diameter. Nonenhanced scans show hypodense masses. Dynamic scanning during intravenous contrast injection reveals peripheral or central foci of enhancement in the nodules (73). In delayed postcontrast scans the lesions become wholly or partly isodense (73). While the CT findings are nonspecific they are consistent with a vascular tumor. Angiographic studies are considered to yield valuable information for angiosarcoma (43,74). The abnormal vascular pattern, with a persistent peripheral tumor stain and a central radiolucent area, is thought to be highly suggestive of angiosarcoma (43).

Gross Findings. The liver involved by angiosarcoma reveals grayish white tumor tissue alternating with hemorrhagic foci; large cavities filled with liquid blood may be observed (figs. 12-26–12-28). A reticular pattern of fibrosis is often seen in cases associated with Thorotrast or prior exposure to vinyl chloride. Typically, the entire liver is involved. The spleen is usually large, except in Thorotrast-related angiosarcoma, when it is atrophic. In cases with previous Thorotrast exposure, sections of the spleen and abdominal lymph nodes have a chalky white appearance. A true cirrhosis, regardless of etiology, is exceptionally rare in our experience.

Microscopic Findings. The tumor cells in angiosarcoma grow along preformed vascular channels: sinusoids, terminal hepatic venules, and portal vein branches (figs. 12-29, 12-30). Sinusoidal growth is associated with progressive atrophy of liver cells and disruption of the plates, with formation of larger and larger vascular channels and eventually, the development of cavitary spaces of varied size (fig. 12-30). These cavities have ragged walls lined by tumor cells, sometimes with polypoid or papillary projections, and are filled with clotted blood and tumor debris. Reticulin fibers and less often, collagen fibers, may support the tumor cells (fig. 12-31). Perithelial cells reactive to alpha-smooth muscle actin antibody may also be present (fig. 12-32). The tumor cells are sometimes packed solidly in nodules that resemble fibrosarcoma (fig. 12-33). Invasion of terminal hepatic venules and portal vein branches (fig. 12-34) leads to progressive obstruction of the lumen, and readily explains the frequently encountered areas of hemorrhage, infarction, and necrosis (fig. 12-35). Hematopoietic activity is observed in the majority of tumors (63), although in one study it was considered to be a feature most typical of Thorotrast-related cases (fig. 12-36) (103).

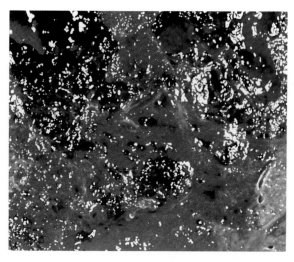

Figure 12-27
ANGIOSARCOMA
Dark, red-brown cavitary lesions formed by the tumor are scattered in this close-up of a liver section. Note also yellowish-tan tumor foci.

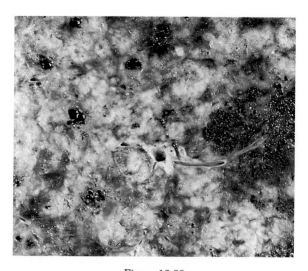

Figure 12-28
ANGIOSARCOMA
This section of the liver has a mottled tan and brown appearance.

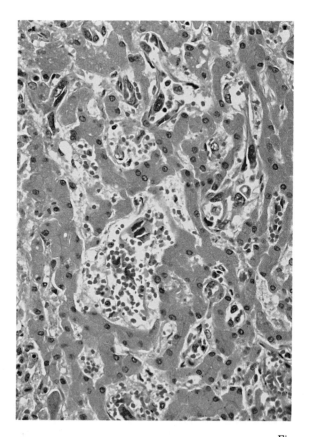

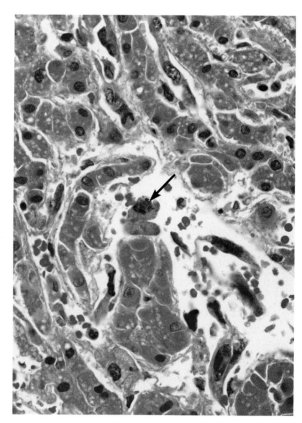

Figure 12-29
ANGIOSARCOMA
Left: Hepatic sinusoids are lined by malignant spindle cells with large hyperchromatic nuclei.
Right: A mitotic figure (arrow) is seen at higher magnification.

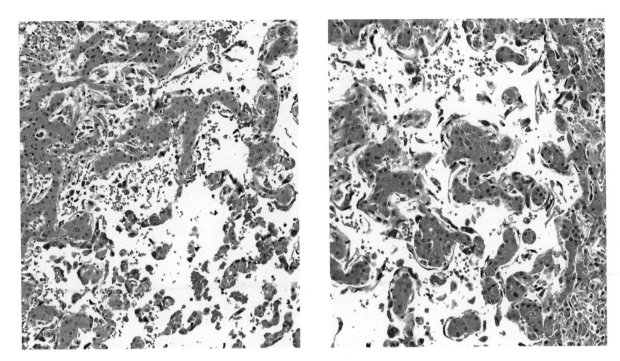

Figure 12-30
ANGIOSARCOMA
Segment of a ragged cavity formed by the tumor (left). Higher magnification of a tumor cavity (right). Detached liver plates surrounded by the tumor cells appear to be suspended in the cavity.

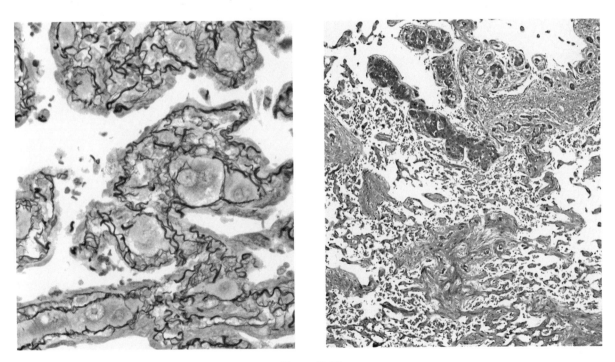

Figure 12-31
ANGIOSARCOMA
Hepatic plates disrupted by the tumor are separated from the tumor cells by irregularly dispersed reticulin fibers (left) (Manuel reticulin stain). This area of a tumor (right) shows collagen scaffolding (Masson trichrome stain).

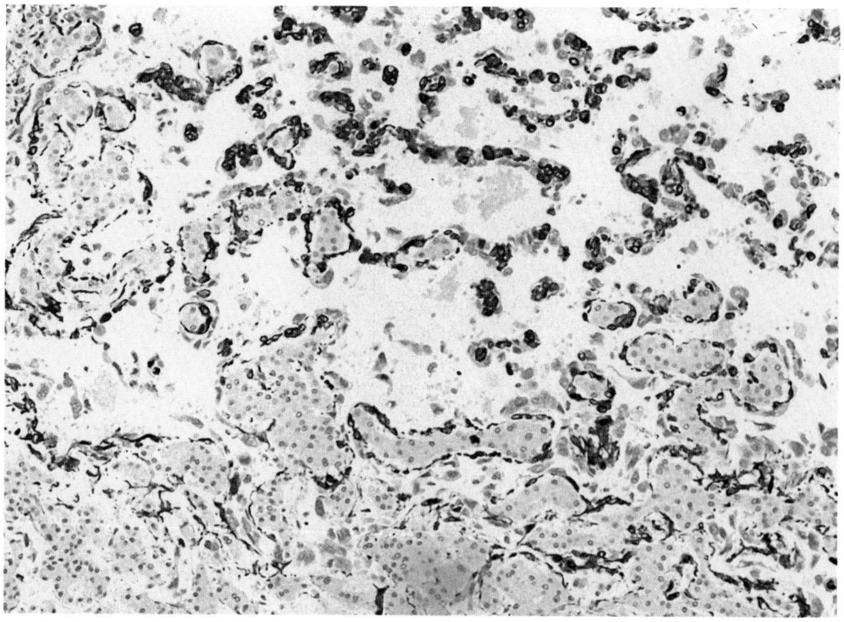

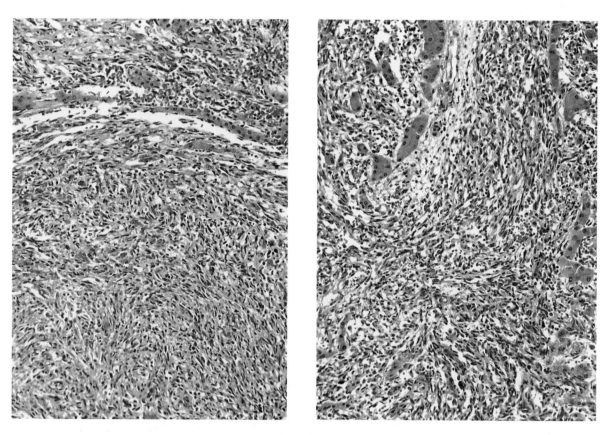

Figure 12-32
ANGIOSARCOMA
Alpha-smooth muscle actin–positive perithelial cells are demonstrated immunohistochemically.

Figure 12-33
ANGIOSARCOMA
Left: Solid fibrosarcoma-like area of the tumor consists of packed, malignant spindle cells. Such areas are never seen in the absence of more typical vascular areas (top).
Right: Higher magnification of same tumor.

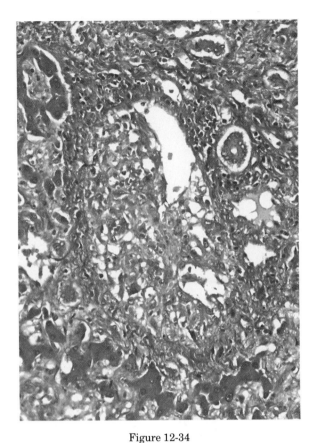

Figure 12-34
ANGIOSARCOMA
Tumor growth within a vein in a portal area (Masson trichrome stain).

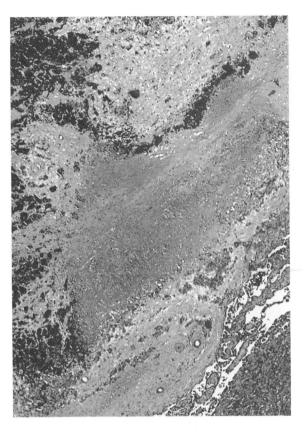

Figure 12-35
ANGIOSARCOMA
Area of infarction and hemorrhage. Viable tumor is present in the lower right corner.

The cells of angiosarcoma are spindle shaped, rounded, or irregular in outline, and often have ill-defined borders (fig. 12-37). The cytoplasm is lightly eosinophilic, and nuclei are hyperchromatic and elongated or irregular in shape. Nucleoli can be small, or large and eosinophilic. Large, bizarre nuclei and multinucleated cells may be seen, and mitotic figures are frequently identified. The spindled cells have ill-defined outlines, a lightly eosinophilic cytoplasm, and vesicular nuclei with blunt ends.

A precursor stage in the development of angiosarcoma has been observed in cases etiologically related to exposure to vinyl chloride, Thorotrast, and arsenic (37,86,100,102). It is characterized by foci of simultaneous activation of both hepatocytes and sinusoidal lining cells, with associated lesions in the sinusoids and perisinusoidal spaces. In our experience, the most striking precursor lesion is that affecting isolated sinusoidal lining cells that are hypertrophied and have large irregular and hyperchromatic nuclei (fig. 12-38). Vinyl chloride–associated lesions in humans are quite comparable to those induced experimentally in rodents (85). Additional light microscopic and ultrastructural studies of hepatic lesions in workers exposed to vinyl chloride (but who did not have angiosarcoma) have been reported (57,93).

Cases related to exposure to Thorotrast and vinyl chloride are often associated with considerable periportal and subcapsular fibrosis, and rarely, cirrhosis has been etiologically related to these two agents, as well as to arsenic. In Thorotrast-induced angiosarcomas the Thorotrast deposits are readily recognized in the reticuloendothelial cells or lying free in portal areas, Glisson's capsule, and the wall of portal vessels or terminal hepatic venules (fig. 12-39). The deposits are colorless and refractile, but in a hematoxylin and eosin–stained section they usually are pink-brown; they are not

299

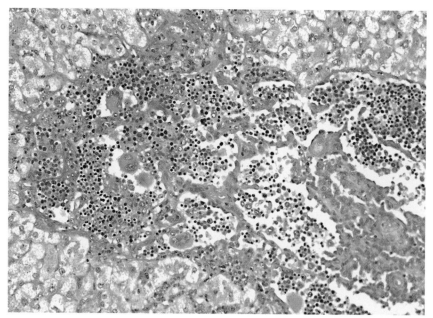

Figure 12-36
ANGIOSARCOMA
Marked extramedullary hematopoiesis (including several megakaryocytes) in the tumor (PAS stain after diastase digestion).

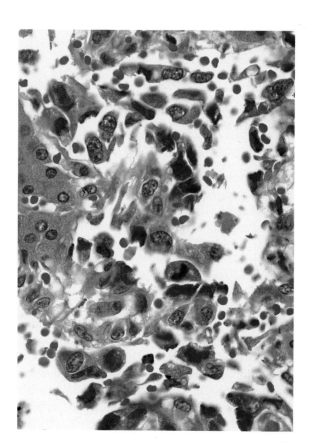
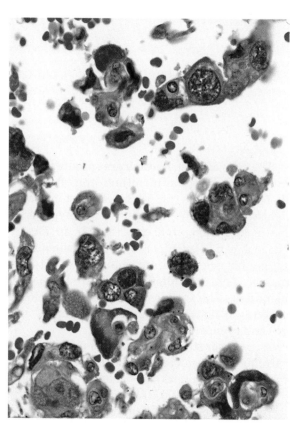

Figure 12-37
ANGIOSARCOMA
Left: Tumor cells exhibiting marked pleomorphism, nuclear hyperchromasia, and a mitotic figure.
Right: Higher magnification shows details of the tumor cells; two of the cells contain multiple nuclei.

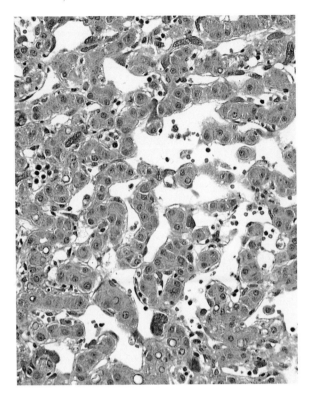

Figure 12-38
ANGIOSARCOMA
Isolated sinusoidal lining cells have enlarged, hyperchromatic nuclei.

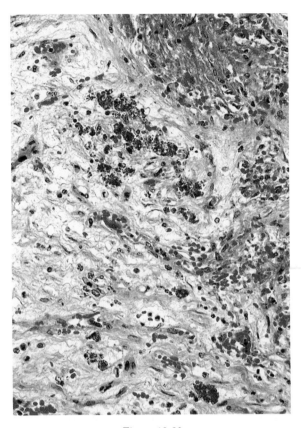

Figure 12-39
ANGIOSARCOMA
Brown, coarsely granular Thorotrast deposits in an area of fibrosis.

birefringent, but can be illuminated by phase contrast microscopy. The alpha emissions of the thorium dioxide in Thorotrast can be captured by autoradiography, appearing as short, dotted tracks. The particles are readily visualized by scanning electron microscopy of paraffin sections (fig. 12-40), and the element thorium can be definitively identified by energy dispersive X-ray microanalysis (fig. 12-41) (39,61,62).

Pediatric Angiosarcoma. This tumor is sufficiently distinct from angiosarcoma of the adult to merit separate consideration. Three small series of pediatric angiosarcomas (51,94,109), as well as a number of case reports, have been published (32,33,62,66,67,90,98). We now consider the type 2 infantile hemangioendothelioma of the liver of Dehner and Ishak (44) to be an angiosarcoma. A gross photograph of a pediatric angiosarcoma is illustrated in figure 12-42. In addition to the histopathologic features of adult angiosarcoma (fig. 12-43), the pediatric cases have a "kaposiform" spindle cell component similar to that of

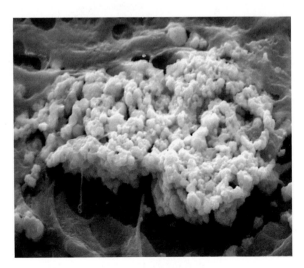

Figure 12-40
ANGIOSARCOMA
Three-dimensional view of Thorotrast aggregate shows particles of varied size (scanning electron micrograph).

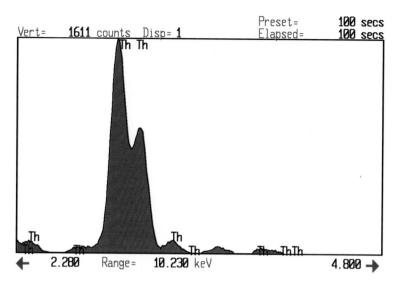

Figure 12-41
ANGIOSARCOMA
X-ray microanalysis of Thorotrast shows several peaks for the element thorium.

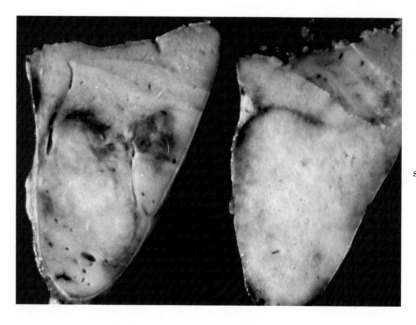

Figure 12-42
KAPOSIFORM ANGIOSARCOMA
A tan and gray-white tumor with scattered hemorrhages.

kaposiform hemangioendothelioma of soft tissues (46,56,82,104,113). Such kaposiform areas are often lobulated and are composed of spindle cells arranged in bundles, with scattered slit-like vascular spaces lined by flat endothelial cells (fig. 12-44). A whorl-like arrangement of cells, described as "glomeruloid foci" by Zukerberg et al. (113) is also seen (figs. 12-45, 12-46). Like Kaposi's sarcoma, the spindle cells express CD31 and CD34 (fig. 12-47) but not von Willebrand factor. Mitotic figures vary from a few to many (fig. 12-44).

Reticulin fibers surround the vascular channels (fig. 12-48) and many perithelial cells express alpha-smooth muscle actin (fig. 12-49). Another feature of the kaposiform areas is the presence of numerous, variably sized eosinophilic (hyaline) globules in the cytoplasm of the spindle cells and occasionally, extracellularly. These globules are PAS positive and resist diastase digestion (fig. 12-50). The cytoplasm of the spindle cells expresses alpha-1-antitrypsin and alpha-1-antichymotrypsin, but the globules do not. By scanning

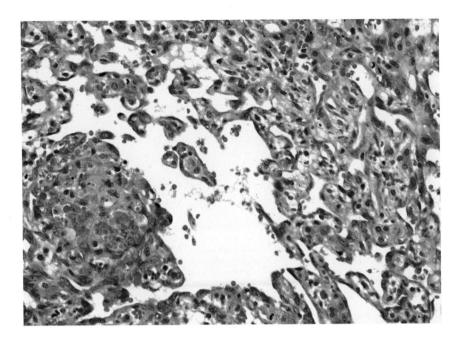

Figure 12-43
KAPOSIFORM
ANGIOSARCOMA
Classic angiosarcoma pattern.

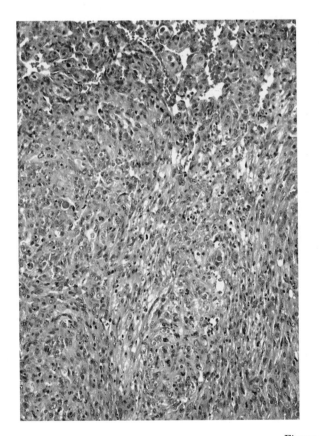
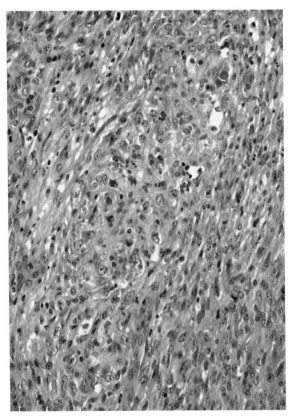

Figure 12-44
KAPOSIFORM ANGIOSARCOMA
Left: Spindle cell kaposiform area with numerous eosinophilic hyaline globules.
Right: Higher magnification of same tumor.

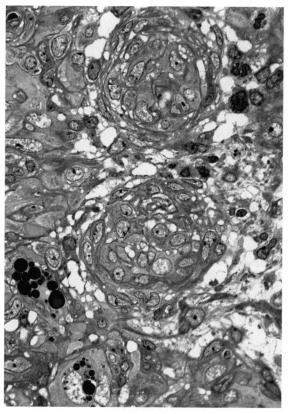

Figure 12-45
KAPOSIFORM ANGIOSARCOMA
Two "glomeruloid" foci with a whorled arrangement of tumor cells. Note the dark blue globules of varied size (1 μm-thick, Epon-embedded section stained with toluidine blue).

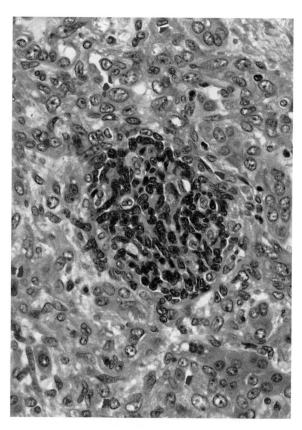

Figure 12-46
KAPOSIFORM ANGIOSARCOMA
Cells of a glomeruloid focus are more closely packed and have denser nuclei than the rest of the tumor.

Figure 12-47
KAPOSIFORM
ANGIOSARCOMA
Spindle cells, as well as the cells of a glomeruloid focus, show strong expression of CD34 (immunostain).

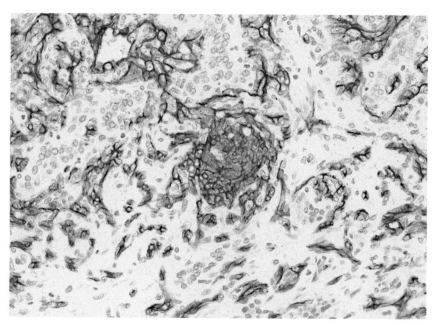

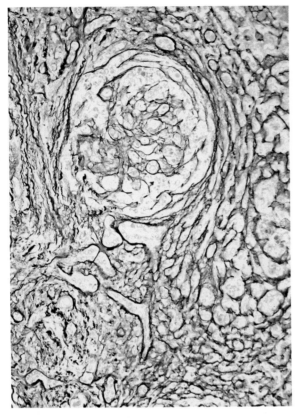

Figure 12-48
KAPOSIFORM ANGIOSARCOMA
A kaposiform area, including a glomeruloid focus, has a well-developed reticulin network (Manuel reticulin stain).

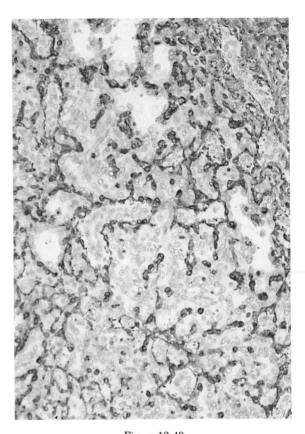

Figure 12-49
KAPOSIFORM ANGIOSARCOMA
A network of alpha-smooth muscle actin–positive cells surrounds the tumor cells in a kaposiform area (immunostain).

Figure 12-50
KAPOSIFORM ANGIOSARCOMA
Globules in the kaposiform areas are intensely PAS positive (PAS after diastase digestion).

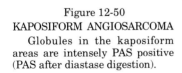
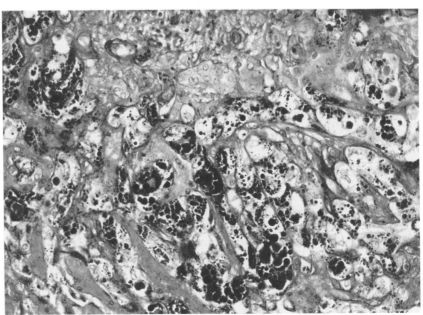

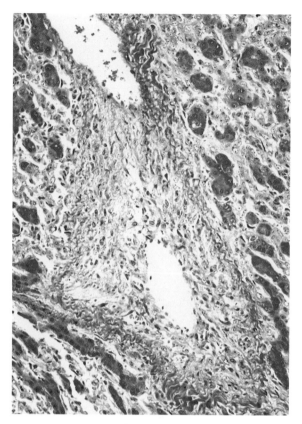

Figure 12-51
KAPOSIFORM ANGIOSARCOMA
A terminal hepatic venule in a kaposiform area is infiltrated by tumor cells (Masson trichrome stain).

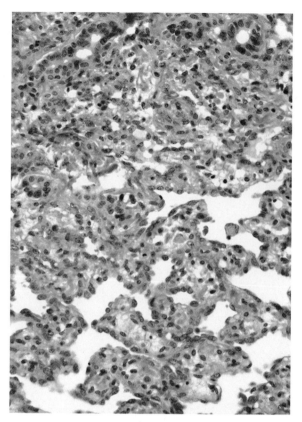

Figure 12-52
KAPOSIFORM ANGIOSARCOMA
An area of infantile hemangioendothelioma.

electron microscopy, the globules have a smooth external surface and a solid interior. Ultrastructurally, they are electron dense and sometimes heterogeneous; they resemble apoptotic bodies.

Kaposiform hemangioendothelioma of the retroperitoneum occurs in infancy and childhood (median age, 2 years; range, 5 months to 19 years) (99). There is, however, at least one report of a similar tumor in a 50-year-old woman (107). The angiosarcomas of the liver (with, in our opinion, kaposiform features) studied by Selby et al. (94) occurred in children between 18 months and 7 years of age (mean, 3.7 years). The retroperitoneal (but thus far not the hepatic) tumors have sometimes been associated with locally aggressive disease, lymphangiomatosis, and the Kasabach-Merritt syndrome (consumption coagulopathy) (113). Distant metastases have not been reported with the retroperitoneal tumors, but have been noted in several of the hepatic cases (94). Vascular inva-

sion is present in some of the tumors (fig. 12-51). Most of the children with angiosarcoma of the liver have died within 2 years; the mean survival period in the series of Selby et al. (94) was 10 months. Therapy, consisting of surgery, radiotherapy, chemotherapy, or combinations thereof, has been ineffective. There is convincing evidence that at least some of the hepatic angiosarcomas arise in a preexisting infantile hemangioendothelioma (fig. 12-52) (51,62,81,98,109).

It is our opinion that the pediatric angiosarcomas resemble the adult angiosarcomas in their morphology and behavior, but have some morphologic "kaposiform" features that are distinctive. We therefore propose calling such tumors, whether they arise in childhood, adolescence, or early adulthood, *kaposiform angiosarcoma*. The etiology of these tumors remains undetermined, but one patient had had heavy exposure to arsenic (2), a recognized cause of adult angiosarcoma.

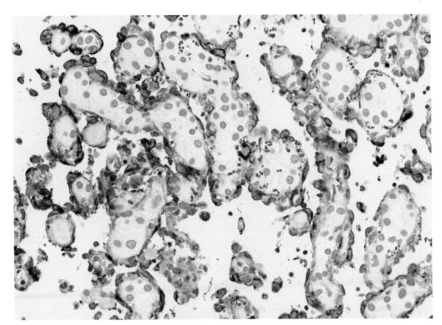

Figure 12-53
ANGIOSARCOMA
Strong expression of CD31 by the malignant cells lining the sinusoidal spaces. There is also strong expression of CD34 by the tumor cells (immunostain).

Immunohistochemical Findings. In our experience and that of others (55,76), von Willebrand factor may be identified in the tumor cells by immunohistologic techniques (fig. 12-53), although it was reported to be negative in the series of Kojiro et al. (69). Immunostaining with *Ulex europaeus* is more sensitive though less specific than that of von Willebrand factor (78). Other useful markers include CD31 and CD34; the former is believed to be the most sensitive immunostain by Miettinen et al. (78) (fig. 12-54).

Differential Diagnosis. Primary angiosarcoma cannot be differentiated from metastatic angiosarcoma. Differentiation from epithelioid hemangioendothelioma is discussed in an earlier section and is outlined in Table 12-2. Kaposi's sarcoma poses no problem in differential diagnosis since the tumor usually occurs in a patient with the acquired immunodeficiency syndrome and the lesions typically are localized to portal areas (see also Table 13-3). Angiosarcoma may require differentiation from other sarcomas, whether primary or metastatic. A needle biopsy specimen obtained from a solid area of angiosarcoma composed of compact malignant spindle cells could be mistaken for fibrosarcoma, or leiomyosarcoma. Other than tumor growth patterns and cytologic features, these tumors do not express endothelial cell markers (e.g., CD34), and leiomyosarcomas express smooth muscle cell markers such as alpha-smooth muscle actin.

Before leaving this section note should be made of the coexistence of angiosarcoma with one or more epithelial malignant tumors (hepatocellular carcinoma and cholangiocarcinoma). This has been reported with both Thorotrast- (64,68,85,108,111) and vinyl chloride-associated (45,83) angiosarcomas.

Pathogenesis. Analysis of angiosarcomas related to vinyl chloride exposure has shown an increased frequency of p53 mutations, with a mutational spectrum (A:T>T:A transversion) characteristic of chloroethylene oxide, a carcinogenic metabolite of vinyl chloride (60,97). Mutations are, however, uncommon in sporadic angiosarcomas (and those associated with Thorotrast), suggesting endogenous mechanisms in the induction of such cases (97). Angiosarcoma cells produce and secrete vascular endothelial growth factor that binds to its receptor on the tumor cells, thus promoting their proliferation (58).

Treatment and Prognosis. The majority of patients with angiosarcoma die in less than 6 months of diagnosis, usually from liver failure or abdominal bleeding. In a recent report of 67 patients and a review of the literature, Mark et al. (77) found that surgery plus radiation therapy offers the best chance for long-term control of angiosarcoma. The role of chemotherapy remains undefined.

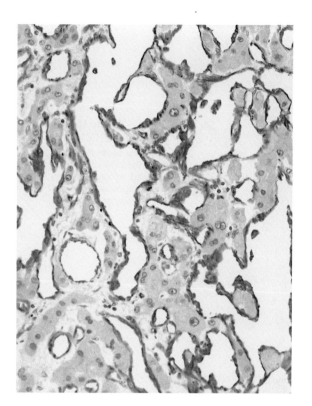
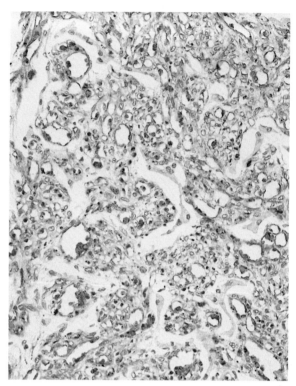

Figure 12-54
ANGIOSARCOMA
Tumor cells lining sinusoids express von Willebrand factor (immunostain).

KAPOSI'S SARCOMA

Definition. A malignant vascular neoplasm, characterized by spindle cells that line blood-filled slit-like spaces, typically portal in location.

Clinical Features. This entity has assumed importance in recent years because of its association with the acquired immunodeficiency syndrome (AIDS), but cases not related to AIDS occur sporadically in Europe and Africa, and in immunosuppressed patients (115). Involvement of the liver has been reported in 12 to 25 percent of fatal cases of AIDS (114,119,127), but does not appear to contribute to the morbidity and mortality of the disease. Definite functional hepatic impairment has not been recorded.

Gross and Microscopic Findings. Kaposi's sarcoma in the liver is visible grossly as irregular, variably sized, red-brown, spongiform lesions that resemble capillary hemangiomas (fig. 12-55). Histopathologically, the lesions are generally confined to the portal connective tissue, but the tumor may infiltrate the adjacent hepatic

parenchyma for short distances (fig. 12-56). Seven histologic patterns of Kaposi's sarcoma, forming a spectrum of cellular differentiation, were described by Ioachim et al. (121). The least differentiated spindle cells have large, plump, and sometimes irregular nuclei with occasional mitoses (figs. 12-57, 12-58). Hyaline globules that are PAS positive (fig. 12-59) and hemosiderin accumulation are found in the majority of cases (fig. 12-60). The nature of the globules is still in dispute; one suggestion is that they represent ingested erythrocytes (117). The spindle cells express the endothelial cell markers CD31 and CD34 (fig. 12-61), the latter being the most sensitive, thrombomodulin and endothelial adhesion molecule-1, and are therefore considered to be of vascular origin (121,130,134). Bcl-2 has been demonstrated immunohistochemically in AIDS-associated and classic Kaposi's sarcoma; the up regulation of Bcl-2 is considered important in the maintenance, growth, and progression of the sarcoma (126). There is also strong

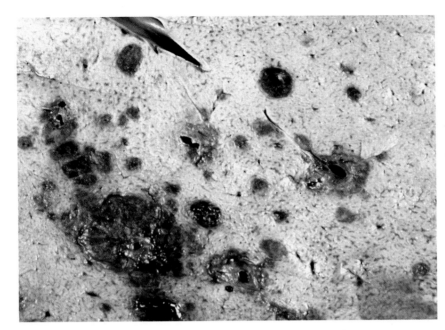

Figure 12-55
KAPOSI'S SARCOMA
This section of liver shows blue-black tumor foci in large portal areas, with confluence of some of the larger foci.

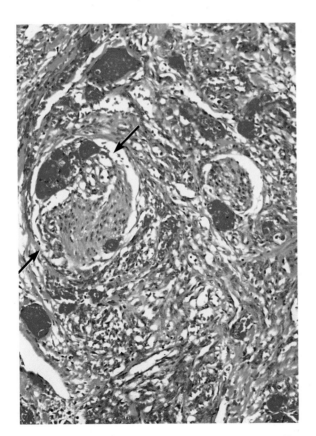
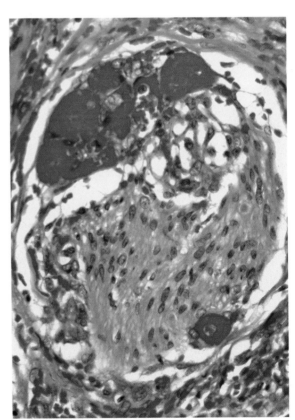

Figure 12-56
KAPOSI'S SARCOMA
Left: The tumor is composed of spindle cells and slit-like spaces. Note the perineural infiltration (arrows).
Right: Higher magnification of a nerve in a portal area infiltrated by the tumor cells.

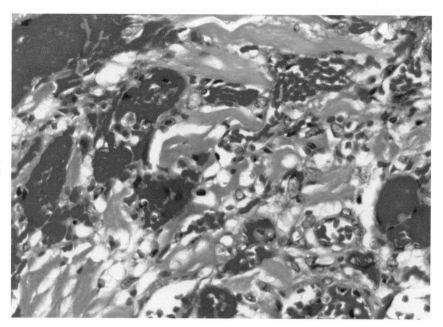

Figure 12-57
KAPOSI'S SARCOMA
High magnification of spindle
cells, some collagen fibers, and
hemosiderin (upper left).

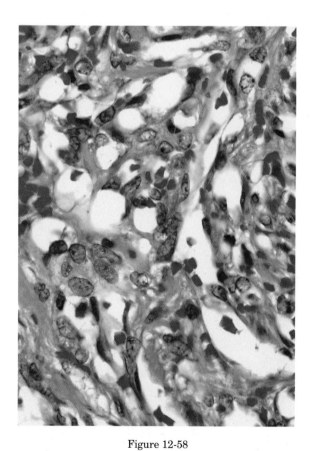

Figure 12-58
KAPOSI'S SARCOMA
Spindle cells have ill-defined outlines and vesicular,
round or ovoid nuclei.

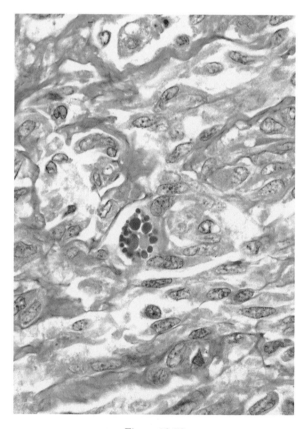

Figure 12-59
KAPOSI'S SARCOMA
Globules in a tumor cell are PAS positive (PAS after
diastase digestion).

expression of kinase insert domain-containing receptor (vascular permeability factor/vascular endothelial growth factor) in AIDS-associated Kaposi's sarcoma (116). This factor is believed to play an important, albeit incompletely understood, role in the pathogenesis of both benign and malignant vascular tumors (116). Also of probable pathogenetic significance is the expression of CD40 antigen by Kaposi's sarcoma tumor cells (120).

Etiology and Pathogenesis. A Kaposi sarcoma-associated herpesvirus (KSHV) has been reported by several groups of investigators; it is thought to play a causative role in the etiology of the disease (120,122,123,125,128,129,133a). It has not been detected in other vascular lesions, such as angiosarcoma (122). Furthermore, in most patients with Kaposi's sarcoma and AIDS, seroconversion to positivity for antibodies against KSHV-related nuclear antigens occurs before the clinical appearance of Kaposi's sarcoma; that

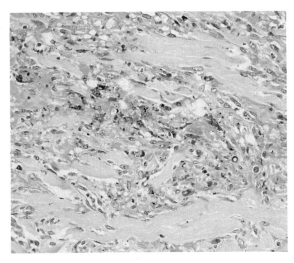

Figure 12-60
KAPOSI'S SARCOMA
Abundant hemosiderin-laden cells (Mallory stain for iron).

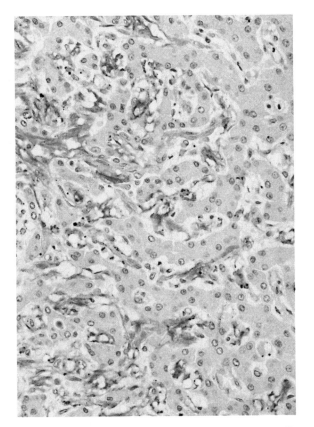

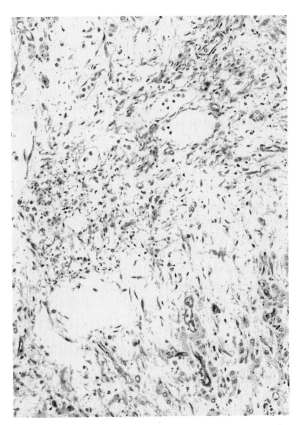

Figure 12-61
KAPOSI'S SARCOMA
Left: Tumor cells, CD34 positive, line vascular spaces (immunostain).
Right: Tumor spindle cells express CD34 (immunostain).

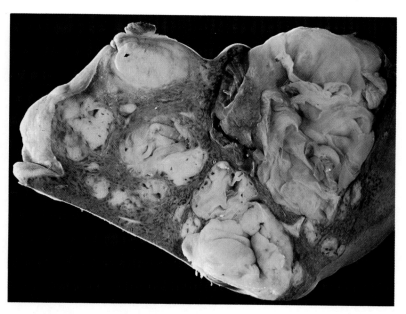

Figure 12-62
EMBRYONAL
RHABDOMYOSARCOMA
Section of liver showing multiple foci of
a light tan-colored tumor. The billowy appearance is due to luminal projections and
folds of the affected bile ducts. The green
discoloration of the liver between the
tumor masses is due to cholestasis.

finding supports the hypothesis that Kaposi's sarcoma results from infection with KSHV (118). Of great interest is the recent demonstration of KSHV-associated herpesvirus DNA sequences in prostate tissue and human semen, lending support to the probable transmission of the virus by sexual contact (124). The recent finding of two lymphatic endothelial cell markers (vascular endothelial growth factor receptor-3 and podoplanin) in Kaposi's sarcoma tumor cells suggests that these cells are related to or even derived from a lymphatic endothelial cell lineage (133).

Treatment. Treatment of Kaposi's sarcoma includes local therapy, radiotherapy, systemic chemotherapy, and use of zidovudine, interferon, granulocyte-macrophage colony-stimulating factor, and other agents (131,132).

The histopathologic features of the malignant vascular tumors of the liver are listed in Table 12-3 and compared with those of the benign vascular tumors.

EMBRYONAL RHABDOMYOSARCOMA

Definition. Embryonal rhabdomyosarcoma is a malignant neoplasm of primitive cells that show skeletal muscle differentiation. This tumor arises in the extrahepatic bile ducts but can involve the large septal ducts within the liver.

Clinical Features. Most patients are less than 5 years of age, but occasional tumors have been

diagnosed in older children and adults (135,136, 139–141,145). A primary intrahepatic rhabdomyosarcoma, forming a "collision" tumor with a hepatocellular carcinoma, was reported in a 62-years-old man (142). In children, embryonal rhabdomyosarcoma affects males and females equally. Patients usually present with intermittent obstructive jaundice, often with fever and hepatomegaly. A mistaken diagnosis of viral hepatitis can lead to delays in definitive therapy (145). In patients with the suggestive symptoms, ultrasonography and CT generally demonstrate a mass in the porta hepatis. Transhepatic cholangiography has been utilized for preoperative diagnosis (137).

Gross Findings. Affected bile ducts have a thick wall and narrow lumen; sections reveal a white glistening tumor (fig. 12-62). In some cases, soft or gelatinous, grape-like masses (sarcoma botryoides) may project into the lumen. Bile ducts proximal to the occluded segment are dilated, and the liver often has a green color from cholestasis.

Microscopic Findings. The polypoid tumor masses projecting into the lumen are covered by bile duct epithelium, but the surface may be ulcerated and inflamed. A dense mass of tumor cells (cambium layer) lies immediately subjacent to the epithelium. Tumor cells may be round, spindled, racquet shaped, or strap shaped (figs. 12-63–12-65). Nuclei are hyperchromatic and elongated, and have blunt ends. Mitotic figures are usually

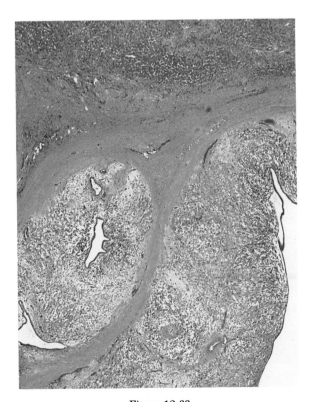

Figure 12-63
EMBRYONAL RHABDOMYOSARCOMA
The wall of the bile duct is extensively infiltrated by tumor, with marked narrowing of the lumen.

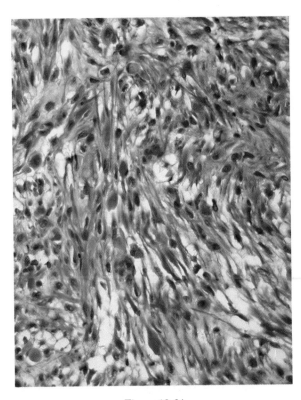

Figure 12-64
EMBRYONAL RHABDOMYOSARCOMA
The tumor cells are spindled or elongated and have an eosinophilic cytoplasm.

abundant. Cross-striations are generally identified with difficulty (fig. 12-66). Tumor cells may undergo marked cytologic differentiation after polychemotherapy (138). The stroma is myxoid with abundant acid mucopolysaccharide, but collagen fibers also may be scattered between tumor cells. Areas of inflammation, necrosis, and hemorrhage are often seen. Ultrastructural studies reveal both thick and thin myofilaments, with recognizable Z bands in some cells (140).

Immunohistochemical Findings. Myoglobin, myosin, muscle-specific actin, and desmin (fig. 12-67) may be identified immunohistologically in tumor cells. The sensitivities and specificities of these markers are discussed in two reviews (143,144). *MYF* (MyoD1) gene expression is the most recently reported and specific marker to date (143,144).

Treatment and Prognosis. Initial therapy is resection of the mass, leaving only microscopic or minimal gross residual tumor; continuity of bile flow is maintained by variations of the Roux-

en-Y jejunostomy (145). Operative cholangiography is invaluable in demonstrating the site of obstruction and verifying a functioning drainage procedure (145). Postoperative therapy includes multidrug chemotherapy and radiotherapy. Second-look surgery evaluates residual or recurrent disease. Of 10 patients treated by the aforementioned multidisciplinary approach, advocated by the Intergroup Rhabdomyosarcoma Study, 3 survived 3, 6 1/4, and 6 1/2 years from diagnosis (145).

EMBRYONAL SARCOMA

Definition. Embryonal sarcoma is a primitive neoplasm, unique to the liver, with characteristic clinical and histologic features. This tumor has most frequently been termed *undifferentiated sarcoma,* but has also been referred to by other synonyms such as *primary sarcoma,* and *malignant mesenchymoma* (151,169,170). The term malignant mesenchymoma, used by a number of authors (151,169,170), is justified only

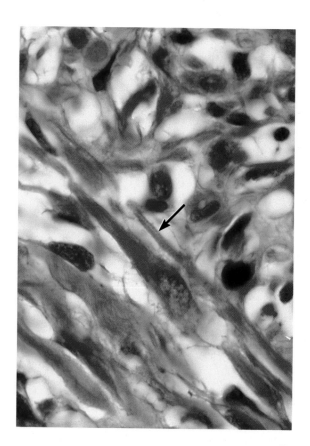

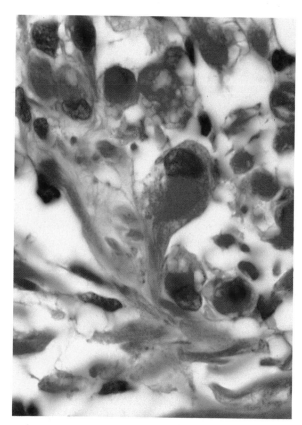

Figure 12-65
EMBRYONAL RHABDOMYOSARCOMA
Left: The cytoplasm of the cells is eosinophilic and the nuclei are hyperchromatic. One cell (arrow) shows faint cross striations.
Right: A tadpole-shaped tumor cell.

Figure 12-66
EMBRYONAL
RHABDOMYOSARCOMA
Cross striations are clearly visible in the cytoplasm of some cells (arrows).

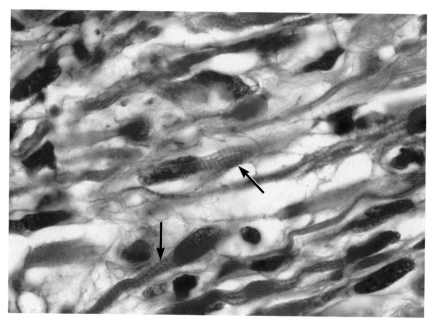

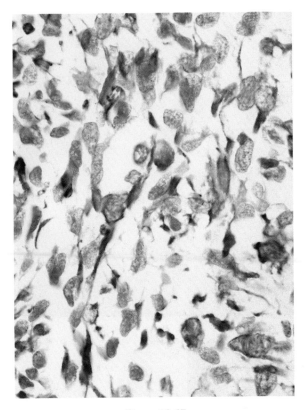

Figure 12-67
EMBRYONAL RHABDOMYOSARCOMA
Tumor cells strongly express desmin (immunostain).

if there is evidence of differentiation into two or more mesenchymal elements (other than fibrosarcoma), which is rarely the case (155,162,163,166).

Clinical Features. Embryonal sarcoma is quite rare. There were 40 cases from 1970 to 1992 in the AFIP files; it constituted 15 percent of all primary hepatic neoplasms in patients 5 to 20 years of age (149). In a survey of 1,237 primary hepatic tumors in childhood culled from the literature (up to 1993) by Weinberg and Finegold (177), 6 percent were sarcomas.

More than half the patients (52 percent) with embryonal sarcoma are between 6 and 10 years of age (171). Cases in adults are rare (153,164, 167,172). Abdominal swelling, with or without a palpable mass, and pain are the usual presenting findings. Some patients complain of various nonspecific gastrointestinal symptoms, fever, and weight loss. Rarely, the tumor invades the inferior vena cava and grows into the right atrium, presenting clinically as a primary intracardiac tumor (155). Leukocytosis with a shift to the left

is a common finding. Liver tests are abnormal in one third to half the patients, the most frequent abnormality being a slight increase of the serum alkaline phosphatase activity. Alpha-fetoprotein values are in the normal range.

Radiologic findings reflect the spectrum of solid and cystic features characteristic of the tumor (168). Sonography typically demonstrates a large mass that may be predominantly solid (with many small anechoic spaces) or cystic. CT reveals a hypodense mass with hyperdense septa of variable thickness, and a dense peripheral rim corresponding to the fibrous pseudocapsule. Angiographically, the tumor is usually hypovascular, but hypervascular and avascular patterns infrequently occur. Differentiation radiologically from mesenchymal hamartoma may be difficult. The older age and more frequent symptomatic presentation of patients with embryonal sarcoma are helpful in diagnosis. A definitive diagnosis requires liver biopsy, which is generally performed at laparotomy. One reported case was diagnosed at peritoneoscopy by guided biopsy (154).

Gross Findings. The majority of embryonal sarcomas are located in the right lobe of the liver. Most measure 10 to 20 cm in diameter, and weigh an average of 1,310 g (171). They are usually globular and well-demarcated, but encapsulation is uncommon. The cut surface is variegated, with solid, glistening, gray-white tumor tissue alternating with cystic gelatinous areas, red and yellow areas of hemorrhage and necrosis, or both (figs. 12-68, 12-69).

Microscopic Findings. A fibrous pseudocapsule may separate the tumor from the adjacent compressed parenchyma. The more peripheral areas typically contain entrapped bile ducts, which can be dilated (figs. 12-70–12-72), and sometimes hepatic parenchymal elements (fig. 12-71). The tumor cells are stellate or spindle shaped and have ill-defined outlines (figs. 12-72, 12-73). They may be compactly or loosely arranged, with an abundant mucopolysaccharide matrix, but areas with a more fibrous stroma are also seen in most tumors. Tumor cells often show marked anisonucleosis with hyperchromasia and sometimes bizarre giant cells; mitoses are usually abundant (figs. 12-74, 12-75). A characteristic feature is the presence of multiple, varying sized eosinophilic globules in the cytoplasm (fig. 12-75); these are PAS positive and resist diastase digestion (fig.

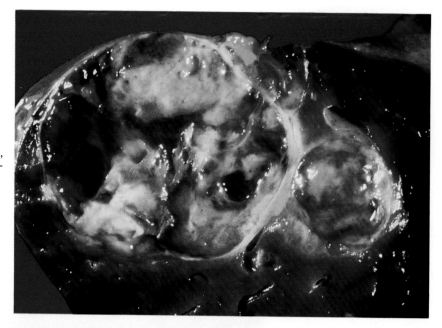

Figure 12-68
EMBRYONAL SARCOMA
A section of liver shows solid, light tan tumor and areas of hemorrhage and cystic degeneration.

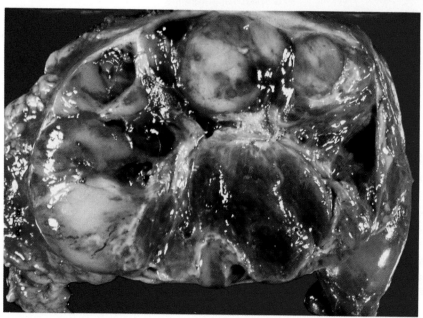

Figure 12-69
EMBRYONAL SARCOMA
This tumor is lobulated and shows solid, yellow-tan areas, as well as necrotic and hemorrhagic foci.

12-75). Ultrastructurally, the globules vary in size and electron density, and are lysosomal. Hematopoietic activity is observed in half the tumors. Hemorrhage and necrosis are often present.

Immunohistochemical Findings. The neoplastic cells may be reactive to antibodies to alpha-1-antitrypsin, alpha-1-antichymotrypsin, and vimentin (fig. 12-76) (146,147,160,161). Occasional tumors express cytokeratin (150,161). Expression of alpha-1-antitrypsin, immunoglob-

ulins, and albumin by the globules in the tumor cells led Abramowsky et al. (146) to conclude that they may represent entrapped serum proteins. On the basis of their ultrastructural characteristics it is our opinion that they represent apoptotic bodies, presumably phagocytosed by the tumor cells.

Ultrastructural Findings. There is no evidence of cellular differentiation under the light microscope, but ultrastructural and immunohistochemical studies in some cases have shown

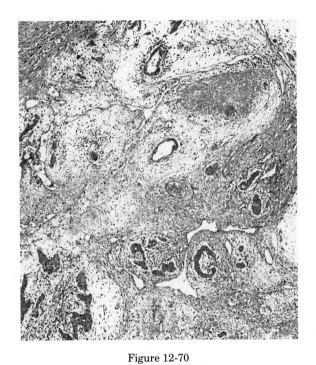

Figure 12-70
EMBRYONAL SARCOMA
Scattered liver plates of varied shapes, as well as bile ducts, are scattered among the sarcomatous elements.

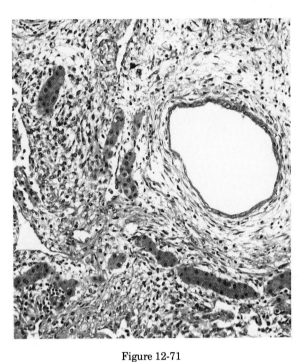

Figure 12-71
EMBRYONAL SARCOMA
Higher magnification of liver plates and bile ducts (asterisks) surrounded by the sarcomatous cells.

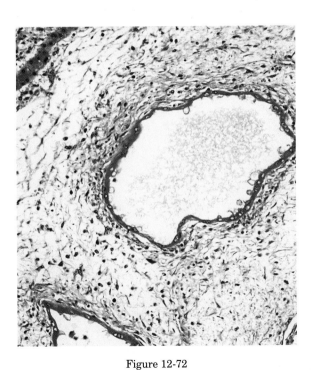

Figure 12-72
EMBRYONAL SARCOMA
Bile ducts in the tumor are cystically dilated; some of the cells have blebs that project into the lumen.

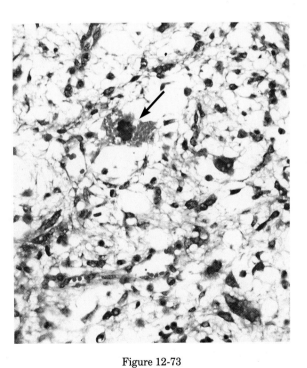

Figure 12-73
EMBRYONAL SARCOMA
The tumor cells are separated by a myxoid matrix. Note the marked anisonucleosis and hyperchromasia. One cell (arrow) contains numerous eosinophilic globules.

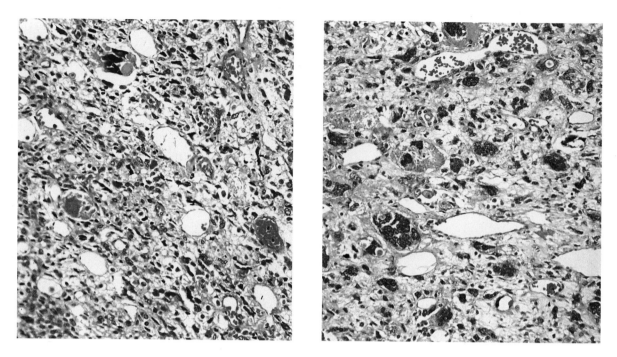

Figure 12-74
EMBRYONAL SARCOMA

Left: Tumor cells exhibit marked nuclear pleomorphism and hyperchromasia, and some are multinucleated.
Right: Higher magnification illustrates multinucleated tumor giant cells.

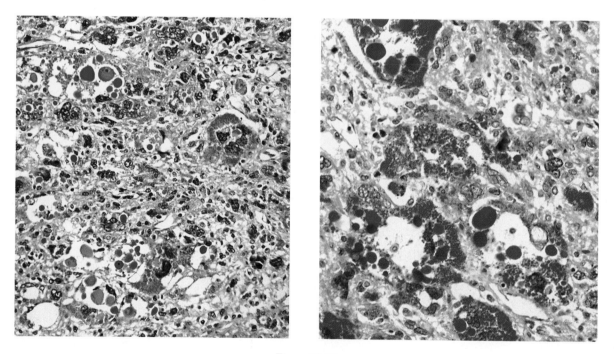

Figure 12-75
EMBRYONAL SARCOMA

Left: Numerous eosinophilic globules of varied size are present in tumor cells and extracellularly; note the nuclear pleomorphism and hyperchromasia.
Right: Globules are intensely PAS positive and exhibit marked variation in size (PAS stain after diastase digestion).

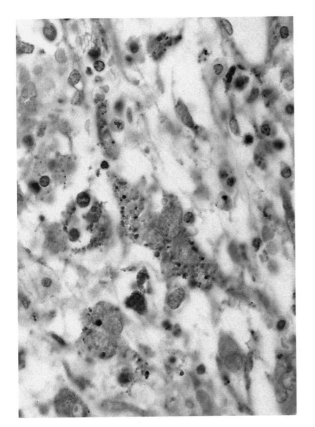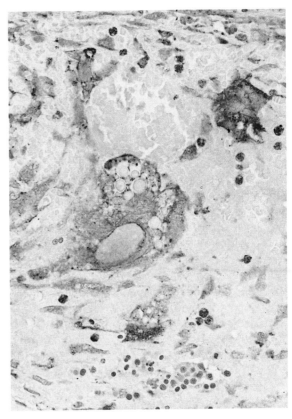

Figure 12-76
EMBRYONAL SARCOMA

Left: Tumor cells express alpha-1-antitrypsin; some of the smaller globules are immunostained by antibodies to alpha-1-antitrypsin (immunostain).

Right: The large globules are not immunoreactive to the antibodies (immunostain).

fibroblastic, rhabdomyoblastic, and leiomyoblastic differentiation (fig. 12-77) (155,156,160, 161,165,166). In view of these findings we concur with the opinion expressed by Parham et al. (165) that the term embryonal sarcoma is preferable to "undifferentiated" sarcoma since these tumors may display partial differentiation.

Etiology. Little is known of possible inducing or promoting factors in embryonal sarcoma, other than one report of a 19-year-old patient who had been exposed prenatally to phenytoin (148). The possibility of origin of embryonal sarcoma from mesenchymal hamartoma (see chapter 4), first suggested by Stanley et al. (170), appears to be confirmed in two cases (152,163a).

Treatment and Prognosis. In the series of Stocker and Ishak (171), the prognosis of patients with embryonal sarcoma was found to be very poor, with a median survival time of less than 1 year after diagnosis. Since then survival

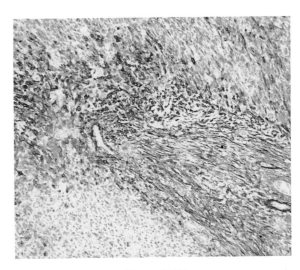

Figure 12-77
EMBRYONAL SARCOMA

Clusters of cells in this tumor express alpha-smooth muscle actin.

has greatly improved, with some patients living 5 or more years after combined modality treatment (157–159,163,169,173–176a).

OTHER MALIGNANT MESENCHYMAL TUMORS

Fibrosarcoma

Fibrosarcoma is a rare tumor of the liver (178–183,184a–190). The ages of the patients have ranged from 30 to 73 years (median, 55 years), most of whom (85 percent) are males. One tumor developed in a donor liver that had been transplanted into a 4-year-old girl 2 years previously, who had been treated with cyclosporine (182). Symptoms and signs are nonspecific and the diagnosis is established by biopsy. The tumor may be associated with severe hypoglycemia (183,188). Hemoperitoneum from rupture is rare. The prognosis is very poor, although several patients have survived from 1 to 3 years following resection with or without radiation therapy.

Fibrosarcoma is often large at the time of diagnosis; one of the largest tumors weighed more than 7 kg (184a). It is firm to rubbery in consistency and has a smooth or irregular surface. The cut surface reveals grayish white tissue, which can display a whorled appearance. Foci of necrosis and hemorrhage, sometimes with cystic degeneration, are often seen. Microscopically, the tumor is composed of spindle-shaped cells arranged in interlacing bundles, with the typical "herringbone" pattern in some areas. Varying numbers of collagen and reticulin fibers arise from, and intermingle with, the tumor cells. The nuclei are hyperchromatic and elongated, and have pointed ends; mitotic activity is variable. The tumor cells express vimentin. Collagen types I and IV have been demonstrated in the neoplastic matrix (184).

Leiomyosarcoma

Leiomyosarcoma is also a rare tumor of the liver. In a review of the literature until 1992, 60 cases were found by Gates et al. (192). These did not include over 50 leiomyosarcomas of the inferior vena cava, tumors occurring in children or adults with human immunodeficiency virus infection (194,199a,199b,204), or tumors developing in liver allografts in pediatric patients (199). Mingoli et al. (196) reviewed 218 leiomyosarcomas of the inferior vena cava in the world literature; 15 other cases have been reported since then (193,200). We believe that tumors previously reported as "leiomyosarcoma" of the ligamentum teres (193b,197, 203) are not leiomyosarcomas but actually related to angiomyolipomas (chapter 4), since they express melanocytic markers (HMB-45 and melan-A) as well as smooth muscle actin (191a,202a).

The intrahepatic leiomyosarcomas occur equally in men and women (192), but those arising in the inferior vena cava are more frequent in women (202). The mean age of presentation is 52 years. Symptoms and signs include an upper abdominal swelling or mass, abdominal pain, and weight loss. Fever at onset is rare. Leiomyosarcomas arising in the hepatic veins or inferior vena cava can lead to the Budd-Chiari syndrome (202). The mean survival time for patients with untreated intrahepatic leiomyosarcoma is less than 1 year. Metastatic disease occurs in about 40 percent of cases (192). The best outcome is that for patients treated with a combination of surgery and chemotherapy, with a mean survival or follow-up period of 3.3 years (192). A reasonably long-term survival was reported recently in a series of 14 patients with leiomyosarcoma of the inferior vena cava (192a): aggressive surgical management combined with adjuvant therapy (chemotherapy and radiation) resulted in a 5-year cumulative survival rate of 53 percent.

Primary leiomyosarcomas of the liver are usually solitary and can attain a large size (fig. 12-78). They are firm to rubbery, with a cut surface that is pinkish white with yellow areas of necrosis or dark red hemorrhagic foci (fig. 12-79). Histopathologically, they are composed of intersecting bundles of elongated, spindle-shaped cells (figs. 12-80–12-83). The lightly eosinophilic cytoplasm may display faint longitudinal striations. Nuclei are hyperchromatic and elongated, and have blunt ends. Mitotic activity is variable. Immunohistochemically, tumor cells express desmin, muscle-specific actin, and alpha-smooth muscle actin (fig. 12-84). Immunoreactivity for cytokeratin and epithelial membrane antigen has also been demonstrated in some leiomyosarcomas (195). Recently, a monoclonal antibody 1H1, anticortactin, has been found useful in diagnosis (198). Ultrastructurally, the cells have thin myofilaments, cytoplasmic dense bodies, marginal dense

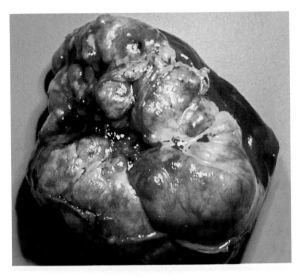

Figure 12-78
LEIOMYOSARCOMA
External surface of bulging, lobulated tumor.

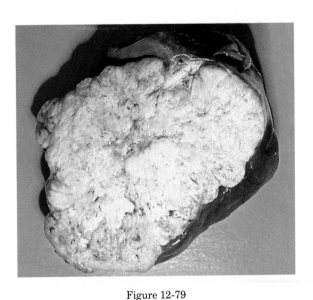

Figure 12-79
LEIOMYOSARCOMA
Section of tumor depicted in figure 12-78. The tumor is sharply demarcated and bulges from the plane of the section. It has a gray-tan, solid surface with a white area of necrosis.

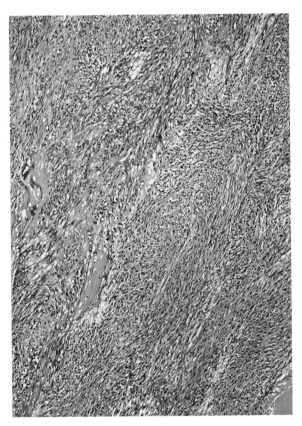

Figure 12-80
LEIOMYOSARCOMA
Intersecting fascicles of spindle cells.

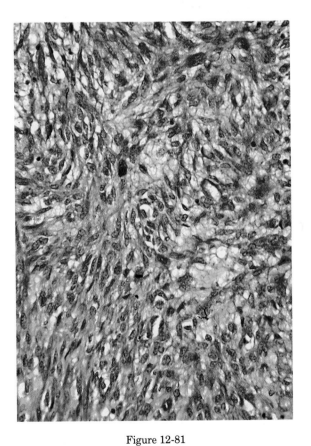

Figure 12-81
LEIOMYOSARCOMA
High magnification shows hyperchromasia and nuclear pleomorphism. The nuclei are oval or elongated with blunt ends.

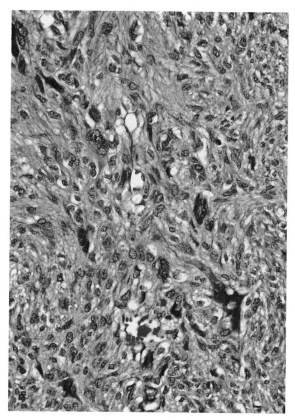

Figure 12-82
LEIOMYOSARCOMA
Another field from the same tumor depicted in figure 12-81 showing marked pleomorphism of the cells, some of which are multinucleated.

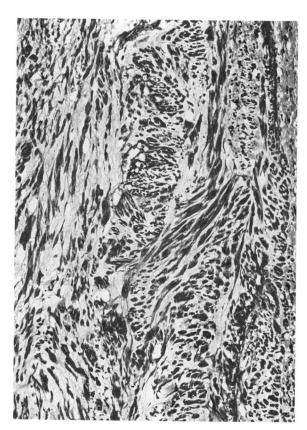

Figure 12-83
LEIOMYOSARCOMA
Intersecting fascicles of tumor cells are well demonstrated in this Masson trichrome-stained section. Note the brick-red color of the cytoplasm of the tumor cells, and the sparsity of collagen fibers in the matrix.

plaques, a basal lamina, and pinocytotic vesicles. Chromosomal abnormalities (both numerical and structural) have been described, but are of little diagnostic relevance (202). Tumor suppressor genes and related molecules in leiomyosarcoma of soft tissues were studied recently by Dei Tos et al. (191). Abnormalities involving the Rb-cyclin D pathway were detected in 90 percent of their cases, in contrast to higher rates of p53 gene and protein, and MDM2 protein abnormalities reported in other types of sarcoma.

Etiologic factors in leiomyosarcoma are largely unknown. The cases in patients with AIDS are believed to be linked to Epstein-Barr virus infection (194,199a). One leiomyosarcoma, arising synchronously with a cholangiocarcinoma, was related to Thorotrast use (201).

Malignant Fibrous Histiocytoma

Malignant fibrous histiocytoma (MFH) is an exceptionally uncommon primary tumor of the liver. Only a few cases have been reported to date (205,206,208,208a,209,210–212). A possible relationship of this tumor to embryonal sarcoma has been raised in one case report (211a). The subtypes described in the soft tissue tumors—storiform, pleomorphic, myxoid, giant cell, inflammatory, and angiomatoid—have been found in primary hepatic MFH. The histogenesis of MFH remains uncertain. In one study, the tumor cells were found to express several types of intermediate filaments, suggesting heterogeneity of the tumor (213). In another study, 15 of 22 MFHs expressed markers of smooth muscle differentiation, again suggesting that the tumor is

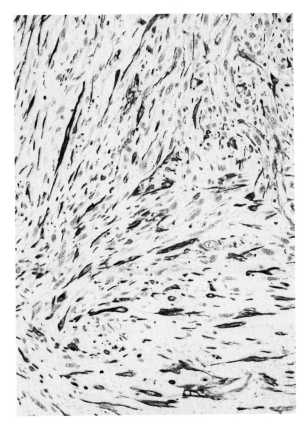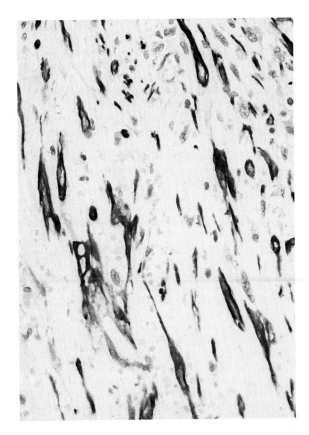

Figure 12-84
LEIOMYOSARCOMA
Left: Tumor cells exhibit strong immunoreactivity to antibodies to alpha-smooth muscle actin (immunostain).
Right: Another field shows similar immunoreactivity to smooth muscle actin (immunostain).

not a unique entity (214). Brooks (207) has hypothesized that MFH is the final common pathway for some types of sarcoma, and is the result of tumor progression or "dedifferentiation." On the basis of experimental data it is now clear that the histiocyte-like cells of MFH are not a neoplastic component; rather, they are macrophages attracted by tumor-derived monocyte chemotactants, while the tumor cells proper are of fibroblastic lineage and are differentiated from mesenchymal cells (215).

Other Primary Sarcomas

Other primary sarcomas, such as *liposarcoma* (79a), *osteogenic sarcoma* (218,220), *malignant mesenchymoma* (217,219), and *malignant schwannoma* (216, 216a,221), are too rare to warrant discussion.

REFERENCES

Introduction

1. Carriaga MT, Henson DE. Liver, gallbladder, extrahepatic bile ducts, and pancreas. Cancer 1995;75:171–90.
2. Edmondson HA, Peters RL. Neoplasms of the liver. In: Schiff L, Schiff ER, eds. Diseases of the liver, 5th ed. Philadelphia: JB Lippincott, 1982:1101–57.
2a. Forbes A, Portmann B, Johnson P, Williams R. Hepatic sarcomas in adults: a review of 25 cases. Gut 1987;28:668–74.
3. Goodman ZD. Nonparenchymal and metastatic malignant tumors of the liver. In: Haubrich WS, Schaffner F, eds. Bockus gastroenterology, 5th ed., vol. 3. Philadelphia: WB Saunders, 1995:2488–500.
4. Shin P, Ohmi S, Sakurai M. Hepatocellular carcinoma combined with hepatic sarcoma. Acta Pathol Jpn 1981;31:815–24.

Epithelioid Hemangioendothelioma

5. Anthony PP, Ramani P. Endothelial markers in malignant vascular tumours of the liver: superiority of QB-END/10 over Von Willebrand factor and Ulex europaeus agglutinin 1. J Clin Pathol 1991;44:29–32.

6. Bancel B, Patricot LM, Caillon P, et al. Hémangioendothéliome épithélioide hépatique. Un cas avec transplantation hépatique. Revue de al littérature. Ann Pathol 1993;13:23–8.

7. Cobden I, Johri S, Terry G, et al. Hepatic epithelioid haemangioendothelioma: difficult name, difficult diagnosis? Postgr Med J 1988;64:128–31.

8. Dail DH, Liebow AA, Gmelich JT, et al. Intravascular, bronchiolar, and alveolar tumor of the lung. An analysis of twenty cases of a peculiar sclerosing endothelial tumor. Cancer 1983;51:452–4.

9. Dean PJ, Haggitt RC, O'Hara CJ. Malignant epithelioid hemangioendothelioma of the liver in young women. Relationship to oral contraceptive use. Am J Surg Pathol 1985;9:695–704.

10. Demetris AJ, Minervini M, Raikow RB, Lee RG. Hepatic epithelioid hemangioendothelioma: biological questions based on pattern of recurrence in an allograft and tumor immunophenotype. Am J Surg Pathol 1997;21:263–70.

11. Dietze O, Davies SE, Williams R, Portmann B. Malignant epithelioid haemangioendothelioma of the liver: a clinicopathological and histochemical study of 12 cases. Histopathology 1989;15:225–37.

12. Ellis GL, Kratochvil FJ. Epithelioid hemangioendothelioma of the head and neck: a clinicopathologic report of twelve cases. Oral Surg, Oral Med, Oral Pathol 1986;61:61–8.

13. Fukayama M, Nihei Z, Takizawa T, Kawaguchi K, Harada H, Koike M. Malignant epithelioid hemangioendothelioma of the liver, spreading through the hepatic veins. Virchows Arch [A] 1984;404:275–87.

14. Furui S, Itai Y, Ohtomo K, et al. Hepatic epithelioid hemangioendothelioma: report of 5 cases. Radiology 1989;171:63–8.

15. Gelin M, Van de Stadt J, Rickaert F, et al. Epithelioid hemangioendothelioma of the liver following contact with vinyl chloride. Recurrence after orthotopic liver transplantation. J Hepatol 1989;8:99–106.

16. Holley MP, Cuschieri A. Epithelioid hemangioendothelioma of the liver: objective response in hepatic intra-arterial 5-FU. Eur J Surg Oncol 1987;15:73–8.

17. Ishak KG, Sesterhenn IA, Goodman ZD, Rabin L, Stromeyer FW. Epithelioid hemangioendothelioma of the liver: a clinicopathologic and follow-up study of 32 cases. Hum Pathol 1984;15:839–52.

18. Kawabe T, Tagawa K, Unuma T, et al. Hepatic epithelioid hemangioendothelioma in a young female. Dig Dis Sci 1987;32:1422–7.

19. Kelleher MB, Iwatsuki S, Sheahan DG. Epithelioid hemangioendothelioma of liver: clinicopathologic correlation of 10 cases treated by orthotopic liver transplantation. Am J Surg Pathol 1989;13:999–1008.

20. Makhlouf HR, Ishak KG, Goodman ZD. Epithelioid hemangioendothelioma of the liver: a clinicopathologic study of 137 cases. Cancer 1999;85:562–82.

21. Marino IR, Todo S, Tzakis AG, et al. Treatment of hepatic epithelioid hemangioendothelioma with liver transplantation. Cancer 1988;62:2079–84.

22. Miettinen M, Lindenmayer E, Chaubal A. Endothelial cell markers CD31, CD34, and BNH9 antibody in H- and Y-antigens—evaluation of their specificity and sensitivity in the diagnosis of vascular tumors and comparison with von Willebrand factor. Mod Pathol 1994;7:82–90.

23. Miller WJ, Dodd GD III, Federle MP, Baron RL. Epithelioid hemangioendothelioma of the liver: imaging findings with pathologic correlation. AJR Am J Roentgenol 1992;159:53–7.

24. Rojter S, Villamil FG, Petrovic LM, et al. Malignant vascular tumors of the liver presenting as liver failure and portal hypertension. Liver Transpl Surg 1995;1:156–61.

25. Scoazec JY, Lamy P, Degott C, et al. Epithelioid hemangioendothelioma of the liver: diagnostic features and role of liver transplantation. Gastroenterology 1988;94:1447–53.

26. Terada T, Nakanuma Y, Hoso M, Kono N, Watanabe K. Hepatic epithelioid hemangioendothelioma in primary biliary cirrhosis [Letter]. Gastroenterology 1989;97:810–1.

27. Terg R, Bruguera M, Campo E, Hojman R, Levi D, Podesta A. Epithelioid hemangioendothelioma of the liver: a report of two cases. Liver 1988;8:105–10.

28. Walsh MM, Hytiroglou P, Thung SN, et al. Epithelioid hemangioendothelioma of the liver mimicking Budd-Chiari syndrome. Arch Pathol Lab Med 1998;122:846–8.

29. Weiss SW, Enzinger FM. Epithelioid hemangioendothelioma: a vascular tumor often mistaken for a carcinoma. Cancer 1982;50:970–81.

30. Weiss SW, Ishak KG, Dail DH, Sweet DE, Enzinger FM. Epithelioid hemangioendothelioma and related lesions. Diagn Histopathol 1986;3:259–87.

31. Yokoyama T, Todo S, Iwatsuki S, Starzl TE. Liver transplantation in the treatment of primary liver cancer. Hepatogastroenterology 1990;37:188–93.

Angiosarcoma

32. Adam YG, Huvos AG, Hadju SI. Malignant vascular tumors of liver. Ann Surg 1972;175:375–8.

33. Alt B, Hafez GR, Trigg M, Shahidi NT, Gilbert EF. Angiosarcoma of the liver and spleen in an infant. Pediatr Pathol 1985;4:331–9.

34. Anonymous. Angiosarcoma of the liver: a growing problem? Br Med J 1981;282:504–5.

35. Baker HC, Paget GE, Davson J. Haemochromatosis of the liver. J Pathol Bacteriol 1956;72:173–82.

36. Baxter PJ, Langlands AO, Anthony PP, Macsween RN, Scheuer PJ. Angiosarcoma of the liver: a marker tumour for the late effects of thorotrast in Great Britain. Br J Cancer 1980;41:446–53.

37. Berk PD, Martin JF, Young RS. Vinyl chloride-associated liver disease. Ann Intern Med 1976;84:717–31.

38. Blendis LM, Smith PM, Laurie BW, Stephens MK, Evans WD. Portal hypertension in vinyl chloride monomer workers: a hemodynamic study. Gastroenterology 1978;75:206–11.

39. Bowen JH, Woodward BH, Mossler JA, Ingram P, Shelburne JD. Energy dispersive X-ray detection of thorium dioxide. Arch Pathol Lab Med 1980;104:459–61.

40. Brady J, Liberatore F, Harper P, et al. Angiosarcoma of the liver: an epidemiologic study. JNCI 1977;59:1383–5.

41. Da Motta CL, Da Silva Horta J, Tavares MH. Prospective epidemiological study of Thorotrast-exposed patients in Portugal. Environ Res 1979;18:152–73.

42. Daneshmend TK, Scott GL, Bradfield JW. Angiosarcoma of liver associated with phenelzine. Br Med J 1979;6:1679.

43. Dannaher CL, Tamburro CL, Yam LT. Occupational carcinogenesis: the Louisville experience with vinyl chloride-associated hepatic angiosarcoma. Am J Med 1981;70:279–87.

44. Dehner LP, Ishak KG. Vascular tumors of the liver in infants and children: a study of 30 cases and review of the literature. Arch Pathol 1971;92:101–11.

45. Delore FC. Association d'un angiosarcome du foie et d'un hepatome, chez un ovrier du chlorure de vinyle. Ann Anat Pathol 1978;23:105–13.

45a. Edmondson HA, Peters RL. Neoplasms of the liver. In: Schiff L, Schiff ER, eds. Diseases of the liver, 5th ed. Philadelphia: JB Lippincott, 1982:1101–57.

46. Ekfors TO, Kujari H, Herva R. Kaposi-like infantile hemangioendothelioma. Am J Surg Pathol 1993;17:314–7.

47. El Zayadi A, Khalil A, El Samny N, et al. Hepatic angiosarcoma among Egyptian farmers exposed to pesticides. Hepatogastroenterology 1986;33:148–50.

48. Falk H, Caldwell GG, Ishak KG, Thomas LB, Popper H. Arsenic-related hepatic angiosarcoma. Am J Ind Med 1981;2:43–50.

49. Falk H, Creech JL Jr, Heath CW Jr, Johnson MN, Key MM. Hepatic disease among workers at a vinyl chloride polymerization plant. JAMA 1974;230:59–63.

50. Falk H, Herbert J, Crowley S, et al. Epidemiology of hepatic angiosarcoma in the United States: 1964–1974. Environ Hlth Persp 1981;41:107–13.

51. Falk H, Hervert JT, Edmonds L, Heath CD Jr, Thomas LB, Popper H. Review of four cases of childhood hepatic angiosarcoma–elevated environmental arsenic exposure in one case. Cancer 1981;47:382–91.

52. Falk H, Telles NC, Ishak KG, Thomas LB, Popper H. Epidemiology of thorotrast-induced hepatic angiosarcoma in the United States. Environ Res 1979;18:65–73.

53. Falk H, Thomas LB, Popper H, Ishak KG. Hepatic angiosarcoma associated with androgenic-anabolic steroids. Lancet 1979;2:1120–3.

54. Forman D, Bennett B, Stafford J, Doll R. Exposure to vinyl chloride and angiosarcoma of the liver: a report of the register of cases. Br J Ind Med 1985;42:750–3.

55. Fortwengler HP, Jones D, Espinosa E, Tamburro CL. Evidence for endothelial cell origin of vinyl chloride-induced hepatic angiosarcoma. Gastroenterology 1981;80:1415–9.

56. Fukunaga M, Ushigome S, Ishikawa E. Kaposiform hemangioendothelioma associated with Kasabach-Merritt syndrome. Histopathology 1996;28:281–4.

57. Gedigk P, Muller R, Bechtelsheimer H. Morphology of liver damage among polyvinyl chloride production workers. A report of 51 cases. Ann NY Acad Sci 1975;245:278–85.

58. Hashimoto M, Ohsawa M, Ohnishi A, et al. Expression of vascular endothelial growth factor and its receptor in RNA in angiosarcoma. Lab Invest 1995;73:859–63.

59. Hoch-Ligeti C. Angiosarcoma of the liver associated with diethylstilbestrol. JAMA 1978;240:1510–1.

60. Hollstein M, Marion MJ, Lehman T, et al. p53 mutations at A: T base pairs in angiosarcoma of vinyl chloride-exposed factory workers. Carcinogenesis 1994;15:1–3.

61. Irie H, Mori W. Long term effects of thorium dioxide (thorotrast) administration on human liver: ultrastructural localization of thorium dioxide in human liver by analytical electron microscopy. Acta Pathol Jpn 1984;34:221–8.

62. Ishak KG. Applications of scanning electron microscopy to the study of liver disease. Prog Liver Dis 1986;8:1–32.

63. Ishak KG. Mesenchymal tumors of the liver. In: Okuda K, Peters RL, eds. Hepatocellular carcinoma. New York: John Wiley & Sons, 1976:247–307.

64. Jansen TL, Meijer JW, Kesselring FO. Synchronous hepatic tumors 60 years after diagnostic thorotrast use. Eur J Gastroenterol Hepatol 1992;4:753–5.

65. Kasper ML, Schoefield L, Strom RL, Theologides A. Hepatic angiosarcoma and bronchioloalveolar carcinoma induced by Fowler's solution. JAMA 1984;252:3407–8.

66. Kauffman SL, Stout AP. Malignant hemangioendothelioma in infants and children. Cancer 1961;6:1186–96.

67. Kirchner SG, Heller RM, Kasselberg AG, Greene HL. Infantile hemangioendothelioma with subsequent malignant degeneration. Pediatr Radiol 1981;11:42–5.

68. Kojiro M, Kawano Y, Kawasaki, H, Nakashima T, Ikezaki H. Thorotrast induced hepatic angiosarcoma, and combined hepatocellular and cholangiocarcinoma in a single patient. Cancer 1982;49:2161–4.

69. Kojiro M, Nakashima T, Ito Y, Ikezaki H, Mori T, Kido C. Thorium dioxide related angiosarcoma of the liver: pathomorphologic study of 29 autopsy cases. Arch Pathol Lab Med 1985;109:853–7.

70. Kwittken J, Tartow LR. Haemochromatosis and Kupffer cell sarcoma with unusual localization of iron. J Pathol Bacteriol 1966;92:571–3.

71. Lander JJ, Stanley RJ, Sumner HW, et al. Angiosarcoma of the liver associated with Fowler's solution. Gastroenterology 1975;68:1582–6.

72. Lee FI, Smith PM, Bennett B, William DM. Occupationally related angiosarcoma of the liver in the United Kingdom 1972–1994. Gut 1996;39:312–8.

73. Levy DW, Rindsberg S, Friedman AC, et al. Thorotrast-induced hepatosplenic neoplasia: CT identification. AJR Am J Roentgenol 1986;146:997–1004.

74. Locker GY, Doroshow JH, Zwelling LA, Chabner BA. The clinical features of hepatic angiosarcoma: a report of four cases and a review of the English literature. Medicine 1979;58:48–64.

75. Mahony B, Jeffrey RB, Federle MP. Spontaneous rupture of hepatic and splenic angiosarcoma demonstrated by CT. AJR Am J Roentgenol 1982;138:965–6.

76. Manning JT, Ordonez NG, Barton JH. Endothelial cell origin of thorium oxide-induced angiosarcoma of liver. Arch Pathol Lab Med 1983;107:456–8.

77. Mark RJ, Poen JC, Tran LM, et al. Angiosarcoma: a report of 67 patients and a review of the literature. Cancer 1996;77:2400–6.

78. Miettinen M, Holhofer H, Lehto VP. Ulex europaeus 1 lectin as a marker for tumors derived from endothelial cells. Am J Clin Pathol 1983;79:32–6.

79. Miyake S, Onoue K, Ueda M, et al. Clinical studies on two cases of hepatic angiosarcoma. Acta Hepatol Jap 1982;23:1326–33.

79a. Nelson V, Fernandez NF, Woolf GM, Geller SA, Petrovic LM. Primary liposarcoma of the liver. A case report and review of the literature. Arch Pathol Lab Med 2001;125:410–2.

80. Nordsten M. Hemangiosarcoma hepatis associeret med brug of androgene steroider. Ugeskr Laeger 1985;147:2615–6.

81. Noronha R, Gonzalez-Crussi F. Hepatic angiosarcoma in childhood: a case report and review of the literature. Am J Surg Pathol 1984;8:863–71.

82. Niedt GW, Greco MA, Blanc WA, Knowles DM II. Hemangioma with Kaposi's sarcoma-like features: report of two cases. Pediatr Pathol 1989;9:567–75.

83. Pialat JM, Pasquier B, Pahn M, Kopp N. Pathologie hepatique du chlorure de vinyle monomere (CVM): Huit observations anatome-cliniques personnelles. Arch Anat Cyto Pathol 1979;27:361–75.

84. Pimentel JC, Menezes AP. Liver disease in vineyard sprayers. Gastroenterology 1977;72:275–83.

85. Popper H, Maltoni C, Selikoff IJ. Vinyl chloride-induced hepatic lesions in man and rodents. A comparison. Liver 1980;1:7–20.

86. Popper H, Thomas LB, Telles NC, Falk N, Selikoff IJ. Development of hepatic angiosarcoma induced by vinyl chloride, Thorotrast and arsenic. Comparison with cases of unknown etiology. Am J Pathol 1978;92:349–69.

87. Regelson W, Kim U, Ospina J, Holland JF. Hemangioendothelial sarcoma of the liver from chronic arsenic intoxication by Fowler's solution. Cancer 1968;21:514–22.

88. Rennke H, Prat GA, Etcheverry RB, et al. Hemangioendothelioma maligno del higado y arsenicismo chronica. Rev Med Chil 1971;99:1582–6.

89. Roat JW, Wald A, Mendelow H, Pataki KI. Hepatic angiosarcoma associated with short-term arsenic ingestion. Am J Med 1982;73:933–6.

90. Ross JM. A case illustrating the effects of prolonged action of radium. J Pathol Bacteriol 1932;35:899–912.

91. Roth F. The sequelae of chronic arsenic poisoning in Moselle vintners. Ger Med Mon 1957;2:211–7.

92. Sakai K, Shiina M, Ishihara N, Kato Y. Thorotrast-induced multiple primary malignant tumors of the liver—cholangiocarcinoma and malignant hemangioendothelioma. Jpn J Clin Oncol 1984;14:411–6.

92a. Salgado M, Sans M, Forns X, et al. Angiosarcoma hepatica: presentacion de un caso asociado al tratamiento con sales de arsenico y revision de la literatura. Gastroenterol Hepatol 1995;18:132–5.

93. Schattenberg PJ, Totovic V, Gedigk P, Marsteller HJ. Die Ultrastruktur der Leberschadigung bei der chronischen Vinylchlorid-Intoxikation. Virchows Arch [A] 1977;373:233–47.

94. Selby DM, Stocker JT, Ishak KG. Angiosarcoma of the liver in childhood: a clinicopathologic and follow-up study in 10 cases. Pediatr Pathol 1992;12:485–98.

95. Shi EC, Fischer A, Crouch R, Ham JM. Possible association of angiosarcoma with oral contraceptive agents. Med J Aust 1981;1:473–4.

96. Smith PM, Crossley IR, Williams DM. Portal hypertension in vinyl-chloride production workers. Lancet 1976;2:602–4.

97. Soini Y, Welsh JA, Ishak KG, Bennett WP. p53 mutations in primary hepatic angiosarcoma not associated with vinyl chloride exposure. Carcinogenesis 1995;16:2879–81.

98. Strate SM, Rutledge JC, Weinberg AG. Delayed development of angiosarcoma in multinodular infantile hepatic hemangioendothelioma. Arch Pathol Lab Med 1984;106:943–4.

99. Sussman EB, Nydick I, Gray G. Hemangioendothelial sarcoma of the liver and hemochromatosis. Arch Pathol 1974;97:39–42.

100. Tamburro CH, Makk L, Popper H. Early hepatic histologic alterations among chemical (vinyl monomer) workers. Hepatology 1984;4:413–8.

101. Telles NC, Thomas LB, Popper H, et al. Evolution of thorotrast-induced hepatic angiosarcomas. Environ Res 1979;18:74–8.

102. Thomas LB, Popper H, Berk PD, et al. Vinyl-chloride induced liver disease. From idiopathic portal hypertension (Banti's syndrome) to angiosarcomas. N Engl J Med 1975;292:17–22.

103. Truell JE, Peck SD, Reiquam CW. Hemangiosarcoma of the liver complicated by disseminated intravascular coagulation. A case report. Gastroenterology 1973; 65:936–42.

104. Tsang WY, Chan JK. Kaposi-like infantile hemangioendothelioma. A distinctive vascular neoplasm of the retroperitoneum. Am J Surg Pathol 1991;15:982–9.

105. Van Kaick G, Muth H, Kaul A, et al. Results of the German Thorotrast study. Prog Cancer Res 1984;26:253–62.

106. Van Kaick G, Siegert A, Luhrs H, Lieberman D. Der Beitrag der Computertomographic zur Quantifizierung der Thorotrastose und zur thorotrastinduzierter Lebertumoren. Radiologe 1986;26:123–8.

107. Vuletin JC, Wajsbort RR, Ghali V. Primary retroperitoneal angiosarcoma with eosinophilic globules. A combined light-microscopic, immunohistochemical, and ultrastructural study. Arch Pathol Lab Med 1990;114:618–22.

108. Wegener K, Leipoz-Angermuller S. Double tumours of the liver following intravenous Thorotrast injection. Patho-anatomic report on two cases. Virchows Arch [A] 1979;382:63–71.

109. Weinberg AG, Finegold MJ. Primary hepatic tumors of childhood. Hum Pathol 1993;14:512–37.

110. White PG, Adams H, Smith PM. The computed tomographic appearances of angiosarcoma of the liver. Clin Radiol 1993;48:321–5.

111. Winberg CD, Ranchod M. Thorotrast induced hepatic cholangiocarcinoma and angiosarcoma. Hum Pathol 1979;10:108–12.

112. Yamada S, Hososda S, Tateno H, Kido C, Takahashi S. Survey of Thorotrast-associated liver cancers in Japan. JNCI 1983;70:31–5.

113. Zukerberg LR, Nickoloff BJ, Weiss SW. Kaposiform hemangioendothelioma of infancy and childhood. An aggressive neoplasm associated with Kasabach-Merritt syndrome and lymphagiomatosis. Am J Surg Pathol 1993;17:321–8.

Kaposi's Sarcoma

114. Antinori S, Ridolfo Al, Esposito R, Vago L, Moroni M. Liver involvement in AIDS-associated malignancies. J Hepatol 1994;21:1145–6.

115. Bergfeld WF, Zemtsov A, Lang RS. Differentiation between AIDS-related and non-AIDS-related Kaposi's sarcoma. Clev Clin J Med 1987;54:315–9.

116. Brown LF, Tognazzi K, Dvorak HF, Harrist TJ. Strong expression of kinase-insert domain-containing receptor, a vascular permeability factor/vascular endothelial growth factor receptor in AIDS-associated Kaposi's sarcoma and cutaneous angiosarcoma. Am J Pathol 1996;148:1065–74.

116a. Fossati S, Proneschi V, Furrcucci S, Brambilla L. Human immunodeficiency virus negative Kaposi sarcoma and lymphoproliferative disorders. Cancer 1999;85:1611–5.

117. Fukunaga M, Silverberg SG. Hyaline globules in Kaposi's sarcoma: a light microscopic and immunohistochemical study. Mod Pathol 1991;4:187–90.

118. Gao SJ, Kingsley l, Hoover DR, et al. Seroconversion to antibodies against Kaposi's sarcoma-associated herpesvirus-related latent nuclear antigens before the development of Kaposi's sarcoma. N Engl J Med 1996;335:233–41.

119. Guarda LA, Luna MA, Smith IL. Acquired immune deficiency syndrome: postmortem findings. Am J Clin Pathol 1984;81:549–57.

120. Huang YQ, Li JJ, Kaplan MH, et al. Human herpes virus-like nucleic acid in various forms of Kaposi's sarcoma. Lancet 1995;345:759–62.

121. Ioachim HL, Adsay V, Giancotti FR, Dorsett B, Melamed J. Kaposi's sarcoma of internal organs. Cancer 1995; 75:1376–85.

122. Jin YT, Tsai ST, Yan JJ, et al. Detection of Kaposi's sarcoma-associated herpesvirus-like DNA sequence in vascular lesions. a reliable diagnostic marker for Kaposi's sarcoma. Am J Clin Pathol 1996;105:360–3.

123. Miller G, Rigsby MO, Heston L, et al. Antibodies to butyrate inducible antigens of Kaposi's sarcoma-associated herpesvirus in patients with HIV-1 infection. N Engl J Med 1996;334:1292–7.

124. Monini P, DeLellis L, Farris M, et al. Kaposi's sarcoma-associated DNA sequences in prostate tissue and human semen. N Engl J Med 1996;334:1168–72.

125. Moore PS, Chang Y. Detection of herpes virus-like DNA sequences in Kaposi's sarcoma in patients with and those without HIV infection. N Engl J Med 1995;332:1181–5.

126. Morris CB, Gendelman R, Marrogi AJ, et al. Immunohistochemical detection of Bcl-2 in AIDS-associated and classical Kaposi's sarcoma. Am J Pathol 1996;148:1055–63.

127. Niedt G, Schinella RA. Acquired immunodeficiency syndrome. Clinicopathologic study of 56 autopsies. Arch Pathol Lab Med 1985;109:727–34.

128. Noel JC, Hermans P, Andre J, et al. Herpesvirus-like DNA sequences and Kaposi's sarcoma: relationship with epidemiology, clinical spectrum, and histologic features. Cancer 1996;77:2132–6.

129. Pammer J, Plettenberg A, Weninger W, et al. CD 40 antigen is expressed by endothelial cells and tumor cells in Kaposi's sarcoma. Am J Pathol 1996;148:1387–96.

130. Regezi JA, MacPhail LA, Daniels TE, De Souza YG, Greenspan JS, Greenspan D. Human immunodeficiency virus-associated oral Kaposi's sarcoma: a heterogeneous cell population dominated by spindle-shaped endothelial cells. Am J Pathol 1993;143:240–9.

131. Tavio M, Vaccher E, Antinori A, et al. Combination chemotherapy with doxorubicin, bleomycin and vindesine for AIDS-related Kaposi's sarcoma. Cancer 1996;77:2117–22.

132. Wang CY, Schroeter AL, Su WP. Acquired immunodeficiency syndrome-related Kaposi's sarcoma. Mayo Clin Proc 1995;70:869–79.

133. Weninger W, Partanen TA, Breiteneder-Geleff S, et al. Expression of vascular endothelial growth factor receptor-3 and podoplanin suggests a lymphatic endothelial cell origin of Kaposis's sarcoma tumor cells. Lab Invest 1999;79:243–51.

133a. Whitby D, Howard MR, Tenant-Flowers M, et al. Detection of Kaposi sarcoma associated herpesvirus in peripheral blood of HIV-infected individuals and progression to Kaposi's sarcoma. Lancet 1995;346:799–802.

134. Zhang YM, Bachmann S, Hemmer C, et al. Vascular origin of Kaposi's sarcoma. Expression of leukocyte adhesion molecule-1, thrombomodulin, and tissue factor. Am J Pathol 1994;144:51–9.

Embryonal Rhabdomyosarcoma

135. Aldabagh SM, Shibata CS, Taxy JB. Rhabdomyosarcoma of the common bile duct in an adult. Arch Pathol Lab Med 1986;110:547–50.

136. Burrig KF, Knauers S. Hepatic rhabdomyosarcoma in adulthood. Case report and literature review. Pathology 1994;15:54–7.

137. Cannon PM, Legge DA, O'Donnell B. The use of percutaneous transhepatic cholangiography in a case of embryonal rhabdomyosarcoma. Br Radiol 1979;52:326–7.

138. d'Amore ES, Tollot M, Stracca-Pansa V, et al. Therapy associated differentiation in rhabdomyosarcomas. Mod Pathol 1994;7:69–75.

139. Davis GL, Kissane JM, Ishak KG. Embryonal rhabdomyosarcoma (sarcoma botryoides) of the biliary tree. Cancer 1969;24:333–42.

140. Lack EE, Perez-Atayada AR, Schuster SR. Botryoid rhabdomyosarcoma of the biliary tract: report of five cases with ultrastructural observations and literature review. Am J Surg Pathol 1981;5:643–52.

141. Mori H, Matsubara N, Fuji M. Alpha-fetoprotein producing rhabdomyosarcoma of the adult liver. Acta Pathol Jpn 1979;29:333–42.

142. Morimoto H, Takade Y, Akita T. A resected case of the collision tumor of hepatocellular carcinoma and primary liver rhabdomyosarcoma. J Jpn Surg Soc 1986;87:456–63.

143. Parham DM. Immunohistochemistry of childhood sarcomas: old and new markers. Mod Pathol 1993;6:133–8.

144. Pinkerton R, Pritchard-Jones K, Carter R, Cooper S. Small-round-cell tumours of childhood. Lancet 1994;344:725–9.

145. Ruymann FB, Raney B, Crist WM, Lawrence W Jr, Lindberg RD, Soule EH. Rhabdomyosarcoma of the biliary tree in childhood: a report from the Intergroup Rhabdomyosarcoma Study. Cancer 1985;56:575–81.

Embryonal ("Undifferentiated") Sarcoma

146. Abramowsky CR, Cebelin M, Choudhury A, Izant RJ. Undifferentiated (embryonal) sarcoma of the liver with alpha-1-antitrypsin deposits: immunohistochemical and ultrastructural studies. Cancer 1980;45:3108–13.

147. Aoyama C, Hachitanda Y, Sato JK, Said JW, Shimada H. Undifferentiated (embryonal) sarcoma of the liver. Am J Surg Pathol 1991;15:615–24.

148. Blattner WA, Henson DE, Young RC, Fraumeni JF. Malignant mesenchymoma and birth defects: prenatal exposure to phenytoin. JAMA 1977;238:334–5.

149. Chandra RS, Stocker JT. The liver, gallbladder and biliary tract. In: Stocker JT, Dehner LP, eds. Pediatric pathology, vol. 2. Philadelphia: JB Lippincott, 1992:703–654.

150. Chou P, Mangkornkanok M, Gonzalez-Crussi F. Undifferentiated (embryonal) sarcoma of the liver: ultrastructure, immunohistochemistry and DNA ploidy analysis of the two cases. Pediatr Pathol 1990;10:549–62.

151. Cozzutto C, De Bernardi B, Comelli A, Soave F. Malignant mesenchymoma of the liver in children: a clinicopathologic and ultrastructural study. Hum Pathol 1981;12:481–5.

152. de Chadarevian JP, Pawel BR, Faerber EN, Weintraub WH. Undifferentiated (embryonal) sarcoma arising in conjunction with mesenchymal hamartoma of the liver. Mod Pathol 1994;7:490–3.

153. Ellis IO, Cotton RE. Primary malignant mesenchymal tumour of the liver in an elderly female. Histopathology 1983;7:113–21.

154. Esposito R, Pollavini G, de Lalla F. A case of primary undifferentiated sarcoma of the liver diagnosed by peritoneoscopy and guided biopsy. Endoscopy 1977;8:108–10.

155. Gallivan MV, Lack EE, Chun B, Ishak KG. Undifferentiated ("embryonal") sarcoma of the liver: ultrastructure of a case presenting as a primary intracardiac tumor. Pediatr Pathol 1983;1:291–300.

156. Gonzalez-Crussi F. Undifferentiated (embryonal) liver sarcoma of childhood: evidence of leiomyoblastic differentiation. Ped Pathol 1983;1:281–90.

157. Harris MB, Shen S, Weiner MA, et al. Treatment of primary undifferentiated sarcoma of the liver with surgery and chemotherapy. Cancer 1984;54:2859–62.

158. Horowitz ME, Etcubanas E, Webber BL, et al. Hepatic undifferentiated (embryonal) sarcoma and rhabdomyosarcoma in children. Results of therapy. Cancer 1987;59:396–402.

159. Kadomatsu K, Nakagewara A, Zaizen Y, et al. Undifferentiated (embryonal) sarcoma of the liver: report of three cases. Jpn J Surg 1992;22:451–5.

160. Keating S, Taylor GP. Undifferentiated (embryonal) sarcoma of the liver: ultrastructural and immunohistochemical similarities with malignant fibrous histiocytoma. Hum Pathol 1985;16:693–9.

161. Lack EE, Schloo BL, Azumi N, Travis WD, Grier HE, Kozakewich HP. Undifferentiated (embryonal) sarcoma of the liver. Clinical and pathological study of 16 cases with emphasis on immunohistochemical features. Am J Surg Pathol 1991;15:1–16.

162. Lagace R, Delage C, Robert J. Le mesenchymome primitif du foie: etude ultrastructurale. Ann Anat Pathol 1974;19:275–86.

163. Leuscher I, Schmidt D, Harms D. Undifferentiated sarcoma of the liver in childhood: morphology, flow cytometry, and literature review. Hum Pathol 1990;21:68–76.

163a. Lauwers GY, Grant LD, Donnelly WH, et al. Hepatic undifferentiated (embryonal) sarcoma arising in a mesenchymal hamartoma. Am J Surg Pathol 1997;21:1248–54.

164. McFadden DW, Kelley DJ, Sigmund DA, Barrett WL, Dickson B, Aron BS. Embryonal sarcoma of the liver in an adult treated with chemotherapy, radiation therapy, and hepatic lobectomy. Cancer 1992;69:39–44.

165. Parham DM, Kelly DR, Donnelly WH, Douglass EC. Immunohistochemical and ultrastructural spectrum of hepatic sarcomas of childhood: evidence for a common histogenesis. Mod Pathol 1991;4:648–53.

166. Pieterse AS, Smith M, Smith LA, Smith P. Embryonal (undifferentiated) sarcoma of the liver. Fine-needle aspiration cytology and ultrastructural findings. Arch Pathol Lab Med 1985;109:677–80.

167. Reichel C, Fehske W, Fisher HP, Hartlapp JH. Undifferentiated (embryonal) sarcoma of the liver in an adult patient with metastasis of the heart and brain. Clin Invest 1994;72:209–12.

168. Ros PR, Olmsted WW, Dachman AH, Goodman ZD, Ishak G, Hartman DS. Undifferentiated (embryonal) sarcoma of the liver: radiologic-pathologic correlation. Radiology 1986;161:141–5.

169. Smithson WA, Telander RL, Carney JA. Mesenchymoma of the liver in childhood: five-year survival after combined modality treatment. J Pediatr Surg 1982;17:70–2.

170. Stanley RJ, Dehner LP, Hesker AE. Primary malignant mesenchymal tumors (mesenchymoma) of the liver in childhood. An angiographic-pathologic study of three cases. Cancer 1973;32:973–84.

171. Stocker JT, Ishak KG. Undifferentiated (embryonal) sarcoma of the liver. Cancer 1978;42:336–48.

172. Tanner AR, Bolton PM, Powell LW. Primary sarcoma of the liver: report of a case with excellent response to hepatic artery ligation and infusion chemotherapy. Gastroenterology 1978;74:121–3.

173. Urban CE, Mache CJ, Schwinger W, et al. Undifferentiated (embryonal) sarcoma of the liver in childhood: successful combined-modality therapy in four patients. Cancer 1993;72:2511–6.

174. Vetter D, Bellocq JP, Amaral D, et al. Sarcomes undifférenciés (ou embryonnaires) hépatiques: Problémes diagnostiques et thérapeutiques à propos dun rhabdomyosarcome botryoide. Gastroenterol Clin Biol 1989;13:98–103.

175. Walker NI, Horn MJ, Strong RW, et al. Undifferentiated (embryonal) sarcoma of the liver: pathologic findings and long-term survival after complete surgical resection. Cancer 1992;69:52–9.

176. Ware R, Friedman HS, Filston HC, et al. Childhood hepatic mesenchymoma: successful treatment with surgery and multiple agent chemotherapy. Med Pediatr Oncol 1988;16:62–5.

176a. Webber EM, Morrison KB, Pritchard SL, Sorensen PH. Undifferentiated embryonal sarcoma of the liver: results of clinical managements in one center. J Pediatr Surg 1999;34:1641–4.

177. Weinberg AG, Finegold MJ. Primary hepatic tumors of childhood. Hum Pathol 1983;14:512–37.

Fibrosarcoma

178. Alrenga DP. Primary fibrosarcoma of the liver: case report and review of the literature. Cancer 1974;36:446–9.

179. Balouet G, Destombes P. A propos de quelques tumeurs mesenchymateuses hépatiques d'apparence primitive. Ann Anat Pathol 1967;12:273–86.

180. Bodker A, Boiesen PT. A primary fibrosarcoma of the liver. Hepatogastroenterology 1981;28:218–20.
181. Cavallo T, Lichewitz B, Rozov T. Primary fibrosarcoma of the liver: report of a case. Rev Hosp Clin Med Sao Paulo 1968;23:44–69.
182. Danhaive O, Ninane J, Sokal E, et al. Hepatic localization of a fibrosarcoma in a child with a liver transplant. J Pediatr 1992;120:434–7.
183. Gen E, Kusuyama Y, Saito K, et al. Primary fibrosarcoma of the liver with hypoglycemia. Acta Pathol Jpn 1983;33:177–82.
184. Hall J, Scheffer C, Tseng G, Timpl R, Hendrix MJ, Stern R. Collagen types in fibrosarcoma: absence of type III collagen in reticulin. Hum Pathol 1995;16:439–46.
184a. Ishak KG. Mesenchymal tumors of the liver. In: Okuda K, Peters RL, eds. Hepatocellular carcinoma. New York: John Wiley & Sons, 1976:247–307.

185. Nakahama M, Takanashi R, Yamazaki I, Machinami R. Primary fibrosarcoma of the liver. Acta Pathol Jpn 1989;39:814–20.
186. Ojima A, Sugiyama T, Takeda J. Six cases of rare malignant tumors of the liver. Acta Pathol Jpn 1964;14:95–102.
187. Smith D, Rele SR. A case of primary fibrosarcoma of the liver. Postgrad Med J 1972;48:62–3.
188. Snapper I, Schraft WC, Ginsberg DM. Severe hypoglycemia due to fibrosarcoma of the liver. Maendschr Kindergenees 1964;32:337–47.
189. Totzke HA, Hutcheson JB. Primary fibrosarcoma of the liver. South Med J 1965;58:236–8.
190. Walter VE, Bodner E, Lederer B. Primares fibrosarkom der Leber. Wein Klin Wochenschr 1972;84:808–10.

Leiomyosarcoma

191. Dei Tos AP, Maestro R, Doglioni C, et al. Tumor suppressor genes and related molecules in leiomyosarcoma. Am J Pathol 1996;148:1037–45.
191a. Folpe AL, Goodman ZD, Ishak KG, et al. Clear cell myomelanocytic tumor of the falciform ligament/ligamentum teres. A novel member of the perivascular epithelioid clear cell family of tumors with a predilection for children and young adults. Am J Surg Pathol 2000;24:1239–46.
192. Gates LK, Cameron AJ, Nagorney DM, et al. Primary leiomyosarcoma of the liver mimicking liver abscess. Am J Gastroenterol 1995;90:649–52.
193. Hines OJ, Nelson S, Quinones-Baldrich WJ, Eilber FR. Leiomyosarcoma of the inferior vena cava. Prognosis and comparison with leiomyosarcoma of the anatomic sites. Cancer 1999;85:1077–83.
193a. Horowitz ME, Etcubaras E, Webber BL, et al. Hepatic undifferentiated (embryonal) sarcoma and rhabdomyosarcoma in children: results of therapy. Cancer 1987;59:396–402.
193b. Ishak KG. Mesenchymal tumors of the liver. In: Okuda K, Peters RL, eds. Hepatocellular carcinoma. New York: John Wiley & Sons, 1976:247–307.
194. McClain KL, Leach CT, Jenson HB, et al. Association of Epstein-Barr virus with leiomyosarcomas in young people with AIDS. N Engl J Med 1995;332:12–4.
195. Miettinen M. Immunoreactivity for cytokeratin and epithelial membrane antigen in leiomyosarcoma. Arch Pathol Lab Med 1988;112:637–40.
196. Mingoli A, Cavallero A, Sapienza P, et al. International registry of inferior vena cava leiomyosarcoma: analysis of a world series of 218 patients. Anticancer Res 1996;16:3201–5.
197. Mital RN, Bazaz-Malik G. Leiomyosarcoma of the ligamentum teres of the liver. Am J Gastroenterol 1971;56:48–51.

198. Parham DM, Reynolds AB, Webber BL. Use of monoclonal antibody IHI, anticortactin, to distinguish normal and neoplastic smooth muscle cells: Comparison with anti-α–smooth muscle actin and antimuscle-specific actin. Hum Pathol 1995;26:776–83.
199. Penn I. Posttransplantation de novo tumors in liver allograft recipients. Liv Transpl Surg 1996;2:52–9.
199a. Prévot S, Néris J, de Saint Maur PP. Detection of Epstein Barr virus in an hepatic leiomyomatous neoplasm in an adult human immunodeficiency virus 1–infected patient. Virchows Arch 1994;425:321–5.
199b. Ross JS, Del Rosario A, Bui HX, Sonbati H, Solis O. Primary hepatic leiomyosarcoma in a child with the acquired immunodeficiency syndrome. Hum Pathol 1992;23:69–72.
200. Shimoda H, Oka K, Otani S, et al. Vascular leiomyosarcoma arising from the inferior vena cava diagnosed by intraluminal biopsy. Virchows Arch 1998;433:97–100.
201. Shurbaji MS, Olson JL, Kuhajda FP. Thorotrast-associated hepatic leiomyosarcoma and cholangiocarcinoma in a single patient. Hum Pathol 1987;18:524–6.
202. Sreekantaiah C, Davis JR, Sandberg AA. Chromosomal abnormalities in leiomyosarcomas. Am J Pathol 1993;142:293–305.
202a. Tanaka Y, Ijiri R, Kato K, et al. HMB-45/Melan-A and smooth muscle actin-positive clear-cell epithelioid tumor arising in the ligamentum teres hepatis. Additional example of clear cell "sugar" tumors. Am J Surg Pathol 2000;24:1295–9.
203. Tomaszewski MM, Kuenster TJ, Hartman K. Leiomyosarcoma of ligamentum teres of liver: case report. Pediatr Pathol 1986;5:147–56.
204. van Hoeven KH, Factor SM, Kress Y, Woodruff JM. Visceral myogenic tumors: a manifestation of HIV infection in children. Am J Surg Pathol. 1991;17:1176–81.

Malignant Fibrous Histiocytoma

205. Alberti-Flor JJ, O'Hara MF, Weaver F, Evans J, McClure R, Dunn GD. Malignant fibrous histiocytoma of the liver. Gastroenterology 1985;89:890–3.

206. Arends JW, Willebrand D, Blaauw AM, Bosman FT. Primary malignant fibrous histiocytoma of the liver—a case report with immunocytochemical observations. Histopathology 1987;11:427–31.

207. Brooks JS. The significance of double phenotypic patterns and differentiation in humans sarcomas: a new model of mesenchymal differentiation. Am J Pathol 1986;125:113–23.

208. Conran RM, Stocker JT. Malignant fibrous histiocytoma of the liver. A case report. Am J Gastroenterol 1985;80:813–15.

208a. Ferrozzi F, Bova D. Hepatic malignant fibrous histiocytoma: CT findings. Clin Radiol 1998;53:699–701.

209. Fukayama M, Koike M. Malignant fibrous histiocytoma arising in the liver. Arch Pathol Lab Med 1986; 110:203–6.

210. Hamasaki K, Minura H, Sato D, et al. Malignant fibrous histiocytoma of the liver: a case report. Gastroenterol Jpn 1991;26:666–73.

211. Katsuda S, Kawahara E, Matsui Y, Ohyama S, Nakanishi I. Malignant fibrous histiocytoma of the liver: a case report and review of the literature. Am J Gastroenterol 1988;83:1278–82.

211a. Keating S, Taylor GP. Undifferentiated (embryonal) sarcoma of the liver: ultrastructural and immunohisto-

chemical similarities with malignant fibrous histiocytoma. Hum Pathol 1985;16:693–9.

212. McGrady BJ, Mirakhur MM. Recurrent malignant fibrous histiocytoma of the liver. Histopathology 1992; 21:290–3.

213. Miettinen M, Soini Y. Malignant fibrous histiocytoma: heterogeneous patterns of intermediate filament proteins by immunohistochemistry. Arch Pathol Lab Med 1989;113:1363–6.

214. Roholl PJ, Elbers HR, Prinsen I, Claessens JA, Van Unnik JA. Distribution of actin isoforms in sarcomas: an immunohistochemical study. Hum Pathol 1990;21:1269–74.

215. Takeya M, Yamashiro S, Yoshimura T, Takahashi K. Immunophenotypic and immunoelectron microscopic characterization of major constituent cells in malignant fibrous histiocytoma using human cell lines and their transplanted tumors in immunodeficient mice. Lab Invest 1995;72:679–88.

Other Sarcomas

215a. Fiel MI, Schwartz M, Min AD, et al. Malignant schwannoma of the liver in a patient without neurofibromatosis. A case report and review of the literature. Arch Pathol Lab Med 1996;120:1145–7.

216. Lederman SM, Martin EC, Laffey KT, Lefkowitch JH. Hepatic neurofibromatosis, malignant schwannoma, and angiosarcoma in von Recklinghausen's disease. Gastroenterology 1987;92:234–9.

217. Nakabayashi H, Aiba H, Sakuma S, et al. An autopsy case of primary malignant mesenchymoma of the liver with various tissue components. Acta Hepatol Jpn 1985;26:369–75.

218. Sumiyoshi A, Nicho Y. Primary osteogenic sarcomas of the liver. Acta Pathol Jpn 1971;21:305–12.

219. Velilla J, Soler G, Munoz JR, et al. Mesenquimoma maligno primitivo hepatico. Gastroenterol Hepatol 1986;9:497–500.

220. von Hochstetter AR, Hattenschwiler J, Vogt M. Primary osteosarcoma of the liver. Cancer 1987;60:2312–7.

221. Young SJ. Primary malignant neurilemoma (schwannoma) of the liver in a case of neurofibromatosis. J Pathol 1975;117:151–3.

❖❖❖

13

PRIMARY HEPATIC LYMPHOMAS AND SUSPECTED LYMPHOMAS

Malignant lymphomas, when they disseminate, frequently involve the liver. A detailed discussion of these tumors is beyond the scope of this text, and the reader who wishes more information on morphology and classification can pursue this in the Fascicle, Tumors of the Lymph Nodes and Spleen (43) and in the publications of the Revised European-American Classification of Lymphoid Neoplasms (REAL Classification) (6,14) and the World Health Organization (WHO) (16). This chapter will deal with primary hepatic lymphomas, and will also discuss types of lesions where lymphoma should be suspected even though diagnostic features are not present.

PRIMARY HEPATIC AND HEPATOSPLENIC LYMPHOMA

Definition. A primary hepatic lymphoma is a malignant neoplasm of lymphoid differentiation that arises in and is initially confined to the liver. As many such tumors also involve the spleen at the time of detection, hepatosplenic lymphoma may be considered synonymous with primary hepatic lymphoma. All cases reported to date have been non-Hodgkin's lymphomas.

General Features. Primary hepatic and hepatosplenic lymphomas are uncommon, with approximately 100 cases reported in the literature. Because they are so rare, etiologic factors are not well understood. Tumors have been reported in patients with acquired immunodeficiency syndrome (AIDS) (24,37), chronic hepatitis B (22), and chronic hepatitis C (31,34), although an etiologic relationship has not been definitely established. Hepatitis C is also associated with nonhepatic extranodal lymphomas (3), and the RNA of this virus has been detected in some tumors (3,31), so it is possible that the hepatitis C virus plays a direct pathogenetic role. Exposure to industrial chemicals has been implicated in a few cases (8), but this association is much less clear.

Clinical Features. There are no clinical findings that distinguish primary hepatic lymphomas from other hepatic malignancies. Lei (22) reviewed 90 cases gathered from the literature and found that there was a male predominance (2.3:1) and

a median age of 53 years (range, 5 to 87 years); only a few occurred in children. Abdominal pain or distention was the presenting complaint in 56 percent, and 82 percent had hepatomegaly. B symptoms of weight loss and fever were present in 40 percent and 22 percent, respectively. Occasional patients presented with fulminant liver failure as the initial manifestation of the disease (13). As with lymphomas of other sites, the response to treatment and prognosis generally reflect the histologic type.

Pathologic Findings and Classification. *Large Cell Lymphoma.* Over half of reported cases of primary hepatic lymphoma are classified as diffuse large cell type. Most, when phenotyped, are *B-cell tumors* (CD20 positive) (7,9,30, 38), but histologically identical T-cell tumors also occur on occasion (17) and are classified as *peripheral T-cell lymphomas.* Large cell lymphomas tend to produce bulky masses that are white to yellow and may be single or multiple (fig. 13-1). Like large cell lymphomas of other sites, they are composed of sheets of loosely cohesive lymphoid cells with large vesicular nuclei, prominent nucleoli, and a moderate amount of cytoplasm (fig. 13-2), although many variants are possible. Most have noncleaved nuclei, but cleaved cell, and mixed large and small cell types have also been seen.

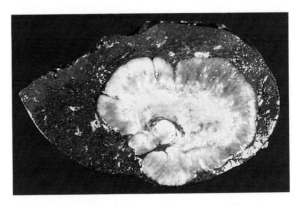

Figure 13-1
PRIMARY HEPATIC LYMPHOMA
The tumor in this right lobectomy specimen is mottled white and yellow.

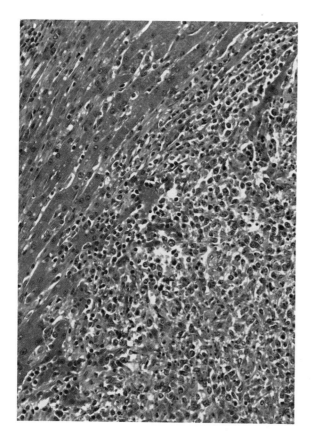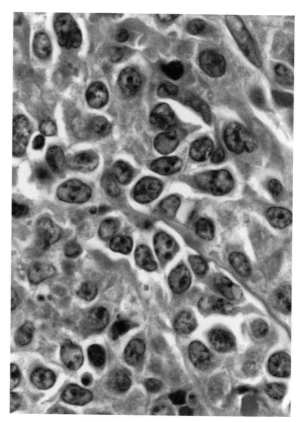

Figure 13-2
PRIMARY HEPATIC LYMPHOMA, LARGE CELL TYPE
Left: The tumor cells have scant cytoplasm with large, vesicular nuclei and prominent nucleoli.
Right: The tumor is an expansile mass of large lymphoid cells.

Some large cell lymphomas diffusely infiltrate the sinusoids and small blood vessels and cause hepatomegaly without a discrete mass. This is more frequent with T-cell lymphoma (see Sinusoidal T-Cell Lymphoma below), but it has also been reported with some primary B-cell lymphomas (28,41). Terms such as "neoplastic angioendotheliomatosis" and "intravascular lymphomatosis" were previously used for such tumors, although these are no longer part of the REAL classification. Nevertheless, such tumors appear to be a form of angiotrophic large B-cell lymphoma, and hopefully they will be recognized in a future classification.

The prognosis of patients with diffuse large cell lymphoma of the liver is generally poor. There have been a few patients who had favorable responses to combination chemotherapy and several who were cured by surgical resection, but the majority of reported patients died of the disease.

Low-Grade B-Cell Lymphoma of Mucosa-Associated Lymphoid Tissue (MALT). Called *extranodal marginal B-cell lymphoma* in the REAL classification, this tumor is well-recognized in the gastrointestinal tract and several other sites, but it is quite rare in the liver (15,19,25,32). MALT lymphomas of the liver are usually solitary but may be multiple. They form discrete tumor-like masses that can be as large as 7.5 cm. Microscopically, they show normal liver architecture that is infiltrated by well-differentiated lymphoid cells forming small spherical masses that coalesce where they are contiguous (fig. 13-3). Germinal centers are present, and there are often lymphoepithelial lesions involving bile ducts (fig. 13-4) that are similar to those seen in MALT lymphomas of the gastrointestinal tract and salivary glands. Some cases contain masses of monocytoid B cells (fig. 13-5). Immunostains typically show a polymorphous population of B cells

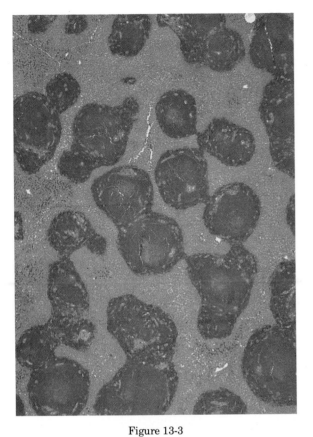

Figure 13-3
MALT LYMPHOMA
Spherical masses of well-differentiated lymphoid tissue surround portal areas, coalescing where they are contiguous. Germinal centers are present in some of the nodules.

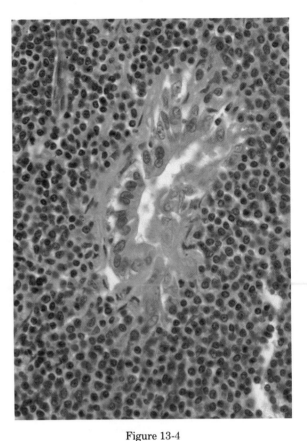

Figure 13-4
MALT LYMPHOMA
A lymphoepithelial lesion of a bile duct is in the center of one of the lymphoid masses.

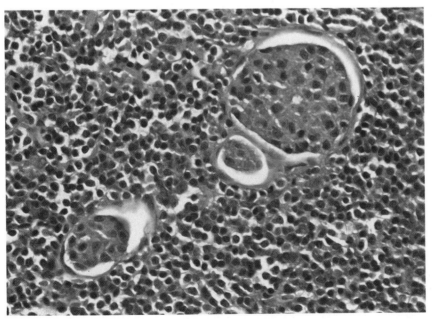

Figure 13-5
MALT LYMPHOMA
Masses of monocytoid B cells appear to be in vessels in this case. Even though they appear epithelial, they are CD20 positive, indicating B-cell differentiation.

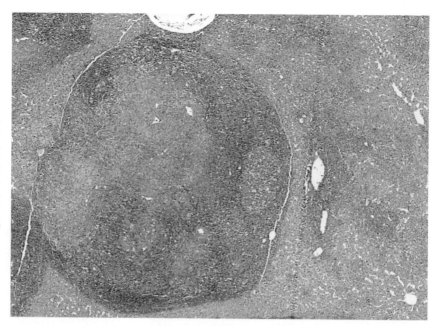

Figure 13-6
T-CELL LYMPHOMA
MIMICKING
MALT LYMPHOMA
Although this lesion is morphologically and immunophenotypically similar to the B-cell MALT lymphomas, it was found to have a monoclonal rearrangement of the T-cell beta gene by PCR. The only difference between this and B-cell MALT lymphoma is the area of granulomatous inflammation, represented by the area of eosinophilia.

and T cells, but molecular studies using PCR demonstrate a monoclonal immunoglobulin heavy chain gene rearrangement, which confirms the diagnosis. The prognosis, as in other sites, is good, and in several cases the tumors appear to have been eradicated by excisional biopsy.

Tumors with apparently identical morphology have been reported as other entities, but it seems likely that they are the actually MALT lymphomas or closely related entities, based on their appearance and eradication by excisional biopsy in two cases and surgery plus chemotherapy in a third. These include one case reported as primary hepatic marginal zone B-cell lymphoma with mantle cell phenotype (42), one reported as pseudolymphoma in a patient with chronic hepatitis C (18), and one that had been classified as follicular small cleaved cell type in a patient with chronic hepatitis B (27). The occurrence of these tumors in patients with chronic liver disease (hepatitis B, hepatitis C, and primary biliary cirrhosis) may mean that they are analogous to MALT lymphomas that occur in the setting of chronic disease of the gastrointestinal tract, thyroid gland, and salivary glands.

We have also observed one patient with multiple lesions having the morphology of a MALT lymphoma in which a clonal rearrangement was detected for the T-cell receptor beta gene, indicating a T-cell neoplasm. Histologically, this had all

the features of MALT lymphoma, as described above, and in addition had areas of granulomatous inflammation within the lesion (fig. 13-6). The patient was not treated and was alive and well at follow up 5 years later. To our knowledge, no other case of a T-cell MALToma has been reported.

T-Cell–Rich B-Cell Lymphoma. This is a rare but distinctive form of large cell lymphoma in which the malignant B cells are few and are scattered among numerous reactive small T cells and variable numbers of histiocytes (fig. 13-7). Some cases are misdiagnosed as T-cell lymphoma, but most are mistaken for inflammatory diseases (8,17). The patients typically have constitutional symptoms, abnormal liver tests, and hepatomegaly, and the liver biopsy usually shows a portal infiltrate with a predominance of small T cells that extend into the surrounding parenchyma, mimicking the interface hepatitis ("piecemeal necrosis") of chronic hepatitis. Histiocytes and even granulomas may be present, and the large, malignant B cells are scattered throughout the infiltrate. Other than the large atypical cells, however, there are clues to the diagnosis of lymphoma in the pattern of tissue infiltration (fig. 13-8): the infiltrates tend to be more irregularly distributed than in any of the usual inflammatory diseases, and there is more extensive tissue destruction, sometimes with areas of infarct-like coagulative necrosis.

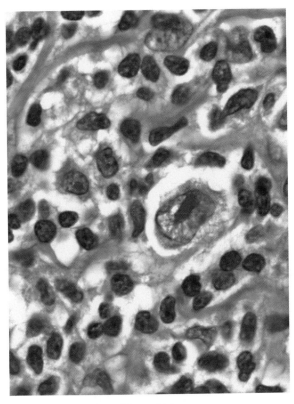

Figure 13-7
T-CELL–RICH, B-CELL LYMPHOMA
Most of the cells are small T cells, but the few malignant cells are large B cells with vesicular nuclei and prominent nucleoli.

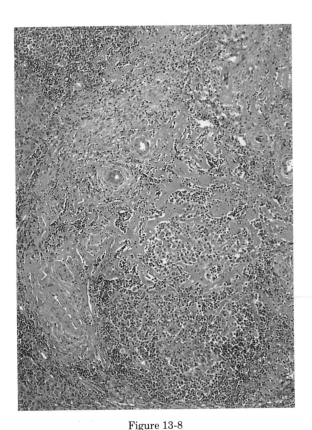

Figure 13-8
T-CELL–RICH, B-CELL LYMPHOMA
Although most of the cells are small, benign-appearing T cells, the tumor infiltrates and destroys liver tissue in a way that non-neoplastic liver diseases never do.

Epstein-Barr Virus (EBV)–Associated Post-Transplant Lymphoproliferative Disorders (PTLD). These occur in patients who are immunosuppressed following liver, kidney, heart, lung, or bone marrow transplantation (4,11,26,29,33). They may take a benign form, either infectious mononucleosis or polyclonal B-cell hyperplasia, both of which resolve with decreased immunosuppression. However, they may take a malignant form, either a polyclonal (polymorphic) or monoclonal (monomorphic) B-cell lymphoma, which does not respond to reduced immunosuppression and rapidly disseminates to involve lymph nodes and viscera.

EBV-associated polyclonal B-cell hyperplasia can be difficult to distinguish from allograft rejection in liver transplant recipients. Both have a portal inflammatory infiltrate with a mixed lymphoplasmacytic infiltrate, but EBV latent membrane protein can be demonstrated in lymphoid cells by immunoperoxidase staining (fig. 13-9) and viral DNA can be demonstrated by in situ hybridization, establishing the diagnosis of an EBV-related PTLD (26,29,33). This is important, as rejection should be treated with increased immunosuppression, while PTLD requires reduced immunosuppression. Monomorphic lymphomas resemble more conventional B-cell neoplasms and may be small or large noncleaved cell lymphomas. Polymorphous B-cell lymphomas typically have a mixture of atypical lymphoid cells (fig. 13-10), which may include immunoblasts and Reed-Sternberg-like cells, while plasma cells and plasmacytoid lymphocytes are not present. They infiltrate the liver parenchyma, often form mass lesions, rapidly disseminate, and have a poor prognosis.

Sinusoidal T-Cell Lymphoma. T-cell lymphomas may diffusely involve the hepatic sinusoids, rather than forming a mass lesion, and they can have a distinctive clinical presentation that mimics acute or chronic liver disease (10,12,20,36,44).

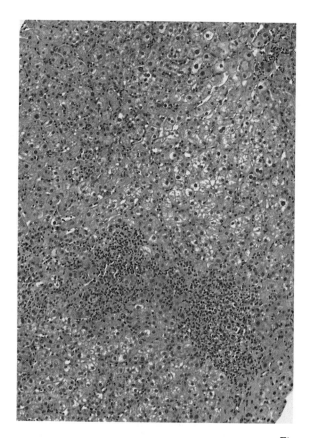

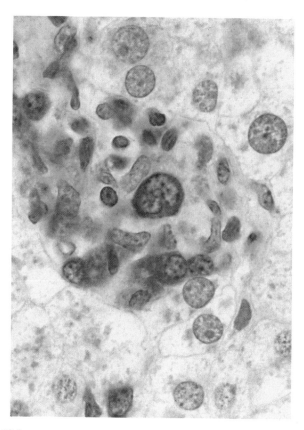

Figure 13-9

EPSTEIN-BARR VIRUS–ASSOCIATED POST-TRANSPLANT LYMPHOPROLIFERATIVE DISORDER

Left: There is a polymorphous lymphoid infiltrate in the portal areas and sinusoids.

Right: Immunoperoxidase stain for EBV latent membrane shows stained lymphoid cells, indicating that this is an EBV driven polyclonal B-cell hyperplasia.

Figure 13-10
EPSTEIN-BARR VIRUS–
ASSOCIATED
POST-TRANSPLANT
LYMPHOPROLIFERATIVE
DISORDER

The atypical mixed lymphoid cells are destroying the bile duct in the center of the field in this EBV-associated polymorphous B-cell lymphoma.

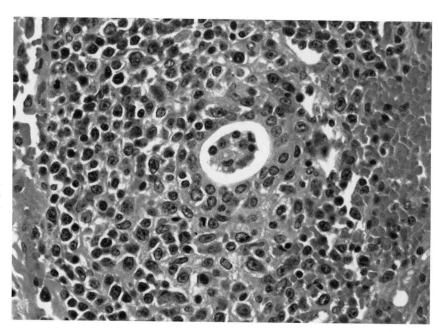

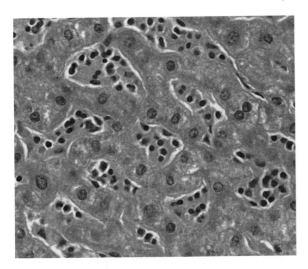
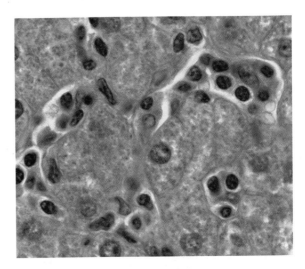

Figure 13-11
SINUSOIDAL T-CELL LYMPHOMA

Left: A γδ T-cell lymphoma shows a diffuse mononucleosis-like sinusoidal infiltrate of small lymphoid cells.

Right: High magnification shows that the infiltrate is composed of uniform cells with minimal atypia. However, molecular studies demonstrated a monoclonal rearrangement of the T-cell gamma receptor gene.

Patients typically have signs and symptoms of systemic disease, such as fever, weight loss, anemia, and thrombocytopenia, along with abnormal liver tests and hepatosplenomegaly that may be quite marked. The disease generally does not respond well to chemotherapy, and most patients die within a few years.

The liver biopsy shows the malignant lymphoid cells in the sinusoids, but the degree of involvement and the cytologic appearance of the cells is quite variable from case to case, and many are initially misdiagnosed as an inflammatory disease rather than a neoplasm. In some cases, there is a diffuse sinusoidal mononucleosis-like infiltrate of small lymphocytes (fig. 13-11) that stain with T-cell markers, such as CD3 and CD45RO. In others, the infiltrate is sparser and easily overlooked. Some cases have a mixture of small and large lymphoid cells, while in a few, there is a predominance of large, atypical, transformed cells resembling those of a large cell lymphoma (fig. 13-12). Erythrophagocytosis by benign sinusoidal Kupffer cells may be present as well, and there may be other secondary changes, such as patchy anoxic zone 3 ("centrilobular") necrosis and resulting inflammation that can make it very difficult to recognize the abnormal lymphoid infiltrate. Molecular studies for T-cell receptor gene rearrangements are extremely helpful

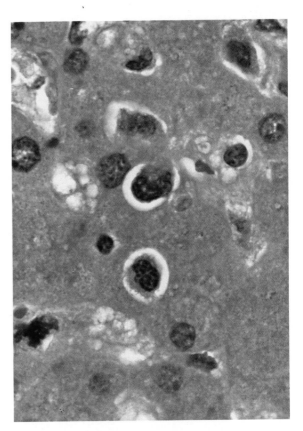

Figure 13-12
SINUSOIDAL T-CELL LYMPHOMA

In this case the malignant T cells are much more atypical than in the case of figure 13-11.

337

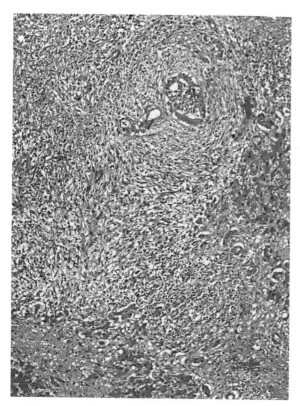

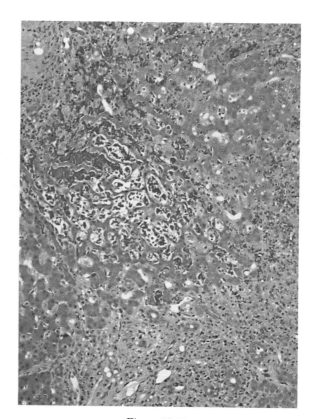

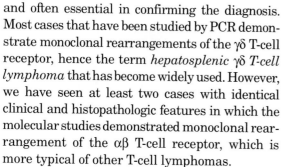

Figure 13-13
ANAPLASTIC LARGE CELL LYMPHOMA
The tumor has invaded along portal tracts, destroyed portal structures, including the bile duct, and infiltrated into the surrounding liver parenchyma.

Figure 13-14
ANAPLASTIC LARGE CELL LYMPHOMA
There is patchy severe congestion, indicating obstruction of hepatic venous outflow.

and often essential in confirming the diagnosis. Most cases that have been studied by PCR demonstrate monoclonal rearrangements of the γδ T-cell receptor, hence the term *hepatosplenic γδ T-cell lymphoma* that has become widely used. However, we have seen at least two cases with identical clinical and histopathologic features in which the molecular studies demonstrated monoclonal rearrangement of the αβ T-cell receptor, which is more typical of other T-cell lymphomas.

Anaplastic Large Cell Lymphoma, T-Cell and Null Cell Type, and Other Peripheral T-Cell Lymphomas. These have only rarely been documented as primary hepatic lymphomas (2,23,35, 40). As with the sinusoidal T-cell lymphomas, patients tend to present with systemic signs and symptoms, liver test abnormalities, sometimes jaundice, and usually hepatomegaly with or without splenomegaly. As with the sinusoidal T-cell lymphomas, these rarely form distinct

tumor masses. Instead, they tend to infiltrate along portal tracts, causing destruction of the portal structures (fig. 13-13). Bile duct involvement is frequent and may cause cholestatic jaundice, while obstruction of portal vessels may produce variable-sized infarctions of hepatic tissue. The infiltrates often extend into the parenchyma surrounding the portal tracts, and there may even be occlusion of small hepatic outflow veins, producing additional injury to the parenchyma (fig. 13-14). Consequently, these cases are frequently misdiagnosed as an inflammatory disease rather than a lymphoma. Even when correctly diagnosed, tumors generally respond poorly to chemotherapy and most prove rapidly fatal, although there have been exceptions (2,22).

Anaplastic large cell lymphoma is defined by the presence of CD30 (Ki-1) antigen and the absence of CD15 (Leu-M1) on the tumor cells (38). The majority also express T-cell markers,

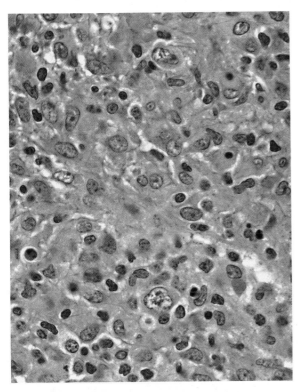

Figure 13-15
ANAPLASTIC LARGE CELL LYMPHOMA
The infiltrates have numerous histiocytes, imparting a vaguely granulomatous appearance that is often mistaken for an inflammatory disease. A few large, atypical mononuclear cells are also present.

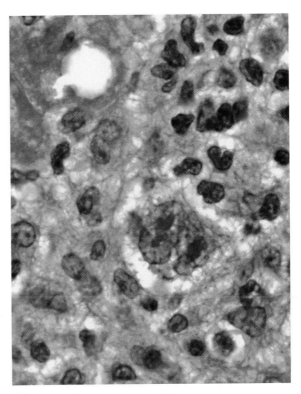

Figure 13-16
ANAPLASTIC LARGE CELL LYMPHOMA
Occasional Reed-Sternberg–like cells can usually be found. A positive immunostain for Ki-1 with a negative stain for Leu-M1 will confirm the diagnosis and separate these tumors from Hodgkin's disease.

but some have no other lymphoid markers or express both B- and T-cell markers; there are rare, morphologically identical tumors that also express B-cell markers and are considered diffuse large B-cell lymphoma in the REAL classification. Histologically, these are polymorphous tumors composed of a mixture of small, benign lymphocytes and often plasma cells and histiocytes, and there is often considerable fibrosis associated with the infiltrates. The histiocytes may be very prominent, giving the lesion a vaguely granulomatous appearance (fig. 13-15), and many cases are misdiagnosed as some type of "granulomatous hepatitis." The malignant, Ki-1–positive cells are a minority of the cellular population. These may have the appearance of large, transformed lymphoid cells or immunoblasts, or they may be binucleate with prominent nucleoli and thus resemble Reed-Sternberg cells (fig. 13-16). Indeed, before recognition of this entity, we at the Armed Forces Institute of Pathology (AFIP) usu-

ally suggested a diagnosis of Hodgkin's disease for cases that we now recognize as anaplastic large cell lymphoma. We strongly suspect that reports in the older literature of hepatic involvement by Hodgkin's disease (5,21) contain many cases of anaplastic large cell lymphoma.

Other peripheral T-cell lymphomas may be primary in the liver and may have a variety of morphologic appearances (1,2,12,35) ranging from small cell to large cell lymphomas. The large cell lymphomas rarely cause diagnostic difficulty; immunohistochemical stains for T-cell markers allow correct classification. Small cell and polymorphous tumors can be more difficult to recognize as lymphoma, since most inflammatory diseases have a predominance of T cells. In such cases, immunostains showing an absence of B cells, supplemented with molecular studies to demonstrate monoclonal T-cell receptor gene rearrangements are often essential in establishing the diagnosis and correct classification.

SUSPECTED LYMPHOMA

Every year at the AFIP we see biopsies that lead us to suspect strongly that the patient has a lymphoma involving the liver, even though the features are not entirely diagnostic. Sometimes in such cases follow-up proves the diagnosis, but often not. Sometimes the patient dies and no autopsy is performed, and sometimes there is an autopsy but the tissue reveals no more than was in the biopsy. The types of lymphoma that we suspect are those that are the most difficult to diagnose, as discussed above. These include, in particular, the various forms of T-cell lymphoma (sinusoidal, peripheral, and polymorphous anaplastic large cell) and occasionally T-cell–rich B-cell lymphoma. Hematopathologists who review these cases, using the strict criteria that apply to the diagnosis of lymphoma in lymph nodes, conclude that there is insufficient evidence to establish a diagnosis of lymphoma in the liver biopsy, and may suggest that the process is reactive. However, since the pattern of tissue destruction and the appearance of the infiltrative process are not those of any known infectious, immunologic, or vascular disease of the liver, or for that matter of any type of non-neoplastic liver disease, we feel confident that conceptual and technical advances in the understanding and diagnosis of lymphoproliferative diseases will eventually allow us to show that these are all indeed lymphomas. At the present time, we report such cases as "atypical infiltrate, probably malignant lymphoma" or as "atypical infiltrate, suggestive of malignant lymphoma," depending on our degree of certainty.

Certain clinical and pathologic features should raise the suspicion of malignant lymphoma in a patient with an undiagnosed liver disease.

1) *Clinical Features.* The patients are almost always middle-aged or elderly and present with the new onset of a grave illness that defies the usual diagnostic evaluation. There is typically fever and other systemic symptoms, hepatomegaly, and abnormal liver tests that lead to a liver biopsy. Although the biopsy is quite abnormal, it is almost always interpreted as inflammatory, often granulomatous, rather than neoplastic. This scenario is so frequent that the history alone makes lymphoma a prime consideration.

2) *Pattern of Tissue Damage Unlike Any Recognized Inflammatory Disease.* This is a concept that is difficult to explain to those who do not have experience with non-neoplastic liver pathology. Infections, biliary and vascular diseases, and various forms of immunologically mediated hepatitis all produce characteristic patterns of liver injury which tend to be regular and often to correspond to the zones of the microscopic hepatic acini. Lymphomas, on the other hand, have an irregular pattern of tissue invasion, often starting in portal areas and expanding in an infiltrative manner, destroying the tissue indiscriminately. When bile ducts and vessels are involved, features of cholestasis and ischemia are superimposed.

3) *Polymorphous Infiltrate, Often with Granulomatous Features.* This is seen especially in anaplastic large cell lymphoma. There may be numerous fibroblasts and histiocytes and sometimes there may be true granulomas, but the features are not those of a recognized granulomatous infection or sarcoidosis. When atypical Reed-Sternberg–like cells are seen and are positive for CD30 (Ki-1), the diagnosis can be made. However, sometimes, none of the malignant cells can be demonstrated. Nevertheless, in the appropriate clinical setting and in the presence of the type of tissue destruction described in the preceding paragraph, this type of infiltrate strongly suggests lymphoma.

Diffuse Sinusoidal Infiltrate that Does Not Look Like a Hepatitis. This characterizes the sinusoidal T-cell lymphomas described previously. If the clinical features are not those of a viral or drug-induced hepatitis, and the degree of hepatocellular injury is not commensurate with the lymphocytic infiltrate, then the possibility of a sinusoidal lymphoma should be considered. Fortunately, molecular studies now make this diagnosis less difficult.

Currently, we report these types of cases as highly suggestive of malignant lymphoma. Hopefully, technological advances will continue to make the diagnosis easier in the future. An example of a suspected lymphoma that was later confirmed is illustrated in figure 13-17.

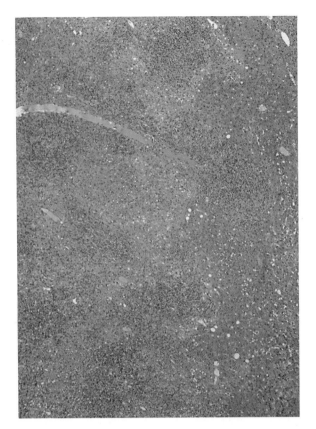
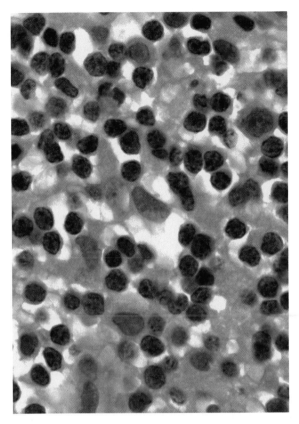

Figure 13-17
SUSPECTED LYMPHOMA

Left: Although lymphoma was strongly suspected on the basis of the pattern of tissue destruction, the infiltrate was not highly atypical and molecular studies were inconclusive.

Right: After the patient died, molecular studies of the autopsy tissue revealed a clonal rearrangement of the T-cell beta gene, confirming the diagnosis of T-cell lymphoma.

REFERENCES

1. Andreola S, Audisio RA, Mazzaferro V, Doci R, Makowka L, Gennari L. Primary lymphoma of the liver showing immunohistochemical evidence of T-cell origin. Successful management by right trisegmentectomy. Dig Dis Sci 1988;33:1632–6.

2. Anthony PP, Sarsfield P, Clarke T. Primary lymphoma of the liver: clinical and pathological features of 10 patients. J Clin Pathol 1990;43:1007–13.

3. Ascoli V, Lo Coco F, Artini M, Levrero M, Martelli M, Negro F. Extranodal lymphomas associated with hepatitis C virus infection. Am J Clin Pathol 1998;109:600–9.

4. Ben-Ari Z, Amlot P, Lachmanan SR, Tur-Kaspa R, Rolles K, Burroughs AK. Posttransplantation lymphoproliferative disorder in liver recipients: characteristics, management, and outcome. Liver Transplant Surg 1999;5:184–91.

5. Cavalli G, Casali AM, Lambertini F, Busachi C. Changes in the small biliary passages in the hepatic localization of Hodgkin's disease. Virchows Arch [A] 1979;384:295–306.

6. Chan JK, Banks PM, Cleary ML, et al. A revised European-American classification of lymphoid neoplasms proposed the International Lymphoma Study Group: a summary version. Am J Clin Pathol 1995;103:543–60.

7. Collins MH, Orazi A, Bauman M, et al. Primary hepatic B-cell lymphoma in a child. Am J Surg Pathol 1993;17:1182–6.

8. Dargent JL, De Wolf-Peeters C. Liver involvement by lymphoma. Identification of a distinctive pattern of infiltration related to T-cell/histiocyte-rich B-cell lymphoma. Ann Diag Pathol 1998;2:363–9.

9. DeMent SH, Mann RB, Staal SP, Kuhajda FP, Boitnott JK. Primary lymphomas of the liver: report of six cases and review of the literature. Am J Clin Pathol 1987;88:255–63.

10. Dommann-Scherrer CC, Kurer SB, Zimmermann DR, et al. Occult hepatosplenic γδ T-lymphoma: value of genotypic analysis in the differential diagnosis. Virchows Arch 1995;426:629–34.

11. Frizzera G. Atypical lymphoproliferative disorders. In: Knowles DM, ed. Neoplastic hematopathology. Baltimore: Williams & Wilkins, 1992:459–95.

12. Gaulard P, Zafrani ES, Mavier P, et al. Peripheral T-cell lymphoma presenting as predominant liver disease: a report of three cases. Hepatology 1986;6:864–8.

13. Ghosh P, Fox IJ, Rader AM, Sorrell MF. Fulminant hepatic failure as the initial manifestation of non-Hodgkin's lymphoma. Am J Gastroenterol 1995;90:2207–9.

14. Harris NL, Jaffe ES, Stein H, et al. A revised European-American classification of lymphoid neoplasms: a proposal from the International Lymphoma Study Group. Blood 1994;84:1361–92.

15. Isaacson PG, Banks PM, Best PV, McLure SP, Muller-Hermelink HK, Wyatt JI. Primary low-grade hepatic B-cell lymphoma of mucosa-associated lymphoid tissue (MALT)-type. Am J Surg Pathol 1995;19:571–5.

16. Jaffe ES, Harris NL, Diebold J, Muller-Hermelink HK. World Health Organization classification of neoplastic diseases of the hematopoietic and lymphoid tissues. A progress report. Am J Clin Pathol 1999;111(Suppl 1):S8–S12.

17. Kahn SM, Cottrell BJ, Millward-Sadler GH, Wright DH. T-cell-rich B-cell lymphoma presenting as liver disease. Histopathology 1993;23:217–24.

18. Kim SR, Hayashi Y, Kang KB, et al. A case of pseudolymphoma of the liver with chronic hepatitis C. J Hepatol 1997;26:209–14.

19. Kirk CM, Lewin D, Lazarchick J. Primary hepatic B-cell lymphoma of mucosa-associated lymphoid tissue. Arch Pathol Lab Med 1999;123:716–9.

20. Krishnan J, Goodman Z, Frizzera G. Primary hepatic sinusoidal presentation of malignant T cell lymphoma. Lab Invest 1992;66:81A.

21. Lefkowitch JH, Falkow S, Whitlock RT. Hepatic Hodgkin's disease simulating cholestatic hepatitis with liver failure. Arch Pathol Lab Med 1985;109:424–6.

22. Lei KI. Primary non-Hodgkin's lymphoma of the liver. Leuk Lymphoma 1998;29:293–9.

23. Lei KI, Chow JH, Johnson PJ. Aggressive primary hepatic lymphoma in Chinese patients: presentation, pathologic features, and outcome. Cancer 1995;76:1336–43.

24. Lisker-Melman M, Pittaluga S, Pluda JM, et al. Primary lymphoma of the liver in a patient with acquired immune deficiency syndrome and chronic hepatitis B. Am J Gastroenterol 1989;84:1445–8.

25. Maes M, Depardieu C, Dargent JL, et al. Primary low-grade B-cell lymphoma of MALT-type occurring in the liver: a study of two cases. J Hepatol 1997;27:922–7.

26. Markin RS, Wright TL. Post-transplant chronic viral infections. In: Bloomer JR, Goodman ZD, Ishak KG, eds. Clinical and pathological correlations in liver disease: approaching the next millennium. Washington, D.C.: Armed Forces Institute of Pathology, 1998;156–71.

27. Matano S, Nakamura S, Annen Y, et al. Primary hepatic lymphoma in a patient with chronic hepatitis B. Am J Gastroenterol 1998;93:2301–2.

28. Nakanuma Y, Kumabashiri I. Neoplastic angioendotheliomatosis with multifocal hemorrhagic necrosis of the liver. Am J Gastroenterol 1988;83:1180–2.

29. Nalesnik MA, Randhawa P, Demetris AJ, Casavilla A, Fung JJ, Locker J. Lymphoma resembling Hodgkin disease after posttransplant lymphoproliferative disorder in a liver transplant recipient. Cancer 1993;72:2568–73.

30. Ohsawa M, Aozasa K, Horiuchi K, et al. Malignant lymphoma of the liver: report of five cases and review of the literature. Dig Dis Sci 1992;37:1105–9.

31. Ohsawa M, Tomita Y, Hashimoto M, Kanno H, Aozasa K. Hepatic C viral genome in a subset of primary hepatic lymphomas. Mod Pathol 1998;11:471–8.

32. Prabhu RM, Medeiros J, Kumar D, et al. Primary hepatic low-grade B-cell lymphoma of mucosa-associated lymphoid tissue (MALT) associated with primary biliary cirrhosis. Mod Pathol 1998;11:404–10.

33. Rizkalla KS, Asfar SK, McLean CA, Garcia BM, Wall WJ, Grant DR. Key features distinguishing post-transplant lymphoproliferative disorders and acute liver rejection. Mod Pathol 1997;10:708–15.

34. Rubbia-Brandt L, Brundler MA, Kerl K, et al. Primary hepatic diffuse large B-cell lymphoma in a patient with chronic hepatitis C. Am J Surg Pathol 1999;23:1124–30.

35. Saito K, Nakanuma Y, Ogawa S, Arai Y, Hayashi M. Extensive hepatic granulomas associated with peripheral T-cell lymphoma. Am J Gastroenterol 1991;86:1243–6.

36. Salhany KE, Feldman M, Kahn MJ, et al. Hepatosplenic γδ T-cell lymphoma: ultrastructural, immunophenotypic, and functional evidence for cytotoxic T lymphocyte differentiation. Hum Pathol 1997;28:674–85.

37. Scarpella EG, Villareal AA, Casanova PF, Moreno JN. Primary lymphoma of the liver in AIDS: report of one new case and review of the literature. J Clin Gastroenterol 1996;22:51–3.

38. Scoazec JY, Degott C, Brousse N, et al. Non-Hodgkin's lymphoma presenting as a primary tumor of the liver: presentation, diagnosis and outcome in eight patients. Hepatology 1991;13:870–5.

39. Stein H, Mason DY, Gerdes J, et al. The expression of the Hodgkin's disease associated antigen Ki-1 in reactive and neoplastic lymphoid tissue: evidence that Reed-Sternberg cells and histiocytic malignancies are derived from activated lymphoid cells. Blood 1985;66:848–58.

40. Suzuki N, Tsujji H, Nakamura S, Asabe H, Sueishi K, Fujishima M. An autopsy case of Ki-1 lymphoma associated with hepatic failure. Am J Gastroenterol 1998;93:115–7.

41. Trudel M, Aramendi T, Caplan S. Large-cell lymphoma presenting with hepatic sinusoidal infiltration. Arch Pathol Lab Med 1991;115:821–4.

42. Ueda G, Oka K, Matsumoto T, et al. Primary hepatic marginal zone B-cell lymphoma with mantle cell lymphoma phenotype. Virchows Arch 1996;428:311–4.

43. Warnke RA, Weiss LM, Chan JK, Cleary ML, Dorfman RF. Tumors of the lymph nodes and spleen. Atlas of Tumor Pathology, 3rd Series, Fascicle 14. Washington, DC: Armed Forces Institute of Pathology, 1995.

44. Wong KF, Chan JK, Matutes E, et al. Hepatosplenic γδ T-cell lymphoma: a distinctive aggressive lymphoma type. Am J Surg Pathol 1995;19:718–26.

14
METASTATIC TUMORS

Because of its location, blood supply, anatomy, and other poorly understood factors, the liver provides a prime location for metastases from malignant tumors. Metastases are by far the most common malignant neoplasms of the liver. In the United States, about 20 percent of deaths are due to cancer. Up to 40 percent of these patients have liver metastases, and 10 percent die from hepatic failure (10). Similar figures have been reported from the United Kingdom, Italy, and Japan (9,13).

Definition. A hepatic metastasis is a malignant tumor that arises in another, discontiguous site and then secondarily spreads to the liver, implants there, and grows. Spread to the liver is usually hematogenous, but tumors can occasionally metastasize through the peritoneal fluid or (theoretically, at least) via lymphatics.

Primary Sites. Lung, breast, colon, and pancreas are the most common primary sites of hepatic metastases (4,9,10,13), but malignant tumors from almost any site can at times metastasize to the liver (Table 14-1). When some tumors disseminate they frequently metastasize to the liver; others do so only rarely. Melanomas, neuroblastomas, and carcinomas of the gastrointestinal tract, biliary tract, pancreas, lung, and breast often metastasize to liver, while cancers of the head and neck and sarcomas of any site seldom do.

Clinical Features. The syndromes produced by metastatic tumors depend on several factors, including the site and type of the primary tumor, the number and location of the metastases within the liver, and the degree of hepatic involvement. Metastases are often detected in presymptomatic patients with known primary lesions during evaluation for stage of disease. Most tumors that cause symptoms are far advanced at the time of presentation. About two-thirds of such patients have clinical signs and symptoms referable to the liver (5). Frequent findings include hepatomegaly (90 percent), anorexia and weight loss (70 to 80 percent), and right upper quadrant abdominal pain, often radiating to the right infrascapular area (30 to 40 percent). Less that 10 percent have a palpable mass. Metastases located near the hilum of the liver may occa-

sionally cause biliary obstruction, and rarely patients may present with acute fulminant liver failure due to massive hepatic replacement by metastases from an occult primary. Metastases from functioning endocrine tumors such as carcinoid, insulinoma, glucagonoma, gastrinoma, or somatostatinoma may result in syndromes of hormonal excess. Liver-associated enzymes, such as alkaline phosphatase and gamma glutamyl transpeptidase, are frequently abnormal in patients with liver metastases.

The gamut of modern radiologic techniques can be employed for detection and characterization of mass lesions in the liver. Each imaging modality has advantages and disadvantages and may be useful in different ways in the diagnosis

Table 14-1

SITES OF ORIGIN OF HEPATIC METASTASES IN 1151 AUTOPSIED PATIENTS FROM LOS ANGELES COUNTY USC MEDICAL CENTER*

Site	Percent of Patients
Lung	24.8
Colon	15.7
Pancreas	10.9
Breast	10.1
Stomach	6.1
Unknown	5.1
Ovary	4.1
Prostate	3.6
Gallbladder	3.3
Cervix	3.0
Kidney	3.0
Melanoma	2.2
Bladder/Ureter	2.2
Esophagus	1.7
Testis	1.7
Endometrium	1.5
Thyroid	1.0

*Data from Table 13 from reference 4.

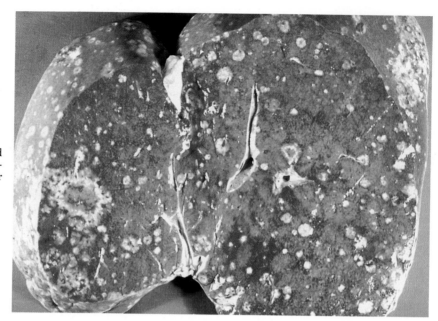

Figure 14-1
METASTATIC CARCINOMA
Multiple nodules scattered throughout both lobes nearly always indicates metastases rather than a primary liver tumor.

of metastases (7). Radionuclide scanning, ultrasonography, computed tomography (CT), magnetic resonance imaging (MRI), and angiography are all successfully employed in various circumstances. The definitive diagnosis of a metastatic neoplasm requires a histologic examination, however, and while percutaneous "blind" needle biopsy is successful in establishing the diagnosis in up to 75 percent of patients (3), guided biopsies utilizing sonography, CT, or one of the other imaging modalities, or during laparoscopy, can improve the yield beyond this. In some cases, especially those with small metastases deep within the liver, guided biopsies may even be superior to direct palpation and biopsy during laparotomy. Fine needle aspiration with a 20 to 23 gauge spinal needle can be performed on deep lesions that are not readily reached with large biopsy needles. When combined with ultrasound, CT, or MRI guidance, over 80 percent of lesions can be adequately sampled, and the material obtained can be smeared for cytologic examination and centrifuged to make cell blocks for histologic study, producing diagnostic specimens in over 90 percent of cases (1).

Gross Findings. Metastases in the liver are only rarely solitary. Typically, there are multiple irregular nodules of varying sizes scattered throughout both lobes (fig. 14-1). Apart from the metastases, the liver is usually otherwise normal.

A tumor in a cirrhotic liver is more likely to be a primary hepatocellular carcinoma (3,9). Metastases may grow to massive size, producing marked hepatomegaly that fills the abdomen and displaces the viscera. We have seen livers with metastases that weighed over 13 kg at autopsy. Areas of necrosis are often present in the center of the metastatic tumor nodules, occasionally causing them to appear cystic. Scarring and retraction can produce an umbilicated appearance that is especially common with metastases from colon cancer and is a differential feature distinguishing these tumors from primary cancers of the liver. A desmoplastic stromal response causes many metastases to be firm or hard. Some tumors infiltrate through the hepatic sinusoids, producing little stromal response, and form soft, "fish flesh" tumor nodules. Occasional tumors, especially metastatic breast cancer, may spread diffusely through the sinusoids rather than forming distinct nodules and may not be grossly visible, even though much of the parenchyma has been replaced by the tumor. Mucinous (colloid) adenocarcinomas may have a slimy, glistening appearance; squamous carcinomas are often white and granular; melanomas are brown or black (fig. 14-2).

Microscopic Findings. Metastases usually resemble the primary tumor, and so if the primary lesion is known and has been biopsied or

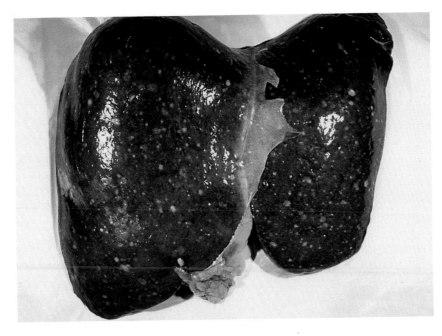

Figure 14-2
METASTATIC MALIGNANT
MELANOMA
The liver is diffusely infiltrated
by a highly pigmented tumor,
turning the entire organ black.

excised, comparison with the microscopic appearance of the tumor in the liver confirms that the hepatic tumor is a metastasis. Many metastatic tumors tend to grow within the hepatic sinusoids. They may fill vascular spaces, grow into the liver cell plates, or displace hepatocytes, giving a false impression of origin from the hepatocytes (fig. 14-3). The degree of stromal response is variable. Tumors that were desmoplastic or scirrhous in their primary sites usually provoke a similar response in their metastases. Metastatic adenocarcinoma may also grow within the intrahepatic bile ducts, mimicking primary cholangiocarcinoma (11).

Experienced pathologists can often suggest the primary site from the microscopic appearance of the metastasis when the primary is not known, and the use of histochemical and immunohistochemical stains can sometimes expand this ability. A few practical considerations and access to the patient's clinical history make this easier than it might seem at first, since some occult tumors are much more likely than others to present with liver metastases as the first sign of disease, as listed below.

Foregut Adenocarcinomas. An adenocarcinoma that is composed of small tubular or tubulopapillary glands, either well, moderately, or poorly differentiated, and that presents in the liver without a known primary is most often of foregut origin

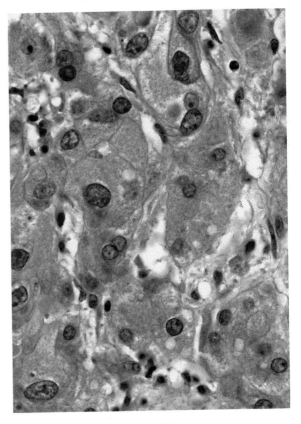

Figure 14-3
METASTATIC ADENOCARCINOMA
The large, basophilic tumor cells are invading the liver cell plates, giving the false impression of an origin from the liver cells.

345

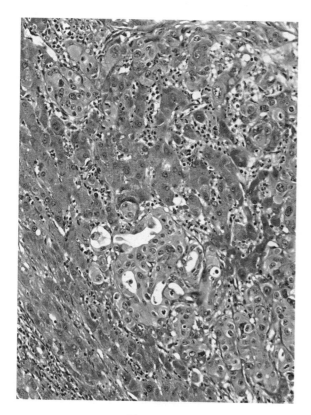

Figure 14-4
FOREGUT ADENOCARCINOMA, METASTATIC
The tumor is moderately differentiated and composed of small, poorly formed glands typical of metastases from the stomach, pancreas, and bile ducts.

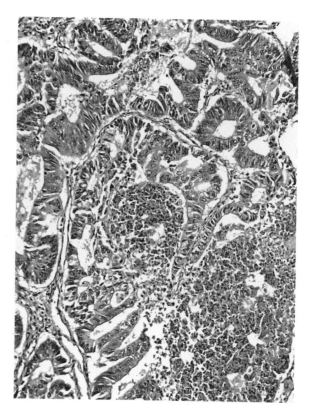

Figure 14-5
COLONIC ADENOCARCINOMA, METASTATIC
The tumor is composed of large, fairly well-formed glands with hyperchromatic nuclei, typical of colon cancer.

(fig. 14-4). That is, it is most likely from the stomach, pancreas, or biliary tract. This is by far the most frequent diagnostic problem for the pathologist. If the tumor arises in an intrahepatic bile duct, it is an intrahepatic cholangiocarcinoma (chapter 10), and the patient may benefit from surgical resection. If it is a metastasis from the stomach, lower esophagus, or pancreas, as is much more likely, then surgical therapy, if any, should be directed to the primary rather than the hepatic metastasis. There is, however, no way to distinguish these from one another on histologic grounds alone or with any immunohistochemical stain, and tumors that arise in other sites can sometimes mimic foregut adenocarcinomas and occasionally present as a liver metastasis.

Colon Cancer. Metastatic colon cancer usually resembles the primary tumor with large, well-formed glands and hyperchromatic nuclei (fig. 14-5). Most are positive with immunostains for cytokeratin 20 and negative for cytokeratin 7, a pattern that is not typical of cholangiocarcinoma or foregut adenocarcinomas. But although colon cancer frequently metastasizes to the liver, it is rare for a case to present with clinically evident liver metastases and an occult primary.

Small Cell Carcinoma. Lung cancer frequently metastasizes to the liver, but it is rare for nonsmall cell tumors to present with clinically evident liver metastases and an occult primary. With small cell carcinoma of the lung, however, the liver may be massively involved with tumor while the primary is still clinically occult (fig. 14-6). Small cell carcinoma may arise in many sites other than the lung (including the gallbladder), but statistically, in an adult, an anaplastic small cell tumor, especially one that is immunohistochemically positive for neuroendocrine markers, is usually from the lung. In a young child, it usually represents metastatic neuroblastoma.

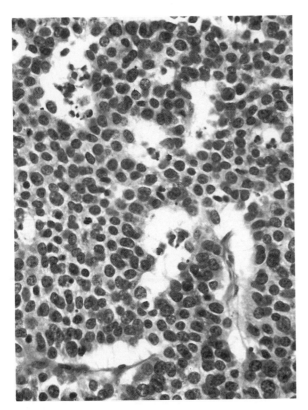

Figure 14-6
SMALL CELL CARCINOMA OF LUNG, METASTATIC
The tumor is composed of cells with scant cytoplasm and hyperchromatic nuclei with frequent mitoses.

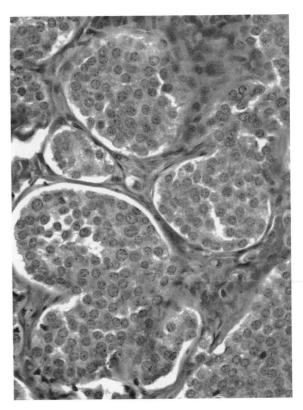

Figure 14-7
CARCINOID TUMOR, METASTATIC
The tumor is composed of nests of uniform cells with prominent nuclei and a moderate amount of cytoplasm, typical of a carcinoid. The primary was in the ileum.

Breast Cancer. This also frequently metastasizes to the liver, but presentation with clinically evident liver metastases and an occult primary is so rare that we have only seen one such case in the past 20 years at the AFIP.

Carcinoid-Islet Cell Tumors and Large Cell Neuroendocrine Carcinoma. Metastatic carcinoid tumors present relatively frequently with liver metastases from an occult primary that is often quite small. Since primary carcinoids of the liver are so rare (see chapter 11), one that is found in the liver should be considered metastatic unless a complete and thorough autopsy has not found another primary. If there is a typical organoid nesting pattern with uniform cells that have a moderate amount of cytoplasm and nuclei with finely granular chromatin pattern (fig. 14-7), stains for neuroendocrine markers such as chromogranin and synaptophysin will nearly always be positive, confirming the diagnosis. Metastatic islet cell tumors are much rarer, and identification

of a pancreatic hormone or clinical evidence of a primary in the pancreas is necessary to distinguish these from carcinoid tumors. High-grade tumors with neuroendocrine features (fig. 14-8) can arise in many sites and sometimes present with liver metastases. Although immunostains can confirm neuroendocrine differentiation in such tumors, a specific site of origin cannot be suggested. Metastatic neuroendocrine carcinomas should be distinguished from carcinoids because of their poorer prognosis.

Melanoma. Malignant melanoma may present with liver metastases years after the primary was excised. Pigmented tumors are usually readily identified, although melanin pigment can be mistaken for bile and prompt a mistaken diagnosis of hepatocellular carcinoma. In amelanotic melanomas, large epithelioid cells with eosinophilic cytoplasm and prominent nuclei with large nucleoli (fig. 14-9) may also suggest a primary hepatocellular carcinoma. If there is no underlying

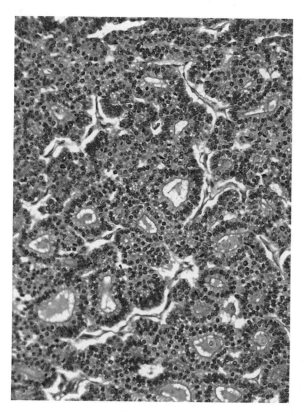

Figure 14-8
NEUROENDOCRINE CARCINOMA
This tumor is forming glands but also has an appearance reminiscent of carcinoid. Immunostains for endocrine markers were positive.

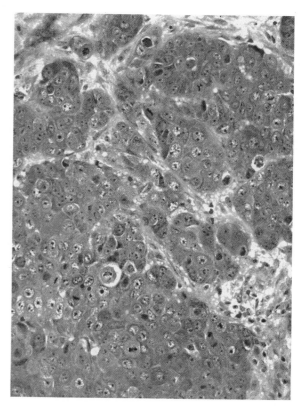

Figure 14-9
MALIGNANT MELANOMA, METASTATIC
This amelanotic melanoma has large epithelioid cells with prominent nuclei and nucleoli, reminiscent of hepatocellular carcinoma, but there are no canaliculi, even with immunostains for CEA, and melanoma markers (HMB-45 and S-100 protein) were positive.

cirrhosis, if the tumor does not have a typical trabecular pattern, and if bile canaliculi are not apparent on routine stains or with immunostains for carcinoembryonic antigen (see chapter 8), metastatic malignant melanoma should be considered. A definitive diagnosis can be made with a positive immunostain for S-100 protein or one of the melanoma antigens such as HMB-45 as long as angiomyolipoma has been excluded (see chapter 4).

Clear Cell Carcinoma. Renal cell carcinoma rarely metastasizes to the liver and imaging studies will virtually always show the primary in the kidney. Nevertheless, a tumor composed of sheets of clear cells raises this in the differential diagnosis of the clear cell variant of hepatocellular carcinoma. If no canaliculi are demonstrated with the carcinoembryonic antigen stain, then renal cell carcinoma should be considered. In general, tumors of the urinary tract and male and female reproductive tracts rarely if ever present with liver metastases from an occult primary.

Spindle Cell Tumors. Most malignant spindle cell tumors in the liver are carcinomas (primary or metastatic) that display spindle cell metaplasia (see chapter 10 for spindle cell cholangiocarcinoma). Leiomyosarcomas/stromal tumors of the gastrointestinal tract may present with liver metastases and an occult primary. A positive stain for actin (smooth muscle actin or muscle-specific actin) or c-kit will confirm that the tumor is of smooth muscle or stromal origin and presumably metastatic. However, a thorough evaluation of the gastrointestinal tract is needed to distinguish this from the rare primary leiomyosarcoma of the liver (chapter 12).

Differential Diagnosis. The major diagnostic problem with metastases is to differentiate them from primary liver tumors. Unfortunately, unless a tumor shows evidence of hepatocellular differentiation, one can never be sure that it is primary in the liver. Bile production, bile canaliculi, and a trabecular growth pattern of tumor cells that resemble liver cells allows one to diagnose hepatocellular carcinoma. Any other malignancy is more likely to be metastatic, and workup for an extrahepatic primary should be done before suggesting that it is primary in the liver. If the tumor resembles a foregut adenocarcinoma, it may well be an intrahepatic cholangiocarcinoma, but radiologic imaging studies to look for a primary in the stomach, lower esophagus, pancreas, or lung should be recommended.

In a patient with a known extrahepatic primary, one should also be cognizant that benign lesions may appear grossly like small metastases on the surface of the liver to a surgeon engaged in abdominal exploration. Peribiliary gland hamartomas ("bile duct adenomas"), characterized by small regular glands lacking atypia, and von Meyenburg complexes, with irregular serpiginous glands with low cuboidal epithelium, should always be in the differential diagnosis of metastatic adenocarcinoma (see chapter 3).

Prognosis and Treatment. The prognosis for patients with metastatic malignancy in the liver is quite poor. Nearly all are dead within 2 years of diagnosis. Patients with rapidly growing tumors or extensive metastatic disease generally die within a few months. Those with fewer metastases or with tumors that are slow growing or respond to therapy may live longer. Survival beyond 5 years is sometimes seen in patients with very slowly growing tumors, such as some carcinoids and low-grade leiomyosarcomas. Reports of spontaneous regression or prolonged survival can be found in the literature, but these are in the realm of medical curiosities.

Treatment of metastases is usually palliative rather than curative (2,6,12). Systemic chemotherapy or direct intra-arterial infusion (via the hepatic artery) of a variety of chemotherapeutic agents has produced favorable responses and prolongation of survival in some patients. Metastases, like primary hepatocellular carcinomas, derive nearly all of their blood supply from the hepatic artery rather than the portal vein, so that angiographic embolization with particles of gelatin sponge (Gelfoam) or iodized oil emulsion (Lipiodol), or even chemoembolization (combining the embolic agent with a chemotherapeutic drug) may produce tumor necrosis and prolong survival. Surgical resection is generally not used, since for most patients the presence of liver metastases is a sentence of doom. The exception is for metastases from colorectal adenocarcinoma, where the liver may be the only site of metastasis. Resection of liver metastases from colorectal cancer has been reported to produce 5-year survival rates ranging from 22 to 45 percent in various series (6,8).

REFERENCES

1. Axe SR, Erozan YS, Ermatinger SV. Fine-needle aspiration of the liver. A comparison of smear and rinse preparations in the detection of cancer. Am J Clin Pathol 1986;86:281–5.
2. Bottles K, Cohen MB. An approach to fine-needle aspiration biopsy diagnosis of hepatic masses. Diagn Cytopathol 1991;7:204–10.
3. Conn HO. Rational use of liver biopsy in the diagnosis of hepatic cancer. Gastroenterology 1972;62:142–6.
4. Craig JR, Peters, RL, Edmondson HA. Tumors of the liver and intrahepatic bile ducts. Atlas of Tumor Pathology. 2nd Series, Fascicle 26, Washington, D.C.: Armed Forces Institute of Pathology, 1989:256–67.
5. Fenster LF, Klatskin G. Manifestations of metastatic tumors of the liver. A study of eighty-one patients subjected to needle biopsy. Am J Med 1961;31:238–48.
6. Fong Y, Blumgart LH. Surgical therapy of liver cancer. In: Zakim D, Boyer TD, eds. Hepatology: a textbook of liver disease, 3rd ed. Philadelphia: WB Saunders Co, 1996:1548–64.
7. Friedman AC, Dachman AH, eds. Radiology of the liver, biliary tract and pancreas. St Louis: Mosby, 1994.
8. Kemeny N, Fong Y. Treatment of liver metastases. In: Holland JF, Bast RC Jr, Morton DL, Frei E III, Kufe DW, Weichselbaum RR, eds. Cancer medicine, 4th ed. Baltimore: Williams & Wilkins, 1997:1939–53.
9. Melato M, Laurino L, Mucli E, Valente M, Okuda K. Relationship between cirrhosis, liver cancer, and hepatic metastases: an autopsy study. Cancer 1989;64:455–9.
10. Pickren JW, Tsukada Y, Lane WW. Liver metastasis: analysis of autopsy data. In: Weiss L, Gilbert HA, eds. Liver metastasis. Boston: GK Hall, 1982:2–18.
11. Riopel MA, Klimstra DS, Godellas CV, Blumgart LH, Westra WH. Intrahepatic growth of metastatic colonic adenocarcinoma: a pattern of intrahepatic spread easily confused with primary neoplasia of the biliary tract. Am J Surg Pathol 1997;21:1030–6.
12. Sugarbaker PH, Kemeny N. Management of metastatic cancer to the liver. Adv Surg 1989;22:1–56.
13. Willis RA. The spread of tumours in the human body. London: Butterworth Co, 1973.

APPENDIX
TNM/pTNM CLASSIFICATION OF MALIGNANT TUMOURS*

LIVER
(ICD-O C22)

RULES FOR CLASSIFICATION

The classification applies only to primary hepatocellular and cholangio- (intrahepatic bile duct) carcinoma of the liver. There should be histological confirmation of the disease and division of cases by histological type.

The following are the procedures for assessing T, N, and M categories:

T categories	Physical examination, imaging, and/or surgical exploration
N categories	Physical examination, imaging, and/or surgical exploration
M categories	Physical examination, imaging, and/or surgical exploration

Note: Although the presence of cirrhosis is an important prognostic factor it does not affect the TNM classification, being an independent prognostic variable.

ANATOMICAL SUBSITES

1. Liver (C22.0)
2. Intrahepatic bile duct (C22.1)

REGIONAL LYMPH NODES

The regional lymph nodes are the hilar nodes (i.e., those in the hepatoduodenal ligament).

TNM CLINICAL CLASSIFICATION

T - Primary Tumour

TX   Primary tumour cannot be assessed
T0   No evidence of primary tumour
T1   Solitary tumour 2 cm or less in greatest dimension without vascular invasion
T2   Solitary tumour 2 cm or less in greatest dimension with vascular invasion; or multiple tumours limited to one lobe, none more than 2 cm in greatest dimension without vascular invasion; or solitary tumour more than 2 cm in greatest dimension without vascular invasion
T3   Solitary tumour more than 2 cm in greatest dimension with vascular invasion; or multiple tumours limited to one lobe, none more than 2 cm in greatest dimension with vascular invasion; or multiple tumours limited to one lobe, any more than 2 cm in greatest dimension with or without vascular invasion
T4   Multiple tumours in more than one lobe; or tumour(s) involve(s) a major branch of the portal or hepatic vein(s); or tumour(s) with direct invasion of adjacent organs other than gallbladder; or tumour(s) with perforation of visceral peritoneum

Note: For classification, the plane projecting between the bed of the gallbladder and the inferior vena cava divides the liver in two lobes.

N - Regional Lymph Nodes

NX Regional lymph nodes cannot be assessed
N0 No regional lymph node metastasis
N1 Regional lymph node metastasis

M - Distant Metastasis

MX Distant metastasis cannot be assessed
M0 No distant metastasis
M1 Distant metastasis

pTNM Pathological Classification

The pT, pN, and pM categories correspond to the T, N, and M categories.

pN0 histological examination of a regional lymphadenectomy specimen will ordinarily include three or more lymph nodes.

G Histopathological Grading

The definitions of the G categories apply to all digestive system tumours. These are:

GX Grade of differentiation cannot be assessed
G1 Well differentiated
G2 Moderately differentiated
G3 Poorly differentiated
G4 Undifferentiated

Stage Grouping

Stage	T	N	M
Stage I	T1	N0	M0
Stage II	T2	N0	M0
Stage IIIA	T3	N0	M0
Stage IIIB	T1	N1	M0
	T2	N1	M0
	T3	N1	M0
Stage IVA	T4	Any N	M0
Stage IVB	Any T	Any N	M1

SUMMARY

Liver

T1 Solitary, ≤ 2cm, without vascular invasion
T2 Solitary, ≤ 2 cm, with vascular invasion
    Multiple, one lobe, ≤ 2 cm, without vascular invasion
    Solitary, > 2 cm, without vascular invasion
T3 Solitary, > 2 cm, with vascular invasion
    Multiple, one lobe, ≤ 2 cm, with vascular invasion
    Multiple, one lobe, > 2 cm, with or without vascular invasion
T4 Multiple, more than one lobe
    Invasion of major branch of portal or hepatic veins
    Invasion of adjacent organs other than gallbladder
    Perforation of visceral peritoneum
N1 Regional

*From Sobin LH, Wittekind C, eds. TNM classification of malignant tumours. 5th ed. New York: John Wiley & Sons, 1997:74–83.

Index*

---

*Numbers in boldface indicate table and figure pages.